Campbell's

Pathophysiology Notes

Campbell's
Pathophysiology Notes

John Campbell

RN (Adult)   RN (Mental Health)   Dip.N   BSc   MSc   Cert Ed.   CNT   NT

Senior Lecturer, Nursing Studies, University of Cumbria, Carlisle Campus.

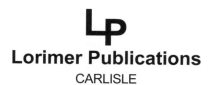

Lorimer Publications

CARLISLE

© 2006 Lorimer Publications

First published in 2006 by Lorimer Publications, Carlisle, Cumbria, U.K.
Second edition published in 2011 by Lorimer Publications, Carlisle, Cumbria, U.K.

Printed and bound in Great Britain by Bell & Bain Ltd., Glasgow

A catalogue record for this book is available from the British Library

ISBN 978-0-9553797-3-4

**Further lesson notes may be downloaded from:
www.campbellteaching.co.uk**

**Further copies of this publication can be ordered from:
orders@campbellteaching.co.uk
or from: TALC (Teaching-aids At Low Cost)**

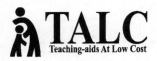

Contents

Acknowledgements

This book would not have been possible without the technical support I have generously received from Jonathan Forsyth and Ed Knapper. They have been responsible for the organisation of the diagrams and text.

I am also very grateful to my proof readers, they have read the text several times to iron out my many errors in the original writing. These people include Caroline Dixon, Lindsay Eplett, Anita Beattie, Erica Dunne, Christine Campbell, Ed Knapper, Barbara Bishop, Jane Bowe, Laura Crellin, David Hepworth, Carol Green, Wendy McManus, Yvonne Halliwell.

I have also enjoyed ongoing support and encouragement from my long term friends and colleagues Cath Boyes, Jean Longrigg, John Houghton and Stephanie Tobin.

My family, Christine, James and Timothy have been central to all of my writing and I realise it has meant there were often times when I was not there.

Introduction

Physiology is vital to give us an understanding of the normal functioning of the body. This knowledge can help us to maintain health in the people we live and work with. Sometimes however, as a result of trauma, disease or degeneration, the body fails to function normally. This means that, by definition, the function has become abnormal. Abnormal body function is termed pathophysiology. An understanding of normal and abnormal body function is necessary if we are to understand what treatments are indicated in a particular situation. This means physiology, pathophysiology and patient management all interlink. Theory will then inform, and provide rationales for interventions. The focus of this text is abnormal function, but this must be considered in the context of physiology and clinical practice. If we understand this linking and interdependence, we can use our knowledge of theory and practice to directly benefit patient care.

This book is intended to be a teaching aid for people who want to understand the causes, pathophysiological changes and clinical features seen in disease processes. Treatment principles are also discussed and should naturally follow on from an understanding of the abnormal processes involved. The topics I have chosen for inclusion in the text are generally those which are most common, or illustrate general principles of pathophysiology. My hope is that this book will allow you to understand what is happening to your patients more fully, and that this knowledge will inform practise. Also I hope it will give you the necessary basic understanding required to comprehend the more detailed texts you will need to gain knowledge about the specific disorders you encounter.

CHAPTER 1

Nature and Aetiology of Disease

Basic Terms

Physiology is the study of normal body function and anatomy is the study of body structure, (ology simply means 'the study of'). Pathology is the study of disease, involving examination of abnormal structure and function. Pathophysiology is the study of abnormal body function, in disease states, and after trauma. Histology and cytology are the study of tissues and cells respectively. Histopathology and cytopathology are therefore the study of abnormal tissues and cells.

Disease literally means any state of not being at ease, there is 'dis-ease'. This definition could include the effects of trauma, as well as disease processes. In practice we tend to use the term disease to refer to abnormal processes occurring within the body and the way in which these manifest in the individual. Pathogenesis is the process whereby the disordered disease state is produced in the body after the causative factor has been introduced.

Causes of disease

The cause of a disease is correctly described as the aetiology. Aetiology is 'that which causes'. Factors which may be involved in disease causation are therefore termed aetiological factors. So the aetiology causes the pathophysiology which in turn generates the clinical features of the disease. Aetiological factors may arise from within the individual, or from the environment the person is exposed to. Factors arising from within are called endogenous; those from the environment are exogenous.

Endogenous aetiology

The only true, absolute, endogenous factors are from the genetics of the person. These are determined from the point of conception; when there is fusion of the chromosomes from the sperm and ovum, into a single fertilized cell called a zygote. This zygote divides repeatedly to form all of the cells in the body. As a result all cells have the same genetic make up as the original zygote. At present there is nothing we can do about the genes we were given at conception. While many experiments are currently being carried out in the field of gene therapy, there are virtually no treatments available using this technique. This means we are to a large extent, 'at the mercy' of our genes.

Genetic disorders

Ultimately, all aspects of anatomy and physiology depend on, and derive from our genes. It is the genes which carry all of the information needed to construct the body, in the genetic code. Genetic disorders are those caused wholly by abnormalities in the genes. Numerous individual genetic disorders exist. They are normally classified by their mode of inheritance, this may be autosomal dominant, autosomal recessive or sex linked.

Autosomal dominant disorders

Autosomes are the 44 non-sex chromosomes present in cell nuclei. Autosomal dominant disorders will be manifest if there is a single copy of the abnormal gene present in the individual's genotype. This means that when one parent is affected by a dominant disorder, any children have a 50% chance of inheriting the condition. For example, achondroplasia which is a form of dwarfism, is transmitted by a dominant gene. Huntington's disease is also dominant and leads to psychiatric symptoms, abnormal movements and eventual dementia. Hypertrophic obstructive cardiomyopathy (HOCM) leads to an abnormal increase in the thickness of the myocardium and is a cause of sudden death. Neurofibromatosis causes numerous small tumours to develop from the sheaths of peripheral and cranial nerves. The BRCA1 and BRCA2 genes significantly predispose to the development of breast and ovarian cancer and are also transmitted in an autosomal dominant pattern.

Autosomal recessive disorders

Autosomal recessive disorders only present if there are 2 copies of the abnormal gene, on each of a pair of chromosomes. In practice these disorders normally occur in the children of two normal parents, who each carry one recessive copy of a particular gene. This means the probability of any child being affected is 1 chance in 4. Examples of diseases caused by this form of inheritance include thalassaemia, which causes abnormalities of the haemoglobin molecule. Phenylketoneuria (PKU) is an enzyme deficiency which means the patient can not process the amino acid called phenylalanine. Sickle cell disease causes abnormal shaped red blood cells and cystic fibrosis leads to viscous secretions from the pancreas and lungs.

Sex linked diseases

Sex linked disorders are virtually always transmitted on the X chromosome, so are sometimes referred to as X linked. Examples include haemophilia which leads to the lack of a clotting factor in the plasma resulting in excessive bleeding. Some forms of muscular dystrophy and colour blindness are also X linked. Females have two copies of the X chromosome and males only have one. This means that women often transmit X linked disorders which their sons suffer from.

Genetic predispositions

The genetic disorders discussed above directly cause a particular abnormality. In a truly genetic disorder the abnormal gene is one hundred percent responsible for the aetiology. This means that life style factors play no part in the pathogenesis. In numerous other disorders there is an environmental and a genetic component in the aetiology. A particular genetic make up can increase the risk that a person will develop a particular disorder. This is described as a genetic predisposition.

However, the genetic predisposition must be acted on by environmental factors in the pathogenesis of the disease process. The degree to which genetic make up places an individual at increased risk of a particular disorder varies from a very slight to a very significant risk. In most disease processes there is at least some genetic predisposition. It has been said, somewhat unhelpfully, that the best way to have a healthy life is to choose your parents carefully.

Implications of genetic knowledge

Often our principle role in dealing with genetic problems is one of health educator. Information should be given to families about the nature of genetic traits and disorders, how they are inherited and the possibilities of future children being affected. Appropriate well communicated information empowers the individual to make informed choices about their lives and reproductive activities at the pre-conceptual stage. It is not the role of nurses or doctors to make these choices on behalf of an individual. All practitioners need to empathise with the anxieties of parents as they decide on issues such as whether to start a pregnancy. In individuals who are at risk of developing a disorder themselves, with a significant genetic component in aetiology, the right of the patient to know, or not to know must be respected. This means that requested information should be given, but information should not be forced on individuals who do not wish to know about aspects of their lives and reproduction. Information exists, but not everyone is obliged to hear it.

Chromosomal disorders

Chromosomal abnormalities may be caused by environmental factors in the parents, such as being exposed to ionizing radiation. Despite this possible aetiology, disorders of chromosome structure are usually also classified as endogenous. Perhaps the best known example of a chromosomal disorder is Down's syndrome. The correct term for this condition is trisomy 21 syndrome. Trisomy 21 means that there are 3 of the 21st chromosome present as opposed to the normal 2 copies. This gives a total number of 47 chromosomes instead of the normal 46.

A variety of features may present as a result of trisomy 21, including characteristic facial features (which gave rise to the old, inaccurate, description of Mongolism), learning difficulties (IQ may be below 50) and possible congenital cardiac abnormalities. The risk of a child being affected by trisomy 21 syndrome increases with the age of the mother. Older women considering a pregnancy should be made aware of this risk. As a general principle it is probably best when mothers have children in their twenties.

Other chromosomal abnormalities include trisomy 18 and 13 syndromes. There may also be abnormalities of sex chromosome numbers. In Klinefelter's syndrome, (XXY syndrome) boys have small testes, are infertile and may have breast development, all caused by an additional X chromosome. Some girls are born with only one X chromosome, so only have a total of 45. This is called Turner's syndrome, these children are usually of short stature with webbing of the neck; they do not menstruate.

Exogenous aetiology

Any factor from the environment which contributes to disease aetiology is exogenous. These factors are also commonly referred to as environmental. This environment includes the one experienced in the uterus, before birth.

Infections

Microorganisms are perhaps the best example of an exogenous factor. We may, or may not be exposed to a particular organism. If we are not exposed, we will not suffer from the corresponding infection. Numerous small organisms (living things) have the potential to cause infective disease including viruses, bacteria, protozoa and larger parasites such as intestinal worms.

Chemical toxins

Numerous chemicals can adversely affect physiological systems leading to disorder. Some affect all of the body, for example cyanide inhibits energy generation in all cells. Others work more locally; mercury and lead for example affect the bones and brain. Dioxins are an important group of dangerous chemical we are exposed to in polluted air as well as from contaminated food. These largely come from the petroleum and plastics industries and can cause cancer.

Physical agents

Numerous physical agents and forms of energy can adversely affect the body. Trauma is usually caused by the effects of kinetic (movement) energy disrupting the integrity of body tissues. Heat and cold can both cause localized tissue damage as well as systemic (whole body) problems. Electrical energy is another agent which can lead to localized burning and can be life threatening if the heart or brain are sufficiently disrupted. Radiation can damage tissue, often by damaging the deoxyribonucleic acid (DNA) which regulates activity of the cell. DNA damage explains why radiation can lead to mutation and malignant changes.

Nutritional factors

Malnutrition means abnormal nutrition and can be caused by too much or too little of a dietary component. If more energy is consumed than the body uses, the excess will be stored as fat, leading to the development of obesity. Excessive ingestion of some foods has been associated with the aetiology of vascular disease, hypertension (high blood pressure), heart disease, stroke, diabetes mellitus type 2 and some cancers.

Deficiency of dietary components can also lead to malnutrition. Lack of protein causes a condition often referred to as kwashiorkor characterized by oedema. Carbohydrate deficiency causes marasmus and a lack of fat in the diet can lead to weight loss and lack of the fat soluble vitamins, A, D, E and K. In practice, lack of protein, carbohydrate and fat usually go together; this causes a condition called protein energy malnutrition (PEM). Lack of water causes dehydration. Diets which are deficient in fibre can lead to constipation, haemorrhoids (piles) and play a role in the development of diverticulitis and cancer of the colon. Deficiency of iron can cause anaemia, as can a lack of folic acid and vitamin B_{12}. Scurvy is caused by lack of vitamin C and iodine deficiency can lead to cretinism and goitre.

Degenerative disorders

These conditions are associated with increasing age and occur as a complication of the degeneration of tissues, often as a result of a decrease in the number of viable cells. Cells are only able to divide a limited number of times; this means that after a limited number of divisions a cell line will die. Degeneration may also occur by a process of 'wear and tear' or as a result of an accumulation of damage sustained over the years.

These ongoing degenerative processes may affect the normal physiology of a cell; this may result in abnormal cell division which partly explains why most cancers become more common in older people. At the level of the tissues, loss of articular cartilage can give rise to osteoarthritis. Loss of brain cells can cause dementia. Decrease in the number of some cells which produce dopamine can cause Parkinson's disease. In the elderly there may be atrophy and degeneration of several organs and tissues which is sometimes severe enough to cause disease. When several disease states occur together in the elderly the term 'senile multiple pathology' is often used.

Abnormal immunity

Normally the immune system is defensive, protecting the body against infections of all types. However the immune system may malfunction leading to disease states. Autoimmunity is when the immune system attacks the body's own tissues, for example in diabetes mellitus type 1, the immune system eradicates the beta cells from the pancreatic islets. Another group of immunological disorders are the hypersensitivity reactions. In these disorders the body reacts in a disproportionate way, often to a foreign material which should generate no immune response at all. This can lead to life threatening states where there is swelling of the airway, bronchospasm and profound shock. Anaphylaxis is an example of one of these hypersensitivity disorders. While the immediate cause of these disorders is exposure to some environmental trigger, (such as nuts) there are also some genetic factors involved in the aetiology.

Neoplasm

'Neo' means new and 'plasm' relates to growth of tissue. A neoplasm is therefore a new tissue. Tumour means 'lump' and these are caused by the presence of new tissue. Tumours may be caused by exposure to environmental agents such as viruses, radiation and chemical carcinogens. A carcinogen is a chemical which can cause cancer, such as tar from tobacco smoke. Essentially, there are two forms of tumour, benign and malignant. A benign tumour is one which does not spread to distant sites in the body by the process of metastasis. Malignant tumours do spread (metastasize) around the body and start to grow at other sites. Many malignancies probably have some genetic component in their aetiology as well as environmental factors.

Psychosomatic factors

'Psych' means to do with the mind and 'soma' the body. Psychosomatic is therefore the effects of the mind on the body. This works the other way around as well, the body is able to affect the mind. The mind and the body are interrelated in numerous intricate ways, and it could be argued that it is not possible to separate them in the complex phenomenon which is a human being.

However, to take simple examples, the mind is affected by the body in many confusional states. If there is a systemic infection or a poor blood supply to the brain it will not be able to work as efficiently as in health. This can interfere with the ability of the brain to generate a clear mind. It is also known that psychological factors such as stress can adversely affect the efficiency of the immune system. Reduced levels of immunity may predispose to infections and arguably other conditions such as some malignancies. The placebo effect is also psychosomatic. This is when a person experiences some physical improvement because they believe an intervention will help them. The benefit of the placebo effect can occur even if a treatment has no physiological effect at all, such as with homeopathy.

Psychiatric disorders

Traditionally psychiatric disorders have been classified as psychotic or neurotic. While this is an over simplification it is often a useful model to use. Neuroses are mental problems caused by adverse environmental factors operating on the mind. For example; if a person gets divorced and loses their job they may become depressed as a reaction to the psychological trauma they have suffered. Excessive stress and things to worry about in the environment of life can lead to anxiety neurosis and panic attacks.

Psychotic illness originates in the mind, not in the environment. In psychotic illnesses the person often may appear to be 'mad'. They may suffer from hallucinations and delusions (false perceptions and beliefs respectively). Behaviour may sometimes, but not always be bizarre. Examples of psychotic illness include all forms of schizophrenia, bipolar disorder and paranoid psychosis.

Iatrogenic disease

These are disorders caused by clinical treatments. 'Iatro' is derived from the Greek for doctor, so literally these disorders begin with the doctor. For example if a patient develops pressure sores, as a result of being nursed in bed, the problem would be iatrogenic. Other causes of iatrogenesis relate to the side effects of drugs; antibiotics may cause iatrogenic diarrhoea, steroids may cause osteoporosis and morphine may cause respiratory depression. Overdose, drug errors and adverse reactions are also iatrogenic. If a nerve was damaged during surgery this would be iatrogenic nerve damage.

Idiopathic disease

The aetiology of idiopathic disease is unknown. Disease occurs, but we are not clear what the aetiology is. In fact idiopathic is a euphemism for 'don't know'. Idiopathic disease is also sometimes described as primary or essential. Although a disease is idiopathic, risk factors may be identified but the mechanism by which the disease is actually caused is unknown.

Multifactorial aetiology

In practice probably most diseases are multifactorial; this means they are caused by several factors which could be genetic and environmental. Many conditions probably involve several genes which give a level of genetic predisposition. This genetic makeup is then acted on by perhaps several environmental factors, which may eventually trigger a genetic predisposition, ultimately resulting in disease. If we are ever asked what causes a particular disease, (and we are not too sure of the answer) we are on fairly safe grounds if we say that 'it is caused by a combination of environmental and genetic factors'.

Congenital disorders

Congenital simply means 'present at birth'. These may therefore have a primarily endogenous or exogenous aetiology. In other words, if a disorder is present at birth, it may have occurred as a result of a genetic disorder or some environmental insult during the developmental process from zygote to baby. Cleft lip and palate is a well known example of a congenital disorder, affecting approximately 1 in a 1000 live births. Severity of this problem varies from a notch in the top lip to complete separation of the lip, up to the nose. There may also be a gap in the hard palate which forms the roof of the mouth.

Teratogenesis

A teratogen is any substance, agent or process which interferes with the normal development of a fetus before birth. Teratogens therefore lead to abnormalities in pre-natal development. The risk associated with exposure to teratogens is greatest during the first 12 weeks of pregnancy; this is the time when most tissue differentiation and generation of form takes place. The generation of form and shape is termed morphogenesis, ('morph' means shape, 'genesis' refers to beginnings). Some drugs and infections can be teratogenic, so is ionizing radiation, such as X rays.

Drugs

Thalidomide affected about 10,000 babies world-wide in the 1960s and caused some very serious developmental abnormalities. Some children were born with massively disrupted limb development. Alcohol is the most common drug leading to teratogenesis today. Fetal alcohol syndrome causes growth deficiencies, mental retardation, microcephaly (small brain) and a characteristic facial appearance with a thin upper lip. Most medicines are not teratogenic, but it is a good principle to avoid drugs in pregnancy if possible, unless we are sure a particular preparation is safe to use.

Adverse effects on the placenta, and therefore on fetal nutrition and oxygenation, are caused by maternal smoking. A mother smoking during pregnancy also increases the incidence of spontaneous abortion and low birth weight babies. Children born to smoking mothers are liable to a measurable delay in their physical and mental development up to the age of 11 years. Paternal (related to the father) drug use is also a bad idea. Cigarette smoking damages DNA in sperm. It has been strongly suggested that up to 14% of childhood cancers can be attributed to fathers smoking before conception.

Intrauterine infections

Some maternal infections in early pregnancy can lead to neurological problems including brain damage, visual impairment, deafness and congenital heart disease. Maternal rubella (German measles) infection is caused by a virus and can lead to disorders of the pulmonary blood vessels, heart, eyes, brain and hearing in affected babies. This is why it is so important to vaccinate girls for rubella before they reach reproductive age. As with other potential teratogens the effects are more serious if the infection is contracted in early pregnancy. Cytomegalovirus (CMV), a member of the herpes group of viruses, is another infection which can be teratogenic.

Radiation

Radiation exposure is a particular risk during pregnancy. Radiation may damage the genetic material in the rapidly dividing cells which are generating the new body in the process of morphogenesis. In addition to the risks of developmental abnormalities children exposed to radiation in the uterus are at increased risk of childhood leukaemia. This is why we must always ensure a woman is not pregnant before she is X-rayed. It is also vital that health care workers stringently avoid X-rays if there is any possibility of pregnancy.

Nutrition

Good maternal nutrition around the time of conception and in pregnancy is important. Neural tube defects, such as spina bifida, affect the development of the spinal cord. Studies have demonstrated that an adequate intake of folic acid has a significant protective effect, greatly reducing the prevalence of this congenital disorder. The practical implication of this are that we should advise prospective mothers to eat foods such as Brussels sprouts, spinach, kale, yeast extracts and cooked black eyed beans. All of these foods are rich sources of folic acid. In some cases supplements may also be advised.

Health care and disease aetiology

If we understand the causation of disease we are then in a position to advise people how to avoid risk factors. This could prevent the formation of disease in some, and delay disease onset in others. It is always better to prevent disease, rather than to treat it once present. Disease prevention may simply involve giving information such as avoiding smoke or eating less fat. It may involve changes in the wider environment to make it healthier; this broader field is the whole area of health promotion. Vaccination is another obvious way that we seek to prevent disease.

Prophylaxis

This term describes any measure which may be taken to prevent or protect against disease or disease complications. As mentioned, vaccination is a prophylactic measure against infectious disease. In some wounds, antibiotics may be given as a prophylactic treatment to prevent infection. A small daily dose of aspirin may be given to reduce platelet stickiness and so reduce the likelihood of developing coronary thrombosis.

Identifying disease

The process whereby a disease is identified, and a conclusion reached, is termed the diagnosis. In order to arrive at a diagnosis there must be an assessment of the clinical features, disease history and often pathological and other investigations are also required.

Clinical features

Recognition of disease comes from discerning the signs and symptoms which present in a particular patient. A sign is something we are able to detect with our senses. For example if we see that the patient is sweating or bleeding this is a sign. Feeling a lump or abnormal pulse are also clinical signs. In fact some signs we may also hear or smell. For example; we may hear noisy, stertorous breathing in a partly obstructed airway or smell acetone on the breath of a patient in a diabetic ketoacidotic coma.

Symptoms are something the patient experiences; we only become aware of them as they are reported to us. For example we cannot see a patient's pain, but they may report it to us as a symptom. Nausea and feelings of sickness are other commonly reported symptoms. Collectively, signs and symptoms are sometimes called clinical features. Together this group of clinical features presents a 'clinical picture' which will indicate the presence of a particular disorder. Another common term is syndrome which describes a group of clinical features which are likely to present together. For example AIDS is acquired immunodeficiency syndrome. There is not a single presentation of the disorder but different individual features from the syndrome may present at a particular time.

History taking

Another essential component of patient assessment is history taking. It is vital that we learn all we can by talking to the patient, or to friends and relatives. This will allow us to build up a picture of the problem itself and how the problem developed. From history taking we learn what the patient has felt and is currently feeling. We learn the background to the individual and to the complaint they have. History taking from a patient is where most information comes from which allows a diagnosis to be made. This is why the ability to communicate with our patients is the most important clinical skill in assessment and diagnosis. Clearly the information gained at this stage will then go on to influence all of the future management the patient will receive. Once the clinical features and history have been assessed, various samples from a patient are often sent to the pathology laboratory. Traditionally these laboratories are divided into sections which study biochemistry, haematology, histology and microbiology.

Pathological investigations

Biochemistry examines the chemical nature of samples and identifies the levels of particular chemicals. Much of the routine work in biochemistry is involved with analysis of blood samples. Common investigations include quantification of serum levels of glucose, cholesterol, urea and electrolytes, cellular enzymes, and thyroid hormone.

Haematology is the study of blood. Common tests will quantify levels of haemoglobin and the proportion of blood volume represented by red cells. Numbers of white cells will be counted and the relative proportion of various forms of leucocytes quantified. This is called a differential white cell count and will give the numbers of neutrophils, lymphocytes, eosinophils, basophils, monocytes and platelets present. Coagulation studies are also carried out in haematology, these determine how long blood takes to clot, a common test in this area is the international normalisation ratio (INR). Reduced numbers of platelets (thrombocytes) will also lead to a reduction in the ability of the blood to clot. The type and form of red and white cells may also be determined using microscopy.

Histology is the study of tissues. Tissue samples from a biopsy or post mortem are usually fixed in wax and mounted on a microscope slide. This is then examined to determine the presence of disease in the tissue or cells. Histology can determine if a particular sample contains malignant or benign cells. Microscopic examination can detect the presence of other tissue abnormalities such as inflammation or pre-malignant change. Histology can also be used to identify where a tissue sample came from. For example after vasectomy it is useful to confirm that the correct tube was cut and ligated. This is done by microscopic examination of a small part of the tissue which is removed.

Microbiology looks for the presence of microorganisms in a sample. This may be done by smearing the sample on a microscope slide and using a stain to identify particular species. However, more commonly bacterial samples are cultured by smearing them onto an agar plate. Agar nourishes any bacteria present and allows them to multiply, forming colonies. Once millions of bacteria are cultured in this way, their identification is relatively straight forward to the experienced eye. As well as studying any organisms present microbiologists also identify which antibiotics a bacterial species is sensitive to. This information can then be passed on to the prescriber who can give the patient the most effective antibiotic for their infection.

Other investigations

Numerous other forms of investigations may be carried out to arrive at a precise diagnosis. X-rays for example can reveal fractures and disorders of bone. They can also identify numerous lung disorders such as asthma and pneumonia. Computerised axial tomography (CAT) scanning also uses X-rays to build up two and three dimensional images of internal body structures. CAT scanning is useful as it can identify and produce images of soft tissues. Magnetic resonance imaging (MRI) uses a very powerful magnetic field to visualise internal structures. This form of scanning is particularly good at imaging neurological tissues and has the advantage of not using potentially dangerous X-rays. Another form of scanning is positron emission tomography (PET) which is a nuclear medicine technique. A radioactive ladled molecule is injected into the patient to allow visualisation of functional processes in the body.

Direct examination using endoscopy is also frequently possible. These flexible devices use fibre optics to transmit an image to an eyepiece and video screen. Specialised instruments may be passed into areas such as the stomach, duodenum, bladder or colon. Direct observation is also possible using 'key hole' techniques such as laparoscopy. Ultrasound scanning can also generate images of internal structures; these can be used to examine any internal organ and are used routinely in pregnancy. Ultrasound can identify numerous disorders including cysts, stones in the bladder or gall bladder and aneurysm development. In cardiology ultrasound can be combined with Doppler to give moving colour images of blood flow.

Differential diagnosis

Sometimes, even after a full assessment of clinical features, history taking and pathological examinations, a definitive diagnosis may not be possible. If there are several possibilities these are called the differential diagnosis. For example, diarrhoea and vomiting may have a differential diagnosis of viral or bacterial gastroenteritis. Headaches are another symptom with multiple differential diagnoses. Headache could be caused by such problems as psychological tension, sinusitis, migraine, head injury, subarachnoid haemorrhage, brain tumours and visual problems. Detailed study of the clinical features, history and investigation results are needed to identify the most likely cause.

Acute and chronic disease

Acute means 'of recent onset' as opposed to chronic which means a disease or disorder has developed slowly or has persisted over a period of time. An acute condition arises rapidly and is usually accompanied by distinctive clinical features which allow it to be recognised. So an acute pneumonia will present quickly, with the patient starting to feel ill over a few hours. There will be fever and malaise. Heart and respiratory rates are both likely to be increased and there may be a reduction in oxygen saturations. Likewise, an acute appendicitis is one which has presented 'all of a sudden'. Acute confusion is a confusional state which has developed abruptly, perhaps overnight. Very often acute conditions require an immediate intervention, for example acute bacterial pneumonia will require immediate treatment with antibiotics. An acute appendicitis may be an indication for the surgical removal of the inflamed appendix. If the cause of the acute confusional state can be identified the condition is fully reversible and the patient will become lucid again.

Examples of chronic conditions include multiple sclerosis, chronic obstructive pulmonary disease, diabetes mellitus, hypertension (high blood pressure), osteoarthritis (wear and tear arthritis) and motor neurone disease. The clinical features typically have an insidious onset and the disorders persist over time. For example, a patient may get vague pains with stiffness in their knee and hip joints which gradually worsen over several years. The condition will progress and eventually osteoarthritis will be diagnosed. Disease progression eventually means that any movement causes severe pain and the joint becomes progressively immobile. These chronic conditions are not usually curable as many acute conditions are. However, symptoms can usually be treated to improve the quality of life. Chronic conditions therefore often require long term follow up and management. For example, a patient with high blood pressure will need to be supervised for life to ensure the blood pressure is controlled on an ongoing basis with appropriate medication. A patient with some neurological deficit after a stroke may need help with the activities of daily living for prolonged periods of time.

Disease severity is how serious the disease is and is a description of how badly a condition is effecting an individual. A mild disease will only generate mild and limited clinical features whereas a severe condition is likely to cause more extreme clinical features and might even be life threatening.

Fulminant disease

Fulminant describes a condition which occurs suddenly and is severe. For example, if there is a sudden severe impairment of liver function after a viral infection or paracetamol overdose, the patient will suffer from confusion, stupor and then coma. This form of acute hepatic failure is fulminant. Lobar pneumonia is another example; the condition can occur acutely and be very severe, even resulting in death.

Complications

A complication is a problem which presents as a result of some previously existing condition. For example a peptic ulcer may digest through the wall of a blood vessel which will start to bleed into the stomach or duodenum. This haemorrhage is a complication. If the ulcer is deep there is a risk that it may erode through the wall of the duodenum and allow gastrointestinal contents to escape in to the peritoneal cavity. In other words peritonitis may complicate peptic ulceration.

If a patient suffers a blood clot in one of the deep veins of the legs this is called deep venous thrombosis (DVT). If part of the clot breaks off and travels to the lungs a pulmonary embolism (PE) will result. This means DVT can be complicated by PE. An important part of patient care is to know what complications may occur in particular conditions and then take measures to prevent them if possible. If a complication cannot be prevented we should be able to recognise it as early as possible to instigate early treatment.

Bed rest, for example may be complicated by pressure sore development if we do not take active measures to prevent their occurrence. Hypostatic bronchopneumonia may also complicate bed rest, especially if the patient spends a lot of time recumbent. Other possible complications of immobility include reduction in metabolic rate, decrease in bone density and muscle mass, urinary tract infection, loss of physical fitness, constipation and psychological depression. Many of these complications can be prevented with good management strategies.

Localised or widespread disease

A localised disease process is restricted to one part of the body, for example conjunctivitis is an inflammation of the conjunctiva which lines the front of the eye. No other tissues or parts of the body are necessarily involved. Other examples of localized infection are an abscess or boil, again only a small area is affected. In contrast to this a widespread disease affects more than one area, the condition may be widespread throughout a whole organ or area of tissue. Systemic disease involves whole body systems, for example a systemic infection can affect almost all of the tissues in the body making the patient feel generally unwell.

Lesion

A lesion is an area of tissue affected by a disease process. There may be a single lesion or many. After a coronary thrombosis there will be an area of dead myocardial muscle. This area is the lesion. In multiple sclerosis there may be multiple small lesions disseminated throughout the central nervous system which give rise to the clinical features of the disease.

Disease evolution

Evolution is a term which simply means 'change'. Any disorder will change and progress over time, this is also described as the natural history of a disorder. We often say that a disorder will 'run its course'. This progression may be in a positive direction, evolving towards resolution. Alternatively the disorder may progress in a negative direction with deterioration and increasing severity.

A typical disease process starts when the individual is exposed to the causative agent of a disease or is injured. For example, a person may be exposed to the virus which causes the common cold. This will be followed by a period of latency, this is an incubation period when the disease will be developing but the patient does not suffer from any signs or symptoms. A good example of this is HIV infection where the period of asymptomatic (without symptoms) latency may last for several years. Next in the progression of a disease process there is a prodromal phase. In this stage the disease process had developed and is starting to make the individual feel unwell with clinical features which are usually mild and non-specific. The prodromal phase will then develop into the acute phase. This is when the presentation of the disease reaches its full intensity. How severe this stage is will vary greatly depending on the disease process and the severity of the disorder. During the acute phase the clinical features usually become more localized and specific, allowing the disease process to be recognised. This is important as specific treatments may be given once the disease is diagnosed. Finally, (unless the condition is terminal) perhaps after some further relapses and remissions, the person will enter the recovery phase. In this stage the patient regains normal health and functionality.

In the ultimate analysis there are three possible outcomes of a disease process. Firstly there may be complete recovery, with a full return to health. This is usually the case after a period of infection. We may be ill with diarrhoea and vomiting for a few days but recover completely. Secondly there may be a degree of recovery but a patient may continue to suffer some adverse effects as a result of the condition. Cerebrovascular accident (stroke) is an example of this. Individuals are often left with a degree of neurological impairment. The term sequela (sequeli in pleural) is often used to describe anything sequel, that is something occurring after a disease process. In this case the neurological impairment is a sequela of the CVA. Thirdly a disease process can lead to death. In some forms of malignant disease, where the cancer cells have spread around the body, death will be the end point of the process.

Relapse, remission and exacerbation

In a disorder that lasts for a period of time there may be relapses and remissions. Multiple sclerosis is a disease which illustrates this principle. A patient may remain fairly well for a time then relapse; this means the condition gets worse. A relapse may be followed by a remission; this is when the condition improves for a time. Remissions may be partial or complete. A partial remission represents an improvement while complete remission would be an apparent return to normal health. Exacerbation is another term which means a condition deteriorates. Patients with chronic bronchitis may suffer an acute exacerbation of the chronic condition as a result of infection. This means the clinical features, which they have all the time to some extent, become rapidly worse.

Convalescence

This describes the time when the active disease process has been treated or has run a natural course. The person no longer has the disease but may be significantly weakened as a result of the condition they have suffered from. Convalescence describes this recovery phase, after the disease, but before they have returned to full health and strength. This period may take days, weeks or months depending on the nature and severity of the disease which the individual has experienced. As a general principle rest, fluids, good nutrition and human company are the most important factors which promote convalescence. Sometimes physiotherapy and other active rehabilitation measures such as those provided by occupational therapists are needed.

Terminal disease and palliative care

A terminal illness is one in which there is no possibility of a cure. The patient's physical condition may decline, rapidly or slowly, but death will be the end result of the disease process. Examples of terminal diseases are severe cardiac failure, hepatic failure, severe obstructive pulmonary disease, degenerative neurological diseases and some malignant disorders. In this situation the focus and philosophy of care changes from curative to palliative. Palliative care is therefore given to patients who have not responded to attempted curative interventions. Palliative care emphasizes control of pain and other distressing features generated by the disease process. There must also be a focus on psychological, social and spiritual aspects of the whole person. The aim is not to hasten death or to prolong life but to improve the quality of life in a positive way. Palliative care is an opportunity to bring the very best of our clinical skills to optimise the time a person has left and to promote human compassion and dignity.

Prognosis

Prognosis is a prediction of the probable course and outcome of a disorder. For an individual a prognosis is not a certain prediction but an expression of what is most likely to occur. The prognosis of a particular disease can be worked out by taking averages from a large number of cases. Typical terms used to describe a prognosis are 'excellent' or 'good' if the outcome is very likely to be favourable. 'Guarded' means the outcome is uncertain. A 'poor' prognosis usually means there is likely to be some ongoing problem as a result of the disease process. 'Grave' means the likely outcome is death.

Epidemiology

Epidemiology studies health and illness in groups and populations, as opposed to individuals. Examples of epidemiological data include mortality and morbidity rates. Mortality rate measures the number of deaths in a population, figures quoted are usually deaths per year per 1000 people. Morbidity measures the levels of illness in a population. This is usually expressed in terms of incidence and prevalence.

Incidence and prevalence

Disease incidence is the number of new cases which present over a period of time, usually measured over one year. Prevalence is the number of cases existing in a population at a particular time, or over a short period of time. This means that acute conditions which are of short duration will have a high incidence and a low prevalence. For example, there will be many new cases of the common cold in any one year, but at any one time, the prevalence may be low. Chronic disorders will have a higher prevalence than incidence. In conditions such as HIV, stable angina or diabetes mellitus, the sufferers may live for tens of years after diagnosis. This means there will be more cases present in a population at any one time than there will be new cases over a year.

Correlation studies

Correlation studies compare two variables in a population. First, health and disease data is collected and then compared with other factors, such as life style. For example, in the 1950s and early 1960s it became obvious that people who smoked were more likely to develop lung cancer than those who were non-smokers. In other words smoking and lung cancer are two variables which are correlated. Later it was discovered that people who smoke also have an increased risk of suffering from coronary heart disease (CHD), in this case the variables are smoking and CHD. Epidemiology can therefore be very useful in identifying environmental aetiological factors of disease. If we know the factors which predispose to a disease state, we can then advise people how to avoid them. Other epidemiological techniques include geographical, cohort (group) and experimental studies.

Screening for disease

Screening involves looking for the early presence of disease in people who appear healthy. If this is done, disease states may be detected at an early stage, when treatment is less traumatic and more likely to be curative than it would be with a late presentation.

Cervical cytology examines cells from the cervix and is able to detect pre-malignant changes. It is possible to remove pre-malignant tissue and therefore prevent cancer from developing. Regular dental check-ups can screen for the early development of oral cancers, and again treatment can be offered. Individuals who are considered to be at increased risk of a disorder can also be monitored closely. For example, testicular cancer is more likely to occur in men who have a childhood history of undescended testes. People who have had polyps in the colon, which can be a pre-malignant condition, may be advised to have a colonoscopy every few years.

In addition, if a disorder is identified at an early stage, further problems caused by the disorder can be prevented. Undiagnosed diabetes mellitus type 2 for example can cause the development of complications such as coronary heart disease, peripheral vascular disease, renal failure and diabetic retinopathy leading to blindness. If diabetes mellitus type 2 is 'picked up' at an early stage it can readily be managed, significantly reducing the risk of long term complications. Undiagnosed hypertension does not generate any clinical features, but it does damage the kidneys, blood vessels and heart. If it is identified it can be managed, greatly reducing the risk of complications. Obesity is another example, it predisposes to diabetes mellitus type 2 and coronary heart disease if present, but if it is identified and weight is lost, the risks are reduced.

CHAPTER 2

Neoplasia

Introduction

Neoplasia is a general term which means 'new growth'. In normal physiology there are mechanisms which regulate cell division and the generation of new tissues. If these physiological mechanisms fail for any reason, cells may then multiply at an increased rate. This will result in the presence of a greater number of cells. These cells take up space and usually form lumps which are called tumours. In leukaemia there is an uncontrolled growth of cells from the bone marrow. These do not form tumours, as the excess numbers of abnormal cells enter the blood. In either case when the increased numbers of cells present are malignant, the condition is described as cancer. Cancer is not a single disease. Over 200 different forms of cancer are recognised, depending on the primary site of the malignancy.

Aetiology of Cancer

Neoplasms and mutations

A mutation describes an alteration in the genetic material of a cell. Factors which contribute to the development of cancer generate mutations in a cell or group of cells. It is believed that many neoplasms develop from a single mutated cell. When the genetic material of a cell is damaged, causing a mutation, the cell will normally die. However, some mutations arise in genes which normally function to stimulate cell division; these are called oncogenes. Other mutations may arise in genes which normally inhibit cell division; these are called tumour suppressor genes. Mutations in oncogenes or tumour suppressor genes may therefore result in greatly increased rates of cell division resulting in a hyperplasia, which describes an increase in the number of cells. Collectively the presence of many new cells generates the new tissue which is the neoplasia.

Chemical carcinogens

A carcinogen is an agent which may cause cancer, literally 'cancer beginning'. Most chemical carcinogens work by altering the chemical composition of the DNA (deoxyribonucleic acid) molecules. This change in the nature of the DNA represents an alteration in the genetic material of the cell, in other words carcinogens cause mutations.

Tobacco smoke as a carcinogen

Tobacco smoke contains numerous carcinogens such as benzopyrene. Cancer risks in smokers are proportional to the number of cigarettes smoked and the duration of smoking. As well as being an independent risk factor for cancer, smoking works synergistically with other risks such as uranium dust, asbestos inhalation or alcohol. Smoking is the single largest cause of cancer in the world. Smoking can clearly cause cancers in the tissues smoke comes into direct contact with; these include cancers of the lips, mouth and larynx. People who smoke 1-14 cigarettes per day have an eight times greater risk of dying from lung cancer compared to non-smokers. At 25 cigarettes per day the risk is 25 times. If a person stops smoking their risk of lung cancer falls by 50% over ten years and by 95% over 15 years after stopping smoking.

Chemical carcinogens from smoke are absorbed through the lungs and excreted via the kidneys and bladder. This has the effect of concentrating carcinogens in these organs explaining why smokers are more likely to develop renal and bladder cancers. Smokers are also more likely to develop cancers of the oesophagus, stomach, pancreas, liver and some forms of leukaemia than non-smokers. Snuff or chewing tobacco can also cause nasal and mouth cancers. Clearly smoking pipes and cigars also increases risk.

Direct and indirect carcinogens

Chemicals which may cause cancer without first being modified in the body are called direct carcinogens. Other chemicals are indirect carcinogens; these are chemicals which only become carcinogenic after they have been metabolically altered in the body. For example, aflatoxin is an indirect carcinogen. Aflatoxins are found in moulds growing on foods, such as grains and peanuts, and contribute to the high incidence of liver cancers in many African regions. Another group of carcinogens are the N-nitroso compounds. These are found in salted, smoked or pickled meat and have a positive correlation with the development of oesophageal, nasopharyngeal, bladder and liver cancer.

Initiation and promotion

Most cancers need to be initiated and then promoted. Exposure to some carcinogens results in a rapid, permanent genetic mutation, as a result of damage to DNA molecules. This is the process of cancer initiation. Chemicals which have this effect are called initiating carcinogens. However this alone does not result in malignant changes. The initiated cells only become malignant if they are subsequently exposed to a promoting carcinogen. This will act on the changes already initiated, leading to the development of a cancer. If cells are exposed to promoters, without having been exposed to an initiating carcinogen, malignant changes will not develop. Promoters work by stimulating increased rates of mitosis in cells already initiated. This promotion completes the process of malignant transformation and gives rise to a population of cancer cells with subsequent tumour formation.

Some tumours only emerge after continued, ongoing exposure to promoters. For example, if a person stops smoking, they will no longer be exposed to promoters in cigarette smoke and so their chances of developing several forms of cancer will progressively decline. Some carcinogens are able to initiate and promote malignant change. These are called complete carcinogens.

Free radicals

Free radicals are highly reactive chemicals produced inside cells as a result of metabolic processes. These molecules are very reactive because they have an unpaired electron in their outer orbital. This means they have a tendency to 'steal' an electron from other molecules around them. If an electron is removed from a molecule this is referred to as oxidation. This means free radicals have the potential to oxidise, and therefore change cellular molecules including the genetic material, DNA. Chemical changes in DNA change the nature of the molecule and are therefore mutations. This is why it is believed free radicals may lead to some cancers.

Radiation

Ionizing radiation may cause cancer. This is radiation which may add or remove electrons from atoms, to generate ions. Ions are chemically reactive. If radiation forms ions in the DNA molecules, subsequent chemical reactions will change the chemical nature of the DNA resulting in mutation. Alternatively, radiation passing into a cell may react with water in the cytosol to convert water into free radical species, such as hydroxyl ions (OH-). Free radicals are reactive species and so may chemically interact with DNA molecules, again leading to mutation

Diagram 2.1
Possible outcomes of DNA damage.
1. This is a healthy cell with an intact complete strand of DNA illustrated.
2. As a result of exposure to a chemical carcinogen or radiation the DNA has been damaged resulting in a change to the genetic material, in other words there has been a mutation.
3. One possible outcome is that the cell is able to repair the DNA.
4. Another possibility is that the mutation triggers cell apoptosis, resulting in cell death. This means the cell is unable to reproduce.
5. Alternatively the damaged cell may survive, carrying the mutation.
6. After mitosis, the damaged cell has divided to produce 2 daughter cells, each with the mutation. These will undergo further mitotic divisions to generate a population of mutated cells.

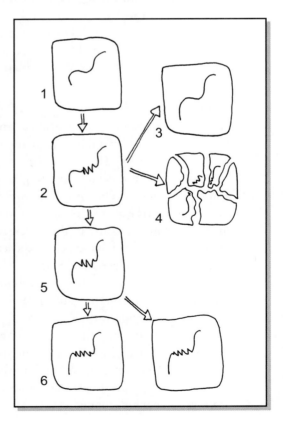

of the cells genetic material. The effects of ionizing radiation were clearly seen after Hiroshima, Nagasaki and Chernobyl. X-rays are also ionizing. The risks of cancers are high when radioactive elements are eaten or inhaled. Such radioactive materials may become lodged in the body and will emit ionizing radiation directly into the body tissues. For example, lung cancer is common in uranium miners who inhale radioactive dust.

Ultraviolet (UV) in sunshine is another form of radiation. Melanin is the dark pigment which skin melanocytes produce as a result of ultraviolet exposure. This melanin will absorb much of the UV, and so gives the skin a significant degree of protection. However, melanin production takes time. This means that if the skin is suddenly exposed to a lot of direct sunshine, there is insufficient time for significant amounts of protective melanin to be synthesized. This leaves the skin vulnerable for a period of time. Ironically the melanocytes themselves are particularly prone to UV damage; this can result in DNA damage, mutation and malignant change causing malignant melanoma.

Radiation damage to cells is cumulative over long periods of time. This is one reason why there should always be a good clinical indication before radiation is used in medical imaging or treatments.

DNA repair

Cells have inbuilt systems to allow repair of damaged DNA. These mechanisms provide a significant degree of protection from cancer development. Specialised intracellular proteins can detect and remove (i.e. excise) damaged sections of DNA. As the DNA molecule consists of a double helix, the damaged strand may be restored, using the undamaged strand as a template. This process is termed excision repair. Other damaged cells commit suicide in the process of apoptosis. These mechanisms can therefore protect against damage to cellular genetic material caused by chemical carcinogens or radiation. However, if

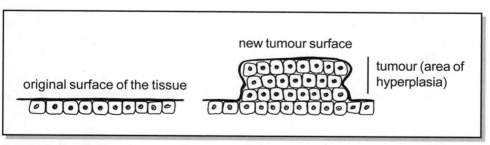

Diagram 2.2
Repeated mitosis of a cell carrying a mutation may generate a population of cells with the same malignant mutation. This will give rise to a group of cells, all with the same genetic material, including the mutation. A group of cells with the same genetic makeup is referred to as a clonal group. Starting with 1 malignant cell, there would be over a million after 20 divisions. The rate of cell division also determines the rate of tumour growth.

damaged DNA cannot be repaired, or the cells fail to undergo apoptosis, the mutated cell may divide to generate a clonal population of mutated cells which then develop into a malignant tumour.

Oncogenic viruses

These are viruses that can cause cancer. Numerous cancer causing (oncogenic) viruses have been identified in animal experiments and several are important in causing human malignancies. Oncogenic viruses may be RNA based retroviruses or DNA viruses. Human papilloma virus (HPV) can cause cervical, skin and anal cancers. Hepatitis B virus may lead to hepatocellular carcinoma. Epstein-Barr virus (EBV) can cause nasopharyngeal cancers as well as an aggressive tumour of B lymphocytes called Burkitt's lymphoma. Hodgkin's disease is another lymphoma and a proportion of cases are also caused by EBV. It is recognised that human T lymphotropic virus 1 (HTLV-1) may cause adult T cell leukaemia. Kaposi's sarcoma is caused by a herpesvirus.

Cancer and immunity

Some cancers, such as lymphoma, are more common in immunosuppressed patients. Also long term immunosuppression leads to more cancers which are virus related. These observations have given rise to the concept of immune surveillance which suggests that the healthy immune system is able to detect and eradicate cancers at an early stage so the person is never aware there has been anything wrong. This line of thinking would suggest that cancer arises as a result of a failure of immune surveillance. The reason the immune system does not always eradicate cancer is that the neoplastic cells derive from the persons own cells. Cancer cells therefore have essentially the same antigens as normal cells. This means the immune system is often unable to identify a cancer cell as being any different from a normal body cell.

Cancer and hormones

Some hormones which stimulate particular tissues are sometimes regarded as promoters. For example, testosterone seems to promote testicular cancer and oestrogen breast cancer. Once a malignancy has developed, the hormone which stimulates the normal tissue also stimulates growth of the malignant cells.

Cancer and age

Most cancers become more common with increasing age. Cancers of the skin, oesophagus, stomach, rectum, prostate and pancreas are generally associated with increasing age. It is sometimes said that everyone will get cancer if they do not die of something else first. Other cancers have a peak age of incidence, such as lymphoblastic leukaemia and those affecting the breast and cervix. Testicular cancers have a peak age of presentation at around 30 years; after this time the incidence of the disease decreases.

Genetic factors

As well as the environmental factors discussed above, genetics can lead to a hereditary predisposition to some cancers. Certain cancers have a clear genetic mode of inheritance. For example, a malignant tumour of the retina called retinoblastoma is often inherited as an autosomal dominant disorder. The same pattern of inheritance is seen in familial adenomatous polyposis, where adenomas of the colon develop. Some specific dominant inherited genes (called the BRCA-1 and BRCA-2 genes) have been shown to strongly predispose to the development of breast and ovarian cancer at an early age.

The concept of 'cancer families' has been known for some time. In these families there are many more cases of cancer than would be normally expected. It could be that some families have been exposed to a common external cancer causing agent, but it seems more likely in most cases that the predisposition is genetic. Members of 'cancer families' often develop malignancies at a much younger age than is normally seen, again indicating a genetic aetiology.

Cancer prevention

It is estimated that about half the cases of cancer in the UK could be prevented with changes in life style. Life style and environmental factors probably play a similar role in the number of cancers caused in different countries. The challenge is to recognise the particular factors operating in our communities and to advise people accordingly.

Never use tobacco

There is no safe level of smoking; any tobacco use will increase cancer risk to some degree. Sniffing or chewing tobacco also increases cancer risk.

Limit alcohol intake

Excessive use of alcohol increases the risk of developing cancers of the mouth, larynx, oesophagus, liver and breast. In several cancers, the risks of alcohol are amplified if the person smokes as well. In other words alcohol and smoking are often synergistic risk factors. Drinking in young people seems to be increasing in the UK with young women being at particular risk. Everyone should be advised to keep below the 'safe' levels of alcohol consumption of 21 units per week for men and 14 for women. All drinkers should therefore be taught the units system and keep a record of their intake. In the UK one unit is equal to 10 mls of pure alcohol.

Have a good diet; avoid 'junk' foods

Dietary factors are probably linked to about a third of UK cancers. Links have been made between diet and cancer of the oesophagus, stomach, bowel, prostate and colon. For example colon cancers are less common in people who eat plenty of fibre and little or no red meat. Eating fish may also offer some protection against bowel cancer. Breast cancer may be linked to a high fat intake.

General dietary advice is to eat at least 5 portions of fruit and vegetables per day. This will provide vitamins, flavanoids and water soluble fibre. We should try to eat a wide variety of foods as these contain different vitamins, micronutrients and flavanoids. Often vegetables are overcooked which degrades many nutrients, we should try to eat vegetables when they are still crunchy. Plenty of non-water soluble fibre, found in brown wheat, brown rice and wholemeal bread is also important. Processed foods generally contain a lot of fat, salt and sugar. Excess of these dietary components is bad for us. Eating well during childhood is probably particularly important; all children should be provided with a balanced, adequate diet.

Several recent studies have suggested good levels of vitamin D in the blood can help to reduce the risk of several cancers. The evidence is probably strongest for vitamin D reducing the occurrence of colorectal cancers, but some studies suggest it may also reduce the likelihood of developing breast, prostate and pancreatic cancers. The body can produce vitamin D when exposed to sunlight, but this depends on latitude and skin colour. People with dark skins produce less vitamin D with sun exposure. It is also found in foods such as liver, eggs and fish oils. More research is needed to clarify the role of vitamin D in preventing, and possibly even in treating some cancers.

Eat enough antioxidants to neutralise free radicals

Oxidation damage caused by free radicals can be reduced by the presence of antioxidants. Antioxidants may donate electrons to free radicals and so neutralise their ability to oxidise other molecules and mutate DNA. Vitamins A, C and E the 'ACE' vitamins all have antioxidant properties. Selenium is a trace element which is incorporated into proteins to make selenoproteins which are antioxidant enzymes. Flavanoids are naturally occurring phenolic compounds. They are powerful antioxidants, found in a wide variety of fruit and vegetables and also found in tea. If people eat a diet with a good variety of fruit and vegetables, they should automatically be eating a variety of antioxidant flavanoids. Most recent trials indicate that taking additional amounts of antioxidants in supplements does not give additional protection and might even be harmful.

Combat and prevent obesity

Being overweight increases the risk of several cancers including uterine, renal, oesophageal and colon. In order to lose weight people need to eat fewer calories, eat healthily and take enough exercise.

Be physically active

Inactivity and obesity increases the risk of colorectal, breast, renal and endometrial cancer. Moderate to high intensity exercise will improve physical fitness and offer some protection against these and possibly other cancers. Current thinking suggests we should all do at least 30 minutes of moderate exercise, such as cycling or brisk walking, at least 5 times per week. Higher levels of exercise probably confer even more benefit.

Avoid too much ultraviolet radiation

Sunlight, and light from sunbeds both contain ultraviolet (UV) radiation. UV causes most cases of skin cancer. Even in tanned people the skin may still be damaged by UV radiation. White people are at much greater risk from UV damage than black or brown people. The darker the colour of the skin the more protective melanin it contains. White children are at most risk, UV exposure in childhood, especially if it leads to sunburn, increases the probability of developing malignant melanoma in later life.

Sunglasses must filter ultraviolet light to be helpful. If they do not filter UV radiation, they will still reduce the amount of visible light reaching the eye, this will cause the pupil to dilate and so will actually increase the amount of UV rays entering the eye.

> The SunSmart code summarises appropriate advice;
> **S**tay in the shade from 11 to 3
> **M**ake sure you never burn
> **A**lways cover up with a hat, shirt and sunglasses
> **R**emember to take extra care with children
> **T**hen use lots of factor 15 or higher sunscreen

Avoid carcinogens

Many people may come into contact with chemical carcinogens at work. Asbestos fibres inhaled into the lungs may cause a malignancy of the pleural membrane called mesothelioma; they may also cause lung cancer. Benzene is a carcinogen found in the petroleum industry, present in oil, petrol and gas. Benzidine dyes may be used to dye textiles. Some organic solvents used in the rubber, textile, paint, printing and cleaning industries are carcinogenic. Some agricultural herbicides, insecticides and fertilizers may also pose a risk. Exposure to chemical carcinogens is a particular risk in developing countries where health and safety regulations are often not enforced. Radiation and nuclear waste are clearly dangerous.

Dioxins are produced by the petroleum and chlorine processing industries. They are also released in large amounts when plastics are burned (this is why we should not burn medical plastic waste in low temperature incinerators). After burning, carcinogenic dioxins fall out onto agricultural land and so are incorporated into the food chain. As dioxins are fat soluble they tend to concentrate in the fatty parts of animals and milk. Humans need to stop releasing dioxins into the environment.

Vaccination

Hepatitis B virus is a major global cause of hepatocellular carcinoma. Health care professionals are at increased risk of being exposed to this virus from blood and body fluids. This is why all nurses and doctors should be vaccinated against hepatitis B. A vaccine against some strains of HPV (human papilloma virus) to protect women from cervical cancer is now available in some countries.

Eradicate Helicobacter pylori

There is a strong link between H. pylori infection and gastric cancer. In this sense H. pylori is a carcinogen. People who have recurrent episodes of gastritis or peptic ulceration are more likely to have this bacterial infection. Once eradication therapy has removed H. pylori bacteria, the risk of gastric cancer is significantly reduced.

Treat chronic gastro-oesophageal regurgitation

Ongoing, unmanaged reflux of gastric contents into the lower oesophagus may lead to the metaplasia of Barrett's oesophagus which strongly predisposes to carcinoma of the oesophagus.

Promote immune function

If it is true that cancer can result from a failure of 'immune surveillance' then factors which promote immunity should offer protection against cancer. Immune function is reduced by psychological stress and malnutrition. It has been strongly argued that exposure to a wide range of microorganisms, especially in childhood, promotes immune function. This may result in less allergies, infections and even malignancies in later life. Clearly there are potential problems associated with this approach as children may suffer from infections. However, it seems clear that children are not designed to live in 'sterile' environments, the immune system needs to be 'trained' in combat with microorganisms.

Epidemiology and incidence of cancer

Over 200 forms of cancer have been recognised and the incidence of particular forms varies between countries. As age is a significant risk factor for cancer, the overall incidence will increase with increasing population age. In the UK, it is estimated that more than a third of people will develop cancer at some stage in their lives.

In the UK the four most common cancers, in order of incidence, are breast, lung, colon and prostate. However in Middle Africa the order is Kaposi's sarcoma, liver, cervix and stomach, in Eastern Asia it is stomach, lung, liver and oesophagus. As well as these geographical variations, incidence varies over time, in the UK cases of breast cancer in women have increased in the recent past while lung cancer in men has decreased. The incidence of malignancy also varies between men and women, usually for obvious reasons such as breast cancer

OVERALL	MEN	WOMEN
Breast	Prostate	Breast
Lung	Lung	Colorectal
Colorectal	Colorectal	Lung
Prostate	Bladder	Ovary
Bladder	Stomach	Body of uterus
Non-Hodgkin lymphoma (NHL)	Head and neck	NHL
Stomach	NHL	Pancreas
Head and neck	Oesophagus	Stomach
Oesophagus	Leukaemia	Bladder
Melanoma	Kidney	Melanoma
Pancreas		
Ovary		
Leukaemia		
Kidney		
Body of uterus		
Brain and CNS		
Multiple myeloma		
Cervix		
Liver		
Testicular		

Table 1
This table lists, in order, the most common primary forms of cancer (excluding NMSC) in the UK. Non-melanoma skin cancer (NMSC) is actually the most common form of primary cancer presentation in the UK but it is usually diagnosed and cured using simple resection by GPs.

being less common in men and women not having a prostate gland. This epidemiology is important as it alerts us to the main problems in our communities. Comparison of the forms of cancers commonly encountered in different areas can also point to the aetiology and so suggest helpful preventative measures which can be taken and specific advice that may be offered.

Naming and classifying cancers

Neoplasms are classified, and named, according to the tissue or cell type of origin. This is the cell or tissue type which undergoes the malignant transformation to become a cancer. Oma means a lump; this suffix usually appears at the end of a name describing a disorder, so a fibroma is a lump in fibrous tissue and a lipoma a lump in fatty tissue. Other useful descriptive words include; adeno – gland, haem – blood, angio – vessel, chondro – cartilage, osteo – bone, endo – inner lining, myo – muscle, leio – unstriated muscle, rhabdo – striated muscle, terat – embryo.

Carcinoma

Carcinomas arise from epithelial tissues. Adenocarcinoma arises from glandular epithelium such as glands lining the gastrointestinal tract. Squamous cell carcinoma arises from squamous epithelium, e.g. lung, oesophagus or cervix. Transitional cell carcinoma arises from transitional epithelium, such as that lining the urinary system. Most malignant tumours are either carcinomas or sarcomas.

Sarcoma

Sarcomas arise from cells in connective tissues. Osteosarcoma develops from bone cells and chondrosarcoma from cartilage. Leiomyosarcoma from smooth muscle and rhabdomyosarcoma from striated muscle. Liposarcoma derives from adipose tissue and a fibrosarcoma from fibrous tissues such as tendons.

Bone marrow derived cells

Leukaemias arise from haemopoietic cells. These are the cells which give rise to the various types of blood cells. Lymphomas are malignancies which arise from lymphocytes. Myeloma describes a malignant proliferation of plasma cells which are derived from B lymphocytes.

Other categories of malignancies

Malignant melanomas arise from melanocytes, such as those in the skin or eye. In the central nervous system, glial cells support the neurones. As neurones do not divide, CNS tumours derive from these dividing glial cells forming gliomas. Malignant teratoma and seminoma arise from germ cells. These forms of malignancy will therefore present in the ovaries or testis.

Hypertrophy and hyperplasia

Swelling in tissues may be caused by hypertrophy. In hypertrophy, the individual cells increase in size, but overall cell numbers remain the same. For example if we exercise, a muscle will increase in size as a result of hypertrophy. This is good, as the enlarged muscle is also stronger. Alternatively hypertrophy may be pathological. If there is a chronic, abnormal increased workload of the left ventricular muscle, this will lead to myocardial hypertrophy. This will result in an enlarged heart, a condition referred to as cardiomegaly.

Stimulation of some tissues results in an increase in the number of cells present. An increase in cell numbers is called a hyperplasia. A tumour is caused by a pathological hyperplasia. In other words there are an increased number of cells present when there should not be. Neoplastic cells do not respond to the signals which normally regulate and inhibit cellular mitosis. This results in cellular proliferation leading to hyperplasia and tumour formation. A tumour may be malignant or benign.

Benign and malignant neoplasms

Characteristics of malignant neoplasms

Malignant neoplasms invade surrounding tissues. Cells from the neoplasm penetrate into the area around, this is termed direct invasion; a previously healthy tissue is 'invaded' by malignant cells. This also means that there is local growth

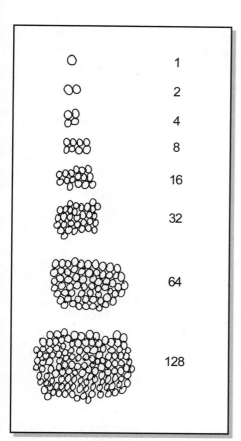

○	1
○○	2
○○	4
○○○○	8
	16
	32
	64
	128

Diagram 2.3
An increase in the number of cells present has resulted in 'new growth'. This neoplasia is caused by a hyperplasia and has resulted in tumour formation.

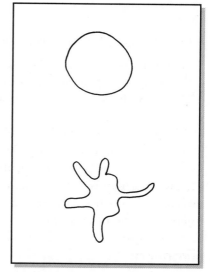

Diagram 2.4
Benign tumours are typically well localised and rounded. They do not invade surrounding tissues but their physical presence may lead to local tissue compression. In contrast, malignant tumours do invade surrounding tissues and form irregular shapes. This is why benign tumours are usually relatively easy to surgically excise and do not recur after removal. However malignant tumours are more difficult to excise completely. If a small part of the tumour is missed, the cells in the remaining area of neoplasm will continue to divide. This will result in recurrence of the tumour.

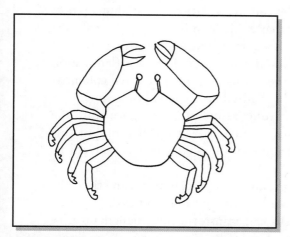

Diagram 2.5
Cancer has been compared with a crab; the legs of a crab are analogous to the 'tentacles' of tumour extension, invading into surrounding tissues.

in the size of the tumour. Another defining characteristic of malignancy is that neoplastic cells spread and generate secondary growths in other parts of the body in the process termed metastasis. Malignant tumours may have areas which do not have an adequate blood supply which can result in areas of necrosis. Also rapidly grown new blood vessels may rupture, resulting in haemorrhage. As malignant cells metastasize, and overall tumour mass increases, the condition will eventually be fatal.

Characteristics of benign neoplasms

Benign tumours may grow, but do not invade surrounding tissues as malignant cells do. Benign tumours do not metastasize. Cells in a benign tumour are usually very similar to the cells in the tissue of origin so are described as being well differentiated.

Benign tumours only cause clinical problems as a result of their physical presence. This means that the risks to the patient depend on where the neoplasm is. For example, if they occur in the central nervous system, they will compress surrounding neurological structures and in the brain they will lead to raised intracranial pressure. Benign tumours may compress other vital structures, e.g. tumours in the neck may compress the trachea or a large blood vessel. Benign tumours of some endocrine glands may result in over secretion of an endocrine hormone.

Metaplastic tissue

Metaplasia describes the conversion of one form of tissue into another form. This transformation is usually caused by chronic irritation or inflammation of a tissue. For example, the normal columnar epithelium in the transitional zone of the cervix may be transformed to squamous epithelium, this is termed squamous metaplasia. This change is often a result of chronic inflammation caused by a viral infection. In smokers, the normal respiratory ciliated columnar epithelium is progressively replaced by non-ciliated metaplastic squamous epithelium. Patients who suffer from chronic reflux of gastric juices into the oesophagus may develop a metaplasia called Barrett's epithelium. In this metaplasia the normal squamous epithelium of the oesophagus is replaced by columnar cells.

Metaplastic tissue is actually benign, and the process may sometimes be reversed if the irritating factor (e.g. smoke or gastric juice) is removed. However, with ongoing irritation metaplastic cells can transform into malignant cells. For this reason metaplasia is usually considered to be a pre-malignant condition. For example, Barrett's oesophagus is associated with a serious risk of transformation into adenocarcinoma. Patients with metaplastic changes may be treated to remove the transformed cells; alternatively they may need to be closely monitored to detect any malignancy at a very early stage.

Invasion and metastasis

Carcinoma in situ

Carcinomas begin as small localised primary growths in the epithelium from which they arise. As long as such early tumours do not penetrate the basement membrane, the condition is called carcinoma in situ. If discovered at this early stage most tumours can be removed and the patient cured. However the stage of carcinoma in situ is usually asymptomatic and a primary tumour usually goes on to enlarge with the risk of spread.

Primary and secondary tumours

A primary tumour is one which occurs at the site where a malignancy originated. A secondary tumour is one which has spread from a primary site in the process of metastasis. Metastasis describes the transfer of malignant cells from one site to another when the two sites are not in direct contact. For example, a primary tumour in the colon may result in secondary spread to the liver. Metastatic spread is the most common cause of death in cancer.

Loss of cell to cell adhesion

In a healthy tissue, cells are stuck together in order to provide integrity and strength. Cells are normally adhered to each other, and surrounding tissue, by specific adhesion molecules. This prevents tissue cells being washed away in the circulation of the blood and lymphatic fluids. Malignant cells do not produce these adhesion molecules normally. This means the cells which comprise a malignant tumour are not properly held together, as a result individual cells or groups of cells may break away. These shed cells are then free to circulate in blood and lymphatic fluids. Malignant cells may spread in four basic ways; by direct invasion, lymphatic spread, blood borne spread, and via body cavities.

Metastasis of malignant cells

Initially a tumour grows by direct invasion of local tissues. This process will be ongoing, resulting in a progressively enlarging primary tumour. Cells which have detached from a primary tumour may enter a blood or lymphatic vessel. From here they passively float in the blood or lymphatic fluid. At some point, the travelling malignant cells become attached to the wall of the vessel and eventually migrate out into the tissue spaces. Initially the malignant cells divide to form a micrometastasis, usually around a small blood vessel. This is because malignant cells need a supply of oxygen and nutrients, the same as any other living tissue. New blood vessels then grow into the tumour by the process of angiogenesis. As the blood supply increases, the tumour may grow to generate a larger metastatic secondary tumour. Another mode of metastasis is via body cavities. For example, a tumour in part of the peritoneal or pleural cavity may spread through the potential space to lodge in other areas. Cerebral tumours may spread through the medium of the cerebrospinal fluid. The

Diagram 2.6
Carcinoma of the bronchus is used as an illustration of how malignancy may spread in the process of metastasis.

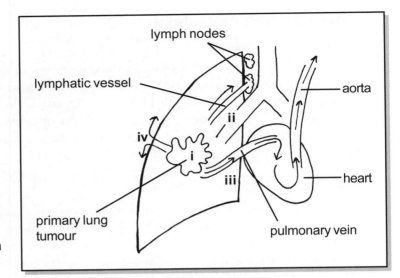

i.   Direct invasion of tissue as the tumour grows locally.

ii. Malignant cells may travel to lymph nodes via afferent lymphatic vessels and then on to the systemic lymphatic system. Ultimately this lymphatic fluid drains back into the venous circulation.

iii. Spread via the blood will return malignant cells to the left atrium, via the pulmonary veins; from here the cells may travel to other organs such as the liver or brain.

iv. Spread may also occur via body cavities, in this case between the visceral and parietal pleural membranes.

Diagram 2.7
The pattern of metastatic spread is partly determined by the nature of the circulatory flow of blood and lymphatic fluid. In this example, some malignant cells have been shed from a gastrointestinal primary. They follow the normal route of the hepatic portal circulation to the liver, where they seed multiple secondary metastatic tumours. As there are no effective treatments for hepatic metastases, the prognosis is poor.

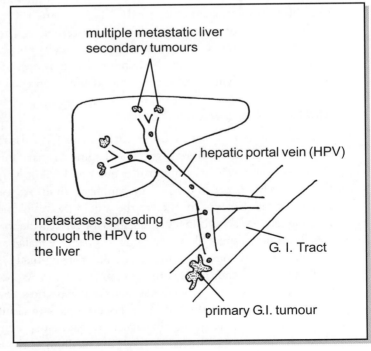

process of metastasis can be repeated many times resulting in hundreds of metastatic tumours. When cancer is widely distributed throughout the body the condition is referred to as carcinomatosis.

The pattern of metastasis is determined by the routes of venous and lymphatic drainage, and the ability of a particular tumour type to grow in a particular 'host' tissue. Gastrointestinal tumours commonly metastasize to the liver, via the hepatic portal circulation, but it is rare for secondary tumours to develop in skeletal muscles despite their copious blood supply. Breast primary tumours often give rise to secondary tumours in the brain and liver. Bone metastases most commonly originate from the prostate, breast, lung, kidney, thyroid or cervix.

Cancer staging

Cancer staging is a useful method of indicating the stage in the disease process and the extent of spread. Different cancers are staged in different ways, however a common useful principle is TNM staging. T stands for tumour and describes the size and extent of local invasion. N is for nodes, i.e. the lymph nodes, this describes the degree of local lymph node involvement. M is for metastases which are found at distant sites of the body. For example $T_1 N_0 M_0$ would describe a small, localized tumour which had not spread to local lymph nodes or distant sites. $T_4 N_3 M_3$ would describe a large primary tumour with significant local invasion which had extensively spread to regional lymph nodes and distant metastatic sites.

Cancer grading

Cancers are graded by their cytological and histological microscopic appearance by a pathologist. Grading is important as an indicator of how aggressive a malignancy is likely to be. Low grade tumours are well differentiated meaning the cells retain many of the appearances of the original tissue from which they derived. Clinically, well differentiated cells are likely to have slower growth rates and be less invasive with less likelihood of metastasis.

Conversely high grade tumours have poorly differentiated cells. This means they lack the differentiating features that indicate the tissue of origin; they are simply recognised as malignant cells. When cancer cells are very poorly differentiated they are described as anaplastic. Tumours containing anaplastic cells are likely to have rapid rates of growth, invasion and metastasis. If cells are seen to be moderately differentiated the tumour is likely to have an intermediate grade and level of aggressiveness.

Tumour markers

Tumour markers are chemicals produced by tumour cells which can be detected in the blood. Unfortunately markers are not specific to malignant cells, but when a larger number of malignant cells are present there is also likely to be more marker found in the blood. This means markers can raise suspicions for diagnostic purposes and can be useful in monitoring the response to a treatment. If a treatment is effective it will reduce the numbers of malignant cells present and so reduce the levels of the marker in the blood. Well known markers include prostate-specific antigen (PSA) in prostate cancer, carcino-embryonic antigen (CEA) in colorectal cancer and CA-125 in ovarian cancer.

Clinical features of neoplasms

As discussed, malignant tumours invade surrounding tissue. This means a tumour has many points of contact in the tissue. As a result the tumour is well fixed and is not easy to move between finger and thumb. Also the irregular shape of a malignant neoplasm means the tumour is ill defined. Malignant tumours consist of cancerous cells and other non-malignant cells. The non-malignant cells and tissues in a tumour are collectively referred to as stroma. Stromal cells include endothelial cells and fibroblasts which form a supportive framework which gives structure to the tumour. Fibroblasts produce fibrous tissue which is rich in collagen. This firm structural protein makes malignant tumours feel hard and firm. The actual clinical features of primary or secondary tumours occur as a result of their direct effect on tissues and as a result of effects which generate paraneoplastic syndromes.

Direct effects

Bulky tumours may have compressive and obstructive effects on surrounding tissues. For example, tumours may compress blood or lymphatic vessels as well as airways or portions of the GI tract. Kidney tumours may compress the normal renal parenchyma and obstruct the flow of urine through the renal pelvis or ureter. Intracranial tumours will compress the brain and peripheral tumours may lead to painful nerve compression. Areas of infarction may develop as tumours compress blood vessels. Also tumours may lead to a twisting of blood vessels (i.e. torsion) which supply the gut, ovaries or testes. Both of these effects can therefore lead to areas of necrosis. Because malignant tumours are invasive, they may directly penetrate blood vessel walls leading to haemorrhage.

Malignant tumours may ulcerate. Ulceration may occur on the skin or internal surfaces. Malignant ulceration of the GI tract, particularly of the stomach or duodenum will disrupt the normal mucus lining which protects underlying layers from hydrochloric acid and digestive enzymes. This may allow digestive enzymes to digest and perforate the gut wall, allowing stomach contents to escape causing peritonitis. Rupture or perforation may occur as a result of a tumour weakening the gut wall, especially if this is combined with an increase in pressure, as may be caused by an obstruction or a tumour growing within the gut lumen. Digestive enzymes may also erode the walls of blood vessels leading to life threatening gastrointestinal haemorrhage.

Pain in cancer may derive from the periosteum or endosteum secondary to bone destruction. There may also be pathological fractures. Other causes of pain include obstruction of lumens, peripheral nerve involvement or compression, pressure effects, ischaemia, necrosis, distension, stretching of organ capsules, inflammation or infection.

Tumours also have generalised systemic effects. There may be lethargy and general malaise caused by metabolic effects, hormonal changes or secondary infections. There is often anaemia with pale mucous membranes and sallow unhealthy looking skin. A hypercoagulable state is often associated with cancer. This means the blood is more likely to clot, leading to thrombus formation. As a result venous thrombosis is more likely, leading to DVT and PE (deep venous thrombosis and pulmonary embolism).

Paraneoplastic syndromes

These are clinical features which may occur in patients with cancer but are not readily explained by the physical presence of primary tumour or metastases. It is thought that most paraneoplastic features are caused by bioactive compounds synthesised and released by malignant cells. Some patients with malignancy present with fever which is not caused by infection. It is likely that this is caused by pryogens released by malignant cells.

Weight loss is common in cancer and cachexia describes a stage of disorder where there is significant weight loss and a 'wasting away' of body tissues. The patient may appear 'skeletal', giving a similar appearance to extreme malnutrition. Cachexia may be partly explained by anorexia and the increased metabolic demand of rapidly dividing malignant cells. However, there are also chemicals called cytokines which are produced by the body's own macrophages. These macrophages can be activated by malignant disease to release cytokines such as tumour necrosis factor (also called cachexin) which induces cachexia.

Endocrine like compounds may be released from malignant cells. For example hypercalcaemia is relatively common and may be caused by a parathyroid like hormone secreted by tumours but may also be associated with bony destruction. Some malignancies of endocrine tissue can result in excessive production of hormones. For example, some tumours of the thyroid produce too much thyroxine. In small cell (oat cell) carcinoma of the lung, excess ACTH may be produced leading to increased release of hydrocortisone and consequent Cushing's syndrome. Cushing's may also be caused by tumours of the adrenal cortex. These may secrete hydrocortisone but do not respond to the normal negative feedback inhibitory mechanisms. Other paraneoplastic effects which do not have well defined explanations include finger clubbing, skin rashes, peripheral neuropathy and cerebral degeneration of the brain.

Early warning signs of cancer

The prognosis in most cases of cancer depends largely on the availability of treatments, and how early the cancer is detected. If a tumour can be detected at an early stage, the possibilities for curative treatment are generally significantly better than if a patient presents with more advanced disease. One approach is therefore to educate the public on the early warning signs of cancer. These are sometimes divided into the following 7 groups of signs and symptoms.

Unusual bleeding or discharge

The cause of any unexplained bleeding should always be ascertained. For example haematuria is commonly caused by infection and may also result from trauma; however it may also be a feature of malignancy. Blood in the urine may derive from any part of the urinary system so may be from the kidneys, ureters, bladder or urethra. Any blood in urine is an abnormal finding. If a trace of blood is detected on a routine dip stick test, this is abnormal and so should be explained. In females blood in the urine during menstruation should not be assumed to be menstrual contamination. This means the test should be repeated in two weeks time when the woman is mid-cycle.

Bleeding from the gastrointestinal tract also has many possible causes, however if haematemesis or melaena are seen, malignancy is a possibility. Detection of occult blood in faeces is also an abnormal finding and should be explained.

Discharges may be a feature of early malignant disease. Discharges themselves usually indicate infection and are composed of inflammatory fluids, bacteria and white blood cells. When a tumour grows it distorts the normal anatomy of an area. This results in a disordered local tissue structure which may increase the probability of infection. For example, a tumour in a bronchial passage may partly obstruct the bronchial lumen. This will inhibit the normal clearance of mucus, leading to an area of stasis in the airways, distal to the tumour. Stasis will lead to infection which may be difficult to clear and is likely to recur. Therefore infection may be an early indicator of malignancy.

Discharges from the urethra may indicate a urinary malignancy. An early sign of breast cancer may be a discharge from the nipple. Vaginal discharges are also abnormal and could indicate infection, secondary to malignancy in the cervix or uterus.

A sore which does not heal

A sore on any part of the body could be a malignant ulceration. These will not heal as a normal lesion does because the malignant process is ongoing, making the condition progressively worse. Warning signs may include a lesion which does not seem to be healing as normal or is getting bigger for no apparent reason. Other potential features of malignancy are increasing pain or a lesion starting to bleed.

A skin lesion which progresses and does not heal may be a basal cell carcinoma (also sometimes called a rodent ulcer). These are normally caused by excessive exposure to direct sunlight and are the most common malignant tumour of the skin. Basal cell carcinomas grow locally but fortunately they rarely metastasize. Squamous cell carcinomas may also arise in the skin and these are highly likely to metastasize if not resected. Collectively these skin lesions are classified as non-melanoma skin cancer (NMSC).

Change in bowel or bladder habits

Potential early warning features could be changes in the frequency of defecation. This could indicate the development of an obstructive tumour within the bowel. Change in the consistency of the faeces may present as constipation or diarrhoea; again this may indicate a change in bowel function as a result of the presence of a tumour or pre-malignant adenoma. If the faeces become dark coloured this may indicate the presence of blood from a bleeding tumour. Pale coloured stools may be caused by a tumour (e.g. in the head of the pancreas) obstructing the bile ducts. Changes in the size and shape of stools may indicate the faecal material is having to squeeze past a distal mass in the colon or rectum.

Changes in bladder emptying habits may indicate a urological malignancy. This may also be a feature of prostatic cancer, although most prostatic conditions which present with urinary alterations are fortunately benign.

Thickening of tissue or a lump in the breast or elsewhere

Some tumours may develop near the surface of the body and so may be palpated at an early stage. Breast lumps are an obvious example. While a breast lump may be a cyst or benign growth, the possibility of malignancy should always be excluded. Lumps in the testes may be felt at an early stage. Some patients with early testicular malignancy complain of a feeling of heaviness in a testis. Tumours in skeletal muscles are rare and can usually be felt at an early stage. Enlarged superficial lymph nodes can easily be palpated and may be an indication of lymphoma or lymphatic spread. Rarely, children may develop a palpable renal mass caused by a malignant neoplasm of the kidney called Wilms' tumour.

Nagging cough or hoarseness

Tumours in the respiratory tract may cause irritation and cough. As discussed, tumours in the bronchial passages may lead to infection and a consequent chronic cough. Hoarseness of the voice is a classical feature of laryngeal cancer. Tumours of the thyroid gland may also affect the voice, by compressing the upper airway or vocal nerves.

Obvious change in a wart or mole

Warts and moles should be observed as they have the potential to become malignant. The ABCDE rule is sometimes helpful in assessing these lesions. A is for asymmetry, does the mole look the same in all parts or are there differences? B is for borders, are the borders of the lesion sharp and well defined or ragged? C is for colour, what are the colours and levels of pigmentation seen in the mole? D stands for diameter, is the size increasing or wider than 6 mm? E is for elevation, does the lesion form a lump, above the level of the normal skin surface?

Malignant melanoma may demonstrate all of the above features. The lesion is asymmetrical, borders between the melanoma and the normal skin are irregular, colour varies over the surface of the lesion due to variable pigmentation, diameter increases beyond 6 mm and the malignancy grows above the skin surface. Malignant melanoma is a serious skin cancer because it may develop in young people and can metastasize at an early stage. As with other forms of skin cancer the incidence is increasing, presumably due to increased exposure of skin to direct sunlight and sun burn. Treatment consists of emergency wide excision of the malignant melanoma.

Indigestion or difficulty in swallowing

Early features of swallowing difficulties may include a feeling of pressure in the throat or chest which make it difficult to swallow. Difficulty in swallowing may indicate the development of a tumour in the oesophagus or fundus of the stomach.

Diagnosis of malignancy

Initial suspicion of a tumour may be generated by any of the above features. Often initial investigations will involve some form of imaging such as X-rays, ultrasound, CT, MRI or isotope scanning. Blood tests for tumour markers or other effects of the malignancy can also be helpful. A definitive diagnosis is usually made by histological examination of a biopsy, i.e. a sample of tissue. As malignant cells have a very different appearance to normal cells, malignancy can then be firmly diagnosed. Superficial tumours may be sampled using fine needle aspiration. In this procedure a hypodermic needle is inserted into the neoplasm and some cells sucked up into a syringe. A biopsy may also be removed during a surgical procedure. Alternatively samples of tissue may be taken during endoscopy, bronchoscopy or colonoscopy.

Screening

Screening refers to mass examination of the public in order to detect the presence of early disease. Screening programmes may be used to pick up cases before clinical features have appeared. Health care workers may therefore pick up cases of disease such as diabetes mellitus type 2, hypertension, hypercholesterolaemia, tuberculosis, heart disease, anaemia and malignancy. In most western countries there are extensive programmes of cervical cytology. These have reduced the death rate from cervical cancer significantly.

Mammography may pick up early cases of breast cancer, and chest X-rays lung cancer. The problem with all examinations using X-rays is that they contribute to an individuals cumulative radiation exposure, which may increase the probability of a cancer developing. Other possible screening tests are safer, such as the examination of stools for the presence of occult blood, or blood testing for tumour markers such as prostate specific antigen. Screening is usually a good idea as long as it does not adversely affect the individual, physically or mentally.

Principles of cancer management

Local excision

Some cancers may be cured by early local excision; skin tumours for example may be detected at an early stage and removed. In situ tumours can also usually be completely removed. For most other solid tumours, surgical removal of the bulk of the primary tumour is possible. However, by the time many primary tumours have been detected there is already microscopic systemic metastatic spread. This means that systemic treatments, such as chemotherapy, are often needed in addition.

Chemotherapy

A wide range of specific chemotherapeutic drugs are available for treating cancers. Unfortunately chemotherapy is not specific to cancer cells and other body tissues may also be adversely affected. Most chemotherapies work by inhibiting the process of mitosis. This inhibiting effect reduces the rate of mitosis in the malignant cells. Typically several drugs are given in combination over several cycles. A cycle consists of giving the drugs for a period of days to attack the cancer, followed by some days without treatment to allow normal tissues to recover. The most common side effects of chemotherapy are nausea and vomiting, tiredness, hair loss, and bone marrow suppression leading to immunosuppression. Hair roots and bone marrow function both depend on rapid rates of cell division but fortunately not all chemotherapy regimes cause hair loss.

The degree to which different cancers respond to systemic chemotherapy is variable. A few cancers respond very well, and even bulky metastatic disease can be cured; this is true of some leukaemias, lymphomas and testicular cancer. However, for most common cancers such as lung, colorectal or breast, there are no effective treatments for bulky metastatic disease. While some patients with early metastatic disease can be effectively treated it remains a sad fact that most systemic malignancy has a disappointing outcome.

Radiotherapy

Radiation is most commonly delivered into tissues in the form of a beam from a linear accelerator. Sometimes radiation is derived by inserting a radioactive source into the body. Both of these approaches are therefore essentially local approaches to therapy. Radiation damages the DNA in cells and this can lead to cell apoptosis. Radiation also generates a lot of free radicals, particularly of oxygen, which damage cell membranes and proteins. Again sufficient cellular damage will lead to cell death. Cells undergoing rapid divisions are more prone to radiation damage than non-dividing cells so hopefully the cancer cells will be disproportionately killed. If beams of radiation are passed through a tumour from various directions, the dose can be focused and concentrated on the malignancy, minimising the harm to healthy tissues. Radiotherapy may be used as a primary treatment in tumours such as those affecting the prostate, cervix, oesophagus, skin or CNS. In addition it may be used as an adjuvant to surgery in tumours such as those of the breast, lung, uterus, bladder and rectum. Some patients may also be given radiotherapy as a palliative measure.

Endocrine related treatment

This involves inhibiting tumour growth by removing hormonal stimulation. For example breast cancer is dependent on ongoing stimulation by oestrogen, in the same way as normal breast tissue. A drug such as tamoxifen will block oestrogen receptors on the breast derived cancer cells and so remove the stimulating hormonal effect. Indeed this inhibition can result in tumour regression and cure of micrometastatic disease. A much more radical approach would be to remove the ovaries, which secrete oestrogen. Similar principles also operate in endometrial cancer. Normal prostatic tissue and cancer of the prostate are both stimulated by testosterone.

Immunotherapy

The immune system is completely capable of eradicating malignant cells from the body, if it were only able to recognise them as foreign cells. The problem is that malignant cells are usually seen as part of the 'self' and so not attacked by the immune system. Despite this difficulty, various immune molecules may have a role in treating some particular malignancies; these include interferons, interleukins, haemopoietic growth factors and monoclonal antibodies. Another approach to immune based therapy is to give BCG bacteria to activate the immune system against some bladder cancers.

Palliative treatment

Palliation refers to treatments which are aimed at improving the quality and duration of life. They are not aimed at curing the patient. Radiotherapy and chemotherapy can both be used as palliative treatments. Surgery is another common palliative measure. Unfortunately in palliative care it is often a matter of balancing the unwanted effects of the disease process with the side effects of treatment. Terminal cancer management depends on high quality nursing care. Attention should be paid to aspects such as hydration, nutrition, preventing complications of immobility, ensuring analgesia and of course psychosocial and spiritual care.

CHAPTER 3

Infectious Disease

Introduction to infection

Infection is a global problem

It has been estimated by the world health organization (WHO) that infectious diseases cause 25% of human deaths worldwide and up to 63% of deaths in children under the age of 4 years. Most of these premature deaths are caused by six major killers. In order of the number of deaths caused these infections are; pneumonia, HIV/AIDS, diarrhoeal diseases, tuberculosis, malaria and measles. The challenge is that all of these major causes of infective deaths can be prevented or treated. This is particularly important as the majority of these preventable deaths occur in our children and young adults. This chapter aims to give the foundational information needed for you to start combating the scourge of infectious disease.

Infection and immunity

Infection describes the presence and reproduction of microorganisms within, or on, a body tissue or tissues. Organism simply means anything which is alive; you may have come across people simply referring to bacteria as 'bugs'. A person who has an infection is described as a host. An infected person may suffer from the clinical features of the disorder. Alternatively an individual may harbor a pathogenic, or potentially pathogenic microorganism, and not have any discernible features of disease; such a person is described as a carrier. Infectious agents may be transferred from a sufferer or a carrier to infect another person, who is then at risk of developing the same disease. This is why infectious conditions are often described as transmissible. In health, people are partly protected against the introduction of infective agents via the mechanisms of innate and specific immunity.

All people are exposed to numerous potentially infective organisms every day. The probability of exposure leading to infection is determined by the virulence of the particular organism, the number of organisms they are exposed to, and the state of the person's immune defenses. Virulence describes the infectiousness or the disease producing power of a microorganism.

Level of host immunity can be affected by several factors. If an individual has been exposed to a particular infection in the past the immune system will have generated specific antibodies to attack the particular antigen. An antigen is anything the immune system recognizes as foreign, such as a bacteria or virus. Previous exposure therefore gives a significant level of immunity to a specific infection; vaccination confers the same immunological benefit. The principle in vaccination is that dead or attenuated (weakened) antigens are injected into the body. The immune system responds by producing specific antibodies which confer acquired immunity if there is subsequent exposure to the living infectious antigens. Good nutrition is vital for adequate immune function. Malnutrition leads to immune compromise and subsequent increased risk of infections. For example, amino acids are needed to synthesise antibodies and acute phase proteins. The very old and very young are at increased risk of contracting infections, reflecting the development and gradual decline of the immune system. Genetic factors may also influence an individual's susceptibility to a particular infection.

Types of human / microbe relationships

Humans have large numbers of bacteria living in association with them; the skin, mouth and vagina for example are all heavily colonized and huge numbers of bacteria live in the lumen of the GI tract. Despite these organisms living in such intimate contact with people, the internal tissues of the body remain sterile, unless of course we have an infection. There are three possible forms of relationship between bacteria and people; these are described as commensalism, mutualism and a parasitic relationship. Bacteria, which live with us but normally cause no harm, comprise the commensal flora. Mutual bacteria derive benefit from us and we from them, for example some organisms in the colon derive nutrients from our faeces and secrete vitamin K which we are then able to absorb. In a parasitic relationship the infecting organism benefits to the host's detriment. The host person becomes ill with an infectious disease as a result of the microorganisms present.

Pathogenic microorganisms

These are often referred to as pathogens and are virulent bacteria or viruses which usually cause disease if present. Other organisms, which may be commensal in normal circumstances, may also cause disease in some situations. For example, normal commensal E. coli causes no harm in the lumen of the colon but if it gets into the bladder it can cause urinary tract infections. Such organisms are sometimes referred to as opportunistic pathogens.

Opportunistic microorganisms

These organisms are usually of low pathogenicity (i.e. innate ability to cause disease) but may cause infections in certain circumstances. Opportunistic organisms typically cause disease when the host's defense mechanisms against infection are low, often as a result of immunosuppression or an underlying disease such as diabetes mellitus or HIV.

Local and systemic infection

In a localised infection, the microorganisms are confined to a particular area of the body and so give rise to localised features. Localised infection usually stimulates a localised inflammatory response, the clinical features of which are heat, pain, redness, swelling and loss of function. For example bacterial infection may lead to conjunctivitis giving a painful inflamed eye. A boil may develop as a result of an infected hair follicle. An abscess is a localised lesion composed of the causative organism, numerous white blood cells and dead tissue cells.

Systemic means relating to a system of the body or the body as a whole. A systemic infection will affect the whole person, they will feel unwell as the infectious agent, or toxins it has produced, circulate around the body. Some localised infections may spread to become systemic. For example cellulitis is an infection of the deep subcutaneous layer and presents as a localised erythema (redness) of the skin. Staphylococcus or streptococcus is the usual cause. The area involved may extend over time and the patient may develop fever and start to feel unwell as there is systemic involvement. In some cases the infection will become life threatening. This explains why it is important to monitor such infections closely and to give treatment at an early stage.

Epidemiology

Epidemiology is the study of the causes, incidence, distribution and control of disease. A condition is described as being endemic if it is established in a geographical area and new cases can be expected. For example, malaria is endemic in many areas of central Africa. An epidemic describes a significant increase in the number of new cases of a disease in a particular area such as the periodic epidemics of meningitis that occur in some areas. If there is a condition which spreads around the world this is described as a pandemic, HIV being a current example. From time to time there are pandemics of influenza.

Mortality rate for a disease describes the number of deaths it causes over one year per 1000 people. The overall mortality rate describes the number of deaths per 1000 of the population per year from all causes. Morbidity describes a state of disease or suffering. The morbidity rate describes the number of people who have a disease compared to the total number of people in a population.

Modes of transmission

Vectors

A vector is a living organism which transmits infection from one host to another. Insects may carry some diseases from infected to previously healthy people, e.g. malaria spread by mosquitoes. If we get bacteria on our hands from an infected wound, and spread this to a wound in another patient, then we too would be a vector.

Fomites

A fomite is any article which transmits infection between hosts. For example a used hypodermic needle may transmit hepatitis virus between drug users. Other classical examples are stethoscopes, telephones, keyboards and pens in hospitals. These can become contaminated with bacteria and tend to get shared and passed around, transmitting the infection with them.

Cross-infection

This occurs whenever an infection is transferred from one person to another. This is sometimes called exogenous infection, as the organisms arrive from without (or outside) the person. Cross infection may also occur as a result of endogenous transfer. This is when organisms are transferred from the patient themselves to another body area, such as a wound, where they cause infection.

Vertical and horizontal transmission

Vertical transmission of an infectious agent occurs from mother to child. If the mother has an infection in the blood there is the possibility that it will be transmitted to the blood of the baby during the process of birth. This is because there is mixing of maternal and fetal blood as the placenta detaches from the uterine wall. Infections which may be transmitted via this vertical route include, syphilis, HIV and hepatitis B. Horizontal transmission describes one member of a species contracting an infection from another member of the same species, who are not in a mother and child relationship. Infection may be directly from one person or indirectly via the environment.

Health-care and community acquired infections

Nosocomial describes infections which are contracted in hospital or as a result of health care interventions. Health-care acquired infection (HAI) is an alternative term which means the same. The combination of the close proximity of compromised patients with health care workers going from patient to patient means any infections present may spread. In addition the extensive use of antibiotics means resistant strains may develop and spread. While vulnerable patients are at particular risk, staff may also contract infections while at work. Commonly encountered hospital acquired infections include Clostridium difficile, viral gastroenteritis and methicillin-resistant Staphylococcus aureus (MRSA). Other risks include viral hepatitis, HIV and tuberculosis. The converse of health-care acquired (or nosocomial) is community acquired. This describes any infection which is contracted, out of the health care setting, in the places where people live and work.

Common sites of HAIs

Health-care acquired infections often affect the urinary tract causing urinary tract infection (UTI). A common cause of UTI in hospitals is urinary catheterisation explaining why this procedure should be reserved for specific essential indications. Pneumonia is another common problem. This may be caused by mechanical ventilation requiring endotracheal intubation. Pneumonia is more likely in patients nursed immobilized or flat (supine) for prolonged periods. This is why all patients should be managed sitting up when possible. Early mobilization after surgery is also important. Deep breathing, coughing and expectoration should be encouraged to promote clearance of sputum. Dehydration and poor nutrition are other risk factors. Smoking should be strongly discouraged.

Surgical site infections (SSIs) are another potential problem. These can occur as a result of contamination during the procedure or in the days after surgery. Infection may be endogenous from the patients own skin or exogenous from other people, possibly vectored by health care staff. Most SSIs are caused by Staphylococcus aureus. Bloodstream infections are less common but have a high case-fatality rate and are often caused by invasive medical devices such as intravenous cannulae. These infections are most commonly endogenous, but may also be transmitted by hospital staff. This is why excellent aseptic technique must be employed when inserting such devices, followed by good after care and patient observation.

Diarrhoea, caused by gastroenteritis, can spread through a ward very rapidly. Common causative agents include Clostridium difficile and noroviruses. Infection with C. difficile is more likely after a patient has received broad spectrum antibiotics. This is because the antibiotics kill the normal flora in the colon, removing the competition from the multiplying C. difficile. Noroviruses are highly contagious and are spread via the faecal-oral route, or as a result of droplets generated during vomiting.

Any time we, as health care workers, cause the spread of an infection we are breaking our prime directive, 'first do no harm'.

Zoonoses

This describes any infections which may be transmitted from animals to humans. Once a human is infected they often have the potential to infect other people. Examples include rabies from dogs, yellow fever from monkeys, leptospirosis from rats and CJD from cows. Influenza viruses may originate from poultry and, after genetic drift or mutation, can spread to humans sometimes via pigs. Avine influenza derives from bird viruses and swine flu partly arose from a pig virus.

Portal of entry

This refers to the route an infection takes to gain access into the host.

Ingestion

Many different forms of viral, bacterial, protozoa or parasitic infection can be taken in through the mouth. Examples include hepatitis A, food poisoning, cholera, typhoid fever and dysentery. Often an infection is derived from the faeces of an infected person, this mode of spread is referred to as the faecal-oral route. For example, if there is poor sanitation there may be contamination of drinking water with sewage. Poor hygiene is another possibility allowing infection to spread from faeces to a new host via the hands of someone preparing food.

Normally, if an infectious agent is eaten it will be attacked by gastric enzymes and hydrochloric acid in the stomach. This will reduce the numbers of microorganisms which survive to go on to start an infection. If all of the potential infection is destroyed then the disease process will not begin. This explains why these ingested organisms must be taken in sufficient numbers to cause disease; this is known as the infectious dose and will vary a lot between individual agents. Host susceptibility will also affect the infectious dose.

Inhalation

Hosts with active infections of their respiratory tract exhale microorganisms in droplets of water when coughing, sneezing, talking or just breathing. These are often described as droplet infections. Examples of diseases spread by inhalation include tuberculosis, pneumonia, meningitis, influenza, the common cold, measles, mumps and chickenpox. Conditions which adversely affect the respiratory tract such as bronchitis, emphysema or damage from smoking, all increase the chances of contracting infections via inhalation.

Penetration

Microorganisms are not usually able to penetrate intact epidermis. Healthy mucous membranes also form a physical barrier to many potential infections. Trauma or disease processes may disrupt the integrity of these integuments and allow the entry of infectious agents. For example burns damage the surface of the skin and are associated with a significant infection risk. Surgical wound infections are another example of a problem caused after skin penetration. Sharp objects and bites may inoculate infection into tissues directly. Bite injuries are associated with a high risk of infection because bacteria from the mouth and teeth are introduced into the tissues directly. Bites inflicted by humans, dogs or other animals are often left open to heal by secondary intention, or closed loosely to reduce infection risk, antibiotics are also often prescribed.

Blood-borne spread

These infections are commonly transmitted via blood or blood products. For example hepatitis, HIV and malaria may all be spread via blood transfusions. This is why blood must always be screened for such potential infections before it is given to a recipient. Penetration of the skin may constitute a significant risk in terms of nosocomial infection. If health care workers have any cuts on their hands, or other skin lesions, they have an increased risk of contracting hepatitis B and C or HIV from contaminated body fluids. Another risk is injury from contaminated sharps or needle stick injuries. These have the potential to introduce bacterial and viral infection directly into our tissues. Post exposure immunoglobulin administration will reduce the risk of contracting viral hepatitis. Anti-retroviral post exposure prophylaxis is also available for HIV.

Direct contact

Some infections are transmitted by close skin contact. These are mostly superficial infections such as scabies or impetigo (usually caused by parasites, staphylococci or streptococci). Some infections may be directly transmitted through intact mucous membranes. For example contact of genital mucous membranes during sex can allow the transmission of human papilloma virus, gonorrhoea, syphilis, chlamydia and herpes. This explains why these disorders are sexually transmitted diseases (STDs or venereal disease). Vertical transmission of these infections, from mother to child may occur during birth.

Infectious agents

Viruses

Viruses may be classified as living or non-living depending on the definitions of life chosen. Some people believe they are not alive because they are obligate intracellular parasites, they can not live independently of living cells. Unlike bacteria they cannot reproduce independently, they can only reproduce inside another living cell. Viruses have a typical diameter of about 30-100nm (there are a thousand nanometres in a micrometre and a thousand micrometres in a millimetre). This makes them very much smaller than bacteria; indeed some viruses may infect and kill bacteria. A viral particle (or virion) consists of a single strand of DNA or RNA (never both) inside a protein shell correctly termed a capsid. Viral particles must first bind onto the cell membrane of a cell they are to infect. The virus then usually triggers a process called endocytosis, meaning the viral particle is taken through the cell membrane into the cytoplasm of the host cell. The viral DNA or RNA then takes over or 'hijacks' the cells genetic and protein synthesising machinery to produce more viral particles. Once produced the new viruses 'bud' from the cell membrane or are released when the cell dies.

Viruses may cause numerous diseases including colds, influenza, mumps, measles, rabies, hepatitis, rubella, poliomyelitis, herpes sores, chickenpox, shingles, and many respiratory and gastrointestinal infections. Viral infections cannot be treated with antibiotics and while more antiviral drugs are being developed, the majority of viral infections remain difficult or impossible to

Diagram 3.1
Individual viral particles as seen under the high power of an electron microscope. (Viral particles have different shapes, these are round rotavirus.)

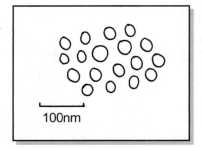

100nm

treat by pharmacological elimination of the virus. Viruses are also involved in the development of some malignancies. For example human papilloma virus can lead to cervical cancer and hepatitis B to hepatocellular carcinoma.

Bacteria

Bacteria are small, single prokaryotic cells, typically about 1 micrometre in diameter. Prokaryotic means the cell does not contain membrane bound organelles, such as mitochondria or a nucleus. (In contrast, eukaryotic animal and plant cells, do contain membrane bound organelles.) In ideal conditions some bacteria can divide every 20 to 30 minutes, this can lead to a massive increase in bacterial numbers over a short period of time.

Bacteria cause clinical features primarily as a result of releasing toxins. Exotoxins are usually proteins secreted as waste products during the life of the bacteria. They are locally released from the bacteria but may also be absorbed into the blood. For example, botulinum toxin is released by Clostridium botulinum and is a powerful neurotoxin which may poison nerves leading to

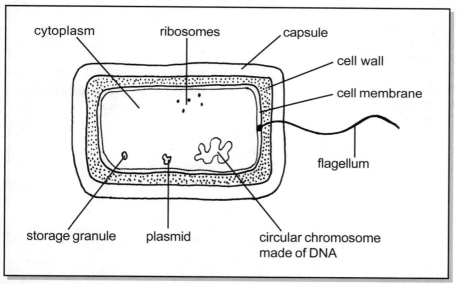

Diagram 3.2
Bacteria are surrounded by a cell wall; this is composed of peptidoglycans which are structural molecules, only found in bacteria. Outside the cell wall some bacteria have a capsule or slime layer. The capsule is often sticky which allows bacteria to stick to surfaces and each other. Encapsulation can also offer some defence against phagocytes. Some bacteria have single or multiple flagella. These waft back and forward to provide motility through fluids. Plasmids are present in some bacteria; they are made of DNA which codes for specific genes. Some bacteria may exchange plasmids, and therefore genetic material, between individual cells. Genetic information carried by plasmids may code for the ability to resist certain antibiotics.

paralysis. Enterotoxins are exotoxins released by pathogens infecting the gastrointestinal tract. For example, Vibro cholerae and some forms of Escherichia coli secrete enterotoxins which cause inflammation and stimulate mucosal cells in the lining of the gut to secrete water, mucus and electrolytes leading to severe diarrhoea. Other exotoxins include cytotoxins which will damage cells, pneumotoxins which will damage the lungs and haemolysins which may break up red blood cells.

Endotoxins are lipopolysaccharides released from the cell walls of Gram-negative bacteria. They are released when the bacteria are destroyed or break up after they have died. When endotoxins enter the blood in significant amounts they cause endotoxaemia or Gram negative severe sepsis. Presence of these endotoxins in the blood greatly stimulates the release of cytokines and other inflammatory mediators. Patients with this condition are very poorly and are likely to initially suffer from fever, tachycardia and increased respiratory rate with a leucocytosis. Later features include hypotension, oedema and haemorrhage as the capillaries become leaky.

Diagram 3.3
Bacteria may be described by looking at their shape. Cocci are roughly spherical, bacilli are rod or comma shaped, spirilla and spirochetes are spiral or helical, (like a corkscrew).

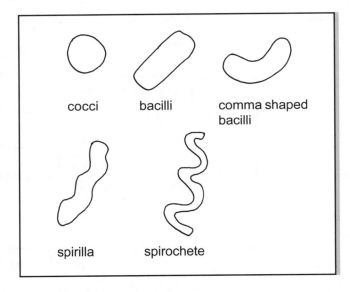

Diagram 3.4
Diplococci occur in pairs, streptococci in strips or lines and staphylococci in clusters.

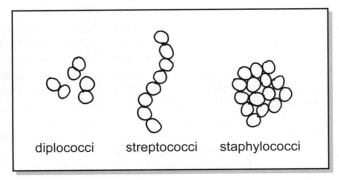

Colonization or infection

Colonization occurs when bacteria inhabit a specific body area. For example, bacteria will always be present on the skin surface, in the bowel or on the surface of a chronic wound. Colonization may be considered normal and the bacteria present do not cause any clinical signs of infection or inflammation. Conversely, in infection there may be a purulent discharge and the local features of an inflammatory response such as heat, pain, redness, swelling and loss of function. In addition there may be systemic features such as pyrexia, malaise and an increased white cell count.

Colonization is not a clinical problem unless bacteria move from the colonized area into another part of the body where they might cause infection. For example bacteria may migrate from the skin into an open wound causing infection. Bacteria may migrate from the anus into the urethra leading to urinary tract infection. Bacteria which are colonizing one patient may spread, via cross infection, to cause infection in another individual. The distinction between harmless colonization and potentially dangerous infection depends primarily on your ability to recognize the clinical features of infection. Once these are recognized appropriate treatment should be given.

Gram-positive or negative

This classification is used by microbiologists to further describe bacteria. Gram's stain (after Christian Gram, 1853-1928) is a simple crystal violet dye which colours some bacteria blue, to make them easy to see. This difference in staining characteristics occurs because of fundamental differences in the nature of the cell walls between the two types. Bacteria which have thick cell walls take up this stain, and therefore appear blue under a light microscope. These are described as gram-positive. Bacteria with thin walls do not take up the blue stain but do however take up a red safranin dye. This means Gram-negative bacteria appear red after this stain has been applied. Common examples include Streptococci which are gram positive and E. coli which are gram negative. This Gram classification has important clinical implications for example, we have seen that Gram negative cells walls may release endotoxins. Also the difference in the nature of the cell wall influences which antibiotics will be needed to treat a particular infection.

Bacterial resistance

Most bacteria can be killed using antibiotics but bacteria may develop resistance. This phenomenon has developed because occasionally a single bacterium arose which was resistant to an antibiotic. This means that when a patient is treated, all of the bacteria which are sensitive to the antibiotic will be killed first, leaving the resistant forms alive for longer. If a patient then fails to complete the whole course of antibiotic, the resistant form will be free to divide and give rise to a resistant population. This resistant strain could then be spread to other people. For example, tuberculosis and some forms of Staphylococcus aureus are resistant to many antibiotics. Development and spread of antibiotic resistance in bacteria is accelerated by short generation times and the exchange of plasmids.

Timing of treatment

The aim of treatment is complete elimination of the pathogen with restoration of the normal physiological function of any tissues affected. This generally means that antibiotic treatment should be started as soon as the diagnosis is clear. This will mean that the infection may be eliminated when bacterial numbers are relatively low which will limit the amount of toxin they are able to release, and so reduce the severity of the clinical features. Also some infections injure healthy tissue. In some tissues this damage cannot be corrected once the injury has occurred. Prompt treatment may therefore prevent tissue or organ damage.

In all forms of infection the patient should rest. Exercise during an active infection may cause permanent damage to organs such as the heart. Plenty of sleep also allows time for the body to recover and regenerate. Adequate hydration should be maintained. The majority of patients should be allowed to eat, or not eat, what they feel like; it seems probable that the body knows what it needs, or does not need, at such times.

Other infectious agents
Fungi

These include moulds and yeasts. Fungi normally live by gaining nutrients from dead plant or animal remains; however they may also live as parasites on living tissues. Fungal infections are called mycoses and may affect superficial or deep tissues. Superficial skin (cutaneous) fungal infections are very common. Fungal tinea infections are often described as ringworm and paratize the dead outer layer of the skin. Tinea capitis infects the scalp, tinea corporis infects the body, tinea curis the groin and the common tinea pedis affects the feet causing athlete's foot. These can all be readily treated with topical antifungal creams.

Candida may cause localized infections of the mouth or vagina. This condition is often referred to as 'thrush', as the mucous membrane has white speckles of fungus, which make it look like the bird. These infections cause pain and burning sensations and can cause significant inflammation. They often develop after antibiotic therapy has killed the commensal bacterial flora, which normally acts as competition for the fungi. While these infections can present in anyone, they are also more common in poorly managed diabetes mellitus and HIV infection. Effective treatments for fungal infections include mouth washes or pessaries of nystatin and systemic preparations such as fluconazole.

Deep fungal infections are typically seen in immuno-compromised patients. For example the fungus Candida albicans may cause serious deep infections of the kidney, liver or brain and may develop into life threatening systemic fungal infection. Cryptococcus meningitis is a life threatening complication of HIV infection caused by a yeast.

Mycoplasma

These organisms are about a third the size of bacteria and do not have a cell wall. In other respects they are like small bacteria. They may cause several diseases in humans including atypical pneumonia, opportunistic urethritis in men and the organism is one of the possible causes of pelvic inflammatory disease. Effective antibiotics include erythromycin and tetracycline.

Helminths

These are multicellular organisms that vary from one centimeter up to ten metres in length. They are usually wormlike parasites and are very common in developing countries and other areas where hygiene is poor. Many forms of worms may live in the gut such as ascariasis round worms. Hookworms infect about 25% of the world's population and are a very common cause of anaemia. Treatments for these infections, such as oral mebendazole, are usually easy, cheap and safe. Other helminths may migrate to infect body tissues, for example filarial worms may live in lymphatic vessels leading to obstruction and swelling of distal tissues with tissue fluid. This may lead to the gross oedematous swelling called elephantiasis.

Arthropods

These are insects including vectors of infectious disease and the ectoparasites which can infest external body surfaces. Examples include scabies, head, body, or pubic lice and fleas. Arthropods can cause inflammation by biting or burrowing into the skin. Infection or infestation on or near the surface of the body caused by arthropods can be readily eliminated. For example scabies can be treated with a scabicide lotion of malathion. Normally the patient's clothes need to be washed at the same time to prevent reinfection.

Protozoa

These are relatively large free living eukaryotic cells. Transmission may be direct from person to person, via infected water or food or via insect vectors. Malaria is probably the most significant condition caused by protozoa and is spread by mosquitoes. Chloroquine and quinine are well established treatments for malaria, although resistance is becoming an increasing problem. Other protozoa cause gastrointestinal infection and liver abscesses. Metronidazole is usually an effective treatment for gastrointestinal or hepatic amoebic infections. Infections with protozoa can also occur in people with reduced immune function; for example, Pneumocystis carinii is a protozoa which may cause pneumonia in HIV infection.

Chlamydiae, rickettsiae, ehrlichieae and coxiella

These organisms are like viruses in that they can only reproduce inside a host cell; however, they also produce peptidoglycan cell walls as do bacteria so are sometimes described as atypical bacteria. Chlamydiae infections can be effectively treated with antibiotics such as tetracycline or doxycycline.

Prions

Prions are rogue infectious proteins. The name derives from **prot**einaceous (protein based) **in**fectious particles. Prions are not organisms, but are still infectious agents because they can spread disease from one person to another. Prions cause spongiform encephalopathies when they cause large vacuoles to develop in the cortex and cerebellum, leaving the brain like a sponge. Conditions caused by prions are sometimes described as transmissible neurodegenerative diseases. In sheep prions cause scrapie and in cows bovine spongiform encephalopathy. In humans the best known disorder caused by prions is Creutzfeld-Jacob disease (CJD). Prions may be spread from animals to humans if we eat infected meat, especially neurological or lymphatic tissues. It is also possible they may be spread from person to person via infected surgical instruments or blood transfusions. They are difficult to remove from surgical instruments by sterilization procedures. There are no specific treatments available for prion disease.

Diagnosis of infection

Koch's postulates

Robert Koch (1843-1910) developed criteria by which it is possible to decide if a condition is infective in nature and for the positive identification of the aetiological organism. Firstly he said that the infectious organism should be found in the lesions of all cases of the disease, and must be absent when there is no disease. Second, it should be possible to isolate and grow pure cultures of the organism outside of the host. Thirdly, it must be possible to produce the same disease by injecting the pure cultured organisms into a healthy subject. In addition he said it should be possible to again isolate the same pathogen from this second host. While Koch's postulates represent an ideal scientific method, and teach us about the nature of transmissible disease, they are not always possible to use in practice.

Clinical diagnosis

In practice, infectious conditions are usually suspected when the patient feels unwell, has localised inflammatory features or is pyrexial. While many infections need to be treated immediately on clinical grounds, absolute diagnosis requires identification of the organism by direct microscopic examination or culture. Some organisms may be seen using direct microscopy of specimens.

However, if available, bacterial culture is standard practice. Culture involves growth of a colony of the aetiological organism outside of the body. This is often done on a small plate of nutrient agar or broth. Once large numbers of the organism have been propagated, microbiologists can readily identify the organism involved. Care must be taken when collecting specimens for culture to prevent bacterial contamination from other areas of the patient themselves, from the environment or from other people. Common forms of specimens colleted for culture in clinical practice include nasal swabs, throat swabs, sputum samples, urine samples, faecal samples, pus or wound exudates, eye swabs, cerebrospinal fluid, blood cultures and biopsy samples. Once bacteria have been cultured it is also possible to carry out sensitivity testing. This identifies which antibiotics the bacteria are sensitive or resistant to. This means the most appropriate antibiotic may then be prescribed.

Serology means the study of serum, i.e. plasma. Identification of specific antibodies in the serum can provide indirect evidence for the presence of the antigen which stimulated its synthesis. (Antigen is a shortened form of antibody generating molecule.) This is often useful for the diagnosis of viral infections. For example, if a patient has antibodies to hepatitis B or HI virus, it is assumed that these infections are present, allowing the patient to be treated. It is also possible to study virions directly using viral studies. Fungal cultures are also possible but these take up to 2 weeks to grow.

Evolution of an infection

Most infectious diseases cause symptoms for a period of time which then resolve. Firstly there is an incubation period which occurs after the agent has entered the host but before clinical features develop. During this period the numbers of infectious agents will increase and the patient will typically become progressively more infectious as the numbers of infecting organisms increase. Incubation periods usually vary from a few hours to months, depending on the pathogen involved. In HIV infection the latent incubation period may last for several years. Next is the prodromal stage, during this time the person starts to feel generally unwell. Features are often fairly general in nature and may include tiredness, headache, mild pyrexia, malaise and myalgia (achy muscles).

After this the acute phase develops. During this phase there is multiplication and possible spread of the causative agent. The patient can feel very unwell due to the presence of microbial toxins, damaged tissues and the body's own response in the generation of inflammation and fever. Often the features at this stage are more specific and can indicate the site and type of infection. The duration of this most unpleasant phase depends on the aetiological organism and the immune response of the patient. If the acute phase continues, and disease severity worsens, death can occur.

Fortunately, in most infections, the numbers and quality of specific antibodies produced by the immune system increases rapidly during the acute phase of the illness. Once there are enough antibodies present these overcome the infection and there is a reduction in the numbers of infecting bacterial or viruses present. This means the patient starts to feel better and they enter the convalescent phase. During convalescence the symptoms improve as the pathogen has been eliminated by immune processes. Damaged tissues can usually be repaired. Convalescence after severe infections may take weeks or even longer, before the person feels fully fit again.

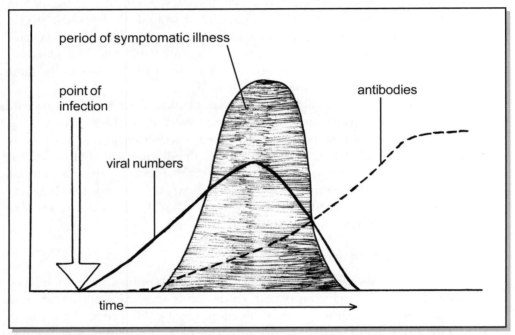

Figure 3.1
The evolution of a typical infection, with a time scale in days, in this case caused by a virus. After a susceptible individual is infected the numbers of virions increases as they reproduce inside the patient. Shortly after infection the immune system recognises the presence of the virus and starts to produce specific antibodies. However, the number of viruses increases rapidly, before this antibody response is adequate to overcome the infection. At first the patient starts to feel generally unwell in the prodromal phase. Then they start to feel worse as the effects of the infection have a systemic effect. During the course of the illness the clinical features usually become more specific allowing the site of the infection to be identified. For example the patient may start to cough, indicating pulmonary involvement. A urinary tract infection is likely to cause urinary symptoms such as dysuria (pain when passing urine). As the numbers of specific antibodies increase they are able to overcome the infecting virus resulting in a reduction in viral numbers. As the viral load in the patient reduces the individual starts to feel better. The numbers of antibodies will continue to increase for a time and the patient will usually enjoy long term immunity to the specific aetiological virus. During convalescence the patient will gradually feel stronger and less tired and will then be able to return to normal duties.

Resolution is said to occur when the pathogen has been completely eliminated and there are no residual clinical features. However, some infections may not resolve completely but go on to become chronic, such as tuberculosis. Other infections are acquired and combated by the immune system, before clinical features develop; these are referred to as subclinical.

CHAPTER 4

Disorders of Immunity

Human immunodeficiency virus infection

HIV (human immunodeficiency virus) is the cause of acquired immune deficiency syndrome (AIDS). This condition is acquired which means the sufferer catches the condition at a point in time. It is a syndrome, as a group of possible clinical features may present, rather than a single small well defined group of signs and symptoms as is the case with many other diseases.

Epidemiology

HIV is a massive global health problem which predominantly affects poorer and developing countries. In sub-Saharan Africa the prevalence may be up to 25% of the total population. Unfortunately many Asian countries, (e.g. India, Thailand and China) are now experiencing significant problems with the infection. However, effective health education programmes in Cambodia have largely contained the epidemic. Incidence is also increasing in Eastern Europe. As the disease is most commonly sexually transmitted, it often affects young adults. Young adults therefore become sick and die in large numbers, so are unable to work and look after their children effectively. This means the condition has the potential to do massive harm to the social and economic well being of individuals and nations.

In many poor countries, prostitution is a big problem, in India and Africa for example, there are millions of prostitutes. Women (and young men) are often forced into prostitution by criminals who organise human slavery. Poverty also forces many to become prostitutes. The problem can be self perpetuating; girls orphaned by AIDS may be forced into prostitution to support other children in the family. As health care workers, we know our own communities best, the question is what are we able, and prepared, to do to help this situation?

HIV/AIDS is a new disease

Recent genetic studies have clarified the origins of the HI virus. It is now known that HIV originated from the simian immunodeficiency virus (SIV) which effects primates in Central and Western Africa. Specifically HIV-1 virus arose from chimpanzees and HIV-2 from sooty mangabey monkeys. This means that HIV is another example of a Zoonoses (an infection derived from animals). HIV-1 was first isolated and identified in 1983, followed by HIV-2 in 1986. Further genetic estimations indicate that HIV-1 first crossed from chimps in 1931 and HIV-2 from sooty monkeys in 1940. After this the viruses were transmitted in the HIV human form from person to person. The term 'AIDS' was not developed until 1982 when the syndrome was first identified in the West. For years the virus was confined to relatively small areas within Africa, then it started to spread over a wider area and then on to Western countries. The first route of large scale transmission in the West was among homosexual men; intravenous drug users and haemophiliacs were other early casualties. HIV then entered the heterosexual community and continued to spread in this way.

HI virus

HIV is a retrovirus; this means it contains an enzyme called reverse transcriptase. This enzyme takes RNA from the virus and codes it into DNA, which is then incorporated into the genetic material of the host cell. There are two forms of the virus, HIV-1 and HIV-2. HIV-2 is mostly found in West Africa and may cause a slightly milder form of the disease. The pandemic form is HIV-1.

During the process of infection, the HI virus first comes into contact with a T helper lymphocyte and binds onto a molecule found on the outer cell membrane called a CD4 receptor. HIV can only bind to cells which have CD4 receptors on their outer membranes. Next the virus inserts its own RNA into the cell. This RNA carries the genetic material of HIV, which contains the information to produce more viral particles. From this RNA, the reverse transcriptase enzyme makes a copy of the viral genes in DNA. This means the information needed to produce more viral particles is now in DNA form. This newly formed DNA then moves into the host cell nucleus and integrates with the rest of the normal DNA.

Using the cells own genetic machinery, the section of DNA which codes for the virus then makes copies in RNA. This process of converting information from DNA into RNA is called transcription. This new RNA then goes into the cell cytoplasm where it codes for the synthesis of new HI viruses. The outer protein coat of the virus is constructed and more viral RNA and reverse transcriptase are incorporated. These new viruses then bud out of the host cell and are released into the blood, where they are free to infect yet more cells.

Once a T helper lymphocyte is infected with HIV, the cell goes on producing more viral particles for about 2 days, then the presence of the virus will kill the cell. It is the T helper lymphocytes which have the CD4 receptor, so this means that the numbers of T helper cells will ultimately decline. Normally it is the T helper cells which stimulate (or help) B lymphocytes to produce antibodies. If T helper cells are not present, then they are unable to stimulate B lymphocytes to produce antibodies. This means there will not be an adequate antibody response to infections. As a result the patient will suffer from infections.

Disease transmission

HI virus can be isolated from a range of body fluids such as urine, saliva and tears. However the main modes of spread are seminal fluid, cervical secretions and blood.

Sexual spread

Heterosexual spread is the most common cause of contagion worldwide. Men can catch HIV from women during vaginal sex. Women are more likely to catch the disease from men, than men are to catch it from women. This is because seminal fluid is deposited high in the vagina and may remain in the female

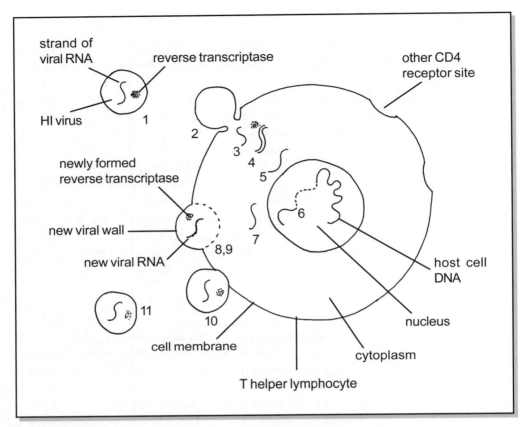

Diagram 3.1

The process of HIV infecting a host cell, taking over the cell and causing it to synthesise more copies of the virus. Viruses are sometimes said to 'hijack' a cell, they take it over for their own purposes.

1. An HI virus approaches the cell.
2. Next the virus combines with the CD4 receptor on the host cell surface.
3. Viral RNA and reverse transcriptase are injected into the cell.
4. Viral RNA is copied, using viral reverse transcriptase, to produce an equivalent length of DNA.
5. The newly formed length of DNA travels to the cell nucleus.
6. This new section of DNA, which codes for making new viruses, is incorporated into the host cell DNA.
7. After the process of transcription, a section of RNA, copied from the viral DNA, enters the cell cytoplasm.
8. Using the cells own protein synthesising machinery, the viral RNA codes for construction of a new viral particle wall, reverse transcriptase and RNA.
9. A new viral particle is being formed.
10. The newly formed virus buds out of the host cell, in reality many viruses will bud from one infected cell.
11. A newly formed HI virus is released into the tissue fluids where it can infect other cells or be transmitted to another person.

genital tract for 5 days. This gives plenty of time for HIV infection to enter her body. The same is true if a homosexual partner accepts seminal fluid into his rectum. Homosexual or heterosexual anal sex carries a significantly increased risk of viral transmission as the simple epithelial lining of the rectum may bleed as a result of the trauma. This provides an open portal for viral entry.

The risk to men and women is increased if they already have a sexually transmitted disease causing disruption or ulceration of the genital mucous membranes. Such lesions provide a ready portal of entry for the virus. If the prevalence of STDs can be reduced in a community, this will reduce the rate of HIV spread. Sexual spread of HIV can also occur during oral sex as seminal fluid or cervical secretions can come into contact with the mucous membranes of the mouth.

Viruses from seminal fluid or cervical secretions will not penetrate healthy intact skin. However if there is a cut or other disruption of the skin this becomes a possibility. Mouth to mouth kissing is considered a low risk activity as the numbers of viral particles found in saliva is low.

Mother to child spread

This is sometimes called vertical transmission and is the most common global cause of HIV infection in children. Figures of how likely a baby is to contract HIV from the mother vary from about 15-40%, depending on the study and geographical area. Most infection of babies occurs during the process of birth. If the child is then breast fed the risk of vertical transmission increases by up to 20%. Caesarean section and not breast feeding both reduces the risk of infecting the child.

Blood borne spread

Blood transfusion with HIV contaminated blood will cause infection. Blood products such as plasma, or clotting factors, have also caused numerous cases of spread. This is why it is essential that all donated blood is HIV (and hepatitis B and C) tested before it is given to a recipient or used in other blood products. Blood ceremonies are another possible form of spread so should be strongly advised against.

Contaminated needles have been a major cause of transmission. Drug users who share needles and syringes expose themselves to a high level of risk. The combination of needle sharing, poor nutrition and selling sex for drugs, explains why HIV infection is so common amongst injecting drug users. It is tragic but true, that many people have been infected with HIV from nurses and doctors reusing needles without proper cleaning and sterilisation. This nosocomial spread can also occur if medical or dental instruments are not cleaned and sterilised between patients. Body piercing and tattoos are another risk. If instruments are not properly sterilised they can act as fomites. There is no evidence that HIV is spread by blood sucking insects.

If you stab yourself with a dirty needle from a HIV positive person the probability of your contracting HIV are about 0.3%. If you do stab yourself with any dirty needle, try to make it bleed as much as possible. Squeeze the blood out and run the injury under a hot tap. Hot water will cause a localised vasodilation and transport more blood to the area for you to squeeze out. As blood is forced out of the wound, it will carry viral particles with it. This will reduce the viral inoculation dose you are exposed to. After this it may be a good idea to soak the wound in an iodine solution as this will kill viruses as well as bacteria. If you get blood splashed in your eye it should immediately be washed out with large volumes of water or saline. Eyes should be irrigated from the inside, pouring the water over the surface of the cornea outwards, (i.e. eyes should be irrigated from the medial to the lateral aspect of the cornea). The risk of contracting HIV from blood splashes to health care workers mucous membranes are much less than blood to blood contact after a needle stick injury. After these immediate measures it is possible to take post exposure prophylactic antiretroviral drugs.

Social contact

HIV is not spread by social contact. It is not spread by shaking hands, hugging or sharing cups or plates. There is no reason why people infected with HIV should not live as fully integrated members of the community. However, razors and tooth brushes should not be shared. Both of these implements can be contaminated with small amounts of blood, which does carry an infection risk.

Clinical features

These can be explained by the developing loss of cellular immunity in AIDS (cellular immunity refers to the production of antibodies by the lymphocytes). Depletion of T helper lymphocytes leaves the patient vulnerable to a wide range of opportunistic, potentially fatal, infections. This means that most patients die from infections rather than the HIV itself. As well as infections, HIV infected people are more prone to developing certain malignant disorders such as Kaposi sarcoma and B cell lymphoma.

Clinical phases in HIV infection

Authorities classify the phases of HIV infection in different ways, but basically there is an initial incubation period followed by seroconversion. There is then a period of latency followed by a period of mildly symptomatic disease called AIDS-related complex (ARC). Finally, in the natural evolution of the syndrome, there is a 'full blown' AIDS related illness. The speed at which the disease progresses varies significantly between individuals, in some the disease progresses rapidly. 'Typical progressors' in developed countries usually develop symptoms about 7-10 years after infection. 'Slow progressors' have not developed AIDS 15 years after infection.

Incubation

For the first 2-6 weeks after infection there are no features of the disease at all. However, during this phase the viral load will progressively increase.

Seroconversion phase

This is when the body first produces HIV antibodies. The HIV antibody test is the normal method used to diagnose infection. Seroconversion describes the change from the patient's serum (i.e. plasma) not having any HIV antibodies to these being present. Most, but not all, patients suffer a so called 'seroconversion illness'. Clinical features in this illness include fever with a rash, headache, painful muscles and joints (myalgia and arthralgia) and possibly some swollen glands (lymphadenopathy) in the neck. These features usually resolve after 1-2 weeks, after which the patient recovers and feels well. Typically, HIV antibodies are detectable in the patient's plasma about 2 months after initial infection. From shortly after infection the patient is probably infectious, this means there is a short time when a patient may pass on HI virus, but is HIV antibody negative.

Latent or asymptomatic infectious phase

This phase typically lasts for 7-10 years. During this time the virus continues to replicate and the patient is infectious. This is perhaps the key issue to grasp when considering HIV/AIDS; patients are infectious for a very long period of time while they are feeling and looking well. It is quite possible for a person to be in the latent phase of HIV infection, and not know they are carrying the virus. During this phase they have the capacity to infect many other people. For example if a person is sexually active they may infect numerous sexual partners. A minority of patients know they are infected but still engage in sex which puts others at risk. Such people need to be taught how dangerous their behaviour is to others. In some countries infected people, who cannot be trusted not to spread the virus around, are controlled forcibly.

During latency, some patients develop persistent generalized lymphadenopathy (PGL). Lymphadenopathy literally means any disease process affecting the lymph nodes. In PGL the lymph nodes swell and may be palpated at sites such as the groin, axilla and neck. PGL usually disappears as the HIV infection progresses; however the presence or absence of swollen lymph nodes does not seem to affect overall disease evolution.

ARC and AIDS phases

This is when the HIV infection becomes symptomatic and manifests itself in clinical immunodeficiency. As the condition develops, CD4 counts (representing T helper lymphocytes) fall and viral load increases. Viral load describes the numbers of viruses present in the blood and body secretions. Firstly there is mildly symptomatic disease caused by reduced levels of cellular immunity. During this period of AIDS-related complex (ARC) the infections suffered from are not severe enough to be classified as AIDS. However as time goes on the patient will develop AIDS defining infections.

The infections a patient suffers from depends partly on where they live and what microorganisms are locally endemic. Some infections are reactivations of previous conditions which had become latent. As the level of immunity falls, these infections may become clinically manifest again. Other infections develop as the patient encounters new pathogens. Microorganisms such as those which cause candidiasis, herpes, pneumococcal pneumonia and tuberculosis are sometimes called high grade pathogens; these are more likely to cause disease even if the patient is only mildly immunocompromised. Clearly, the more immunosuppressed the patient, the wider a range of possible infections they are at risk of suffering from. Organisms which cause infection in immunosuppression are said to 'take the opportunity' to multiply in the host causing infection. This is why they are referred to as opportunistic organisms or OIs (opportunistic infections).

Clinical presentations in HIV infection

Weight loss, mostly caused by anorexia, is a common feature which may progress onto serious wasting in later phases. Chronic diarrhoea is common and malabsorption may present. As well as affecting T helper cells, HIV can directly affect other tissues, such as the nervous system. Damage to the CNS can lead to AIDS dementia complex, which is a form of encephalopathy. The meninges and peripheral sensory nerves may also be involved. Infections can also affect the skin, eyes, blood, gut, lungs, heart, kidneys and endocrine system.

Candida

Infection of mucous membranes with candida is very common and may be one of the infections which present at a relatively early stage. Creamy plaques or reddened inflamed areas may develop in the mouth, pharynx, oesophagus and vagina. Systemic antifungal drugs will probably be indicated.

Pneumocystis carinii pneumonia (PCP)

The Pneumocystis organism which causes this condition has characteristics in common with both protozoa and fungi. PCP is a progressive form of pneumonia which is often fatal without treatment. It is not seen clinically in people with normal immune systems. This is one of the most common OIs in AIDS; about 80% of patients develop it at some stage in their illness. The patient has malaise, fever and progressive shortness of breath which may develop over a few weeks, there is a non-productive cough. There will be rapid breathing, tachycardia and hypoxia which may manifest as cyanosis. Treatment is with intravenous sulfamethoxazole and trimethoprim for 21 days. In severe cases corticosteroids and ventilatory support may be needed.

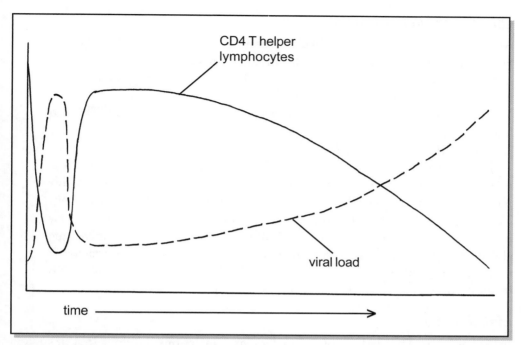

Figure 4.1
The natural evolution of HIV infection in the absence of antiretroviral treatment. Initially the viral load in the blood increases rapidly. It is this viral load which may give rise to the seroconversion illness. During this phase the increasing viral load decreases the number of CD4 T helper lymphocytes from 1000 to 300-400 per ml of blood, or even lower. Then as antibodies develop the spread of the virus between cells is reduced allowing a degree of recovery in CD4 lymphocyte numbers. This allows the patient to enter the latent asymptomatic phase. Typically, over 7-10 years the condition deteriorates and the viral load increases, decreasing the CD4 count. The reduction in CD4 numbers leaves the patient vulnerable to more and more infections, which will eventually prove fatal.

Cryptococcal meningitis

This condition is acquired by inhalation of cryptococcal fungal spores. There are many possible sources of the infection including bird faeces. Typically there is a slow, insidious onset of headache, nausea and fever; later there will be reduced levels of consciousness. Classical features of meningitis such as photophobia, neck and back stiffness are caused by the generation of an inflammatory response to the presence of an antigenic organism. However in HIV this inflammatory response may be significantly inhibited. This means these features may be mild or absent. To be sure of the diagnosis a sample of cerebrospinal fluid (CSF) needs to be examined, in positive cases the organism can be directly observed. It is also possible to culture cryptococcus from CSF. Some patients respond to oral systemic antifungal drugs such as fluconazole, others require intravenous treatment with amphotericin or fluconazole.

Other possible forms of OI

AIDS patients are much more likely to develop several protozoal infections. For example toxoplasmosis causes localized, focal neurological lesions with headache, fever and possible convulsions. Treatment is with systemic anti-toxoplasmosis drugs such as pyrimethamine.

Viral infections such as cytomegalovirus pose a risk in later disease. This can lead to eye disease and blindness. Reactivation of herpes virus can lead to nasty cold sores which can usually be treated with local acyclovir.

Perhaps the most significant global bacterial infection in HIV/AIDS is tuberculosis. Respiratory transmission of Mycobacterium tuberculosis is highly prevalent in many parts of the world where there is a lot of HIV. Unfortunately, TB is prone to develop even if there is only slight immunocompromise, so may present early in the evolution of HIV. Multidrug resistant TB is an increasing global problem. Clearly any patient with active TB, whether HIV is a factor or not, can infect other previously healthy people. Treatment is with normal TB medication but may need to be continued for longer.

Malignancies

In Kaposi's sarcoma dark coloured malignant skin lesions develop. It seems immunosuppression caused by AIDS allows increased activity of a form of herpesvirus, which in turn gives rise to these tumours. Giving HAART may cause the lesions to become smaller and radiotherapy is helpful. Lymphoma is another potential problem and is associated with Epstein-Barr virus.

Management principles in HIV

Highly active antiretroviral therapy (HAART)

This does not eradicate the HI virus from a patient so is not a cure. However, therapy can reduce viral load in the blood to almost undetectable levels and will allow a partial recovery of CD4 lymphocytes. These two changes should prevent OIs from developing. In essence, it means HIV infection can be managed on a long term basis, rather than leading to a very premature death. HAART normally uses 3 antiretroviral drugs in combination and dramatically improves the morbidity and mortality caused by HIV infection. Ongoing use of HAART inhibits viral replication. If the therapy is stopped HIV will again progress. One of the current challenges to the world is to give HAART to every human being who needs it.

HIV and pregnancy

The key point to grasp is that the risk of a baby contracting HI virus is proportional to the viral load in the blood of the mother. Lower maternal viral load reduces the chances of baby contracting HIV. Pregnant women may be given a range of possible antiretroviral treatments which significantly reduce the probability the baby will contract HIV infection. After delivery the baby should receive treatment for a further 4-6 weeks.

HIV and you

As health care workers we are at some risk from contracting HIV from infected patients. If you are exposed to HIV at work, a 4 week course of antiretroviral therapy will reduce the probability of infection becoming established. This post exposure treatment may also be used after a patient has had unprotected sex with a HIV positive partner.

Preventing opportunistic infections (OIs)

As the CD4 T lymphocyte numbers fall, the patient becomes increasingly prone to more infections. Some infections can be prevented by avoiding potentially infecting organisms. Good food hygiene can prevent food poisoning. People with active respiratory infections such as pulmonary tuberculosis or influenza should be avoided. Sometimes vaccinations may be a good idea, but HIV patients should not be given live vaccines such as oral polio or yellow fever vaccine. Some infections are less likely if prophylactic medications can be given. In the absence of HAART, morbidity and mortality can be much improved with simple secondary prophylaxis with septrin (co-trimoxazole) or antifungals.

Prevention of HIV

Ideally HIV infection should be prevented; however there is controversy as to how this should be achieved. There are many underlying social problems which also contribute to contagion. For example in many countries men work away from home for long periods of time. During their time away from home they may use local prostitutes. After a few months they go home and infect their wives, and possibly any future children. Men from developed countries may travel to developing countries as sexual tourists, infecting or becoming infected by local people they pay for sex.

Condom use is an effective method of preventing the spread of HIV, but to be safe, condoms need to be available and used on every sexual occasion. Condom use may be adversely affected by personal preference, cultural influences and cost and availability issues. If monogamy between non-infected people is maintained the risk of HIV being acquired via the sexual route is zero. There is some evidence that male circumcision slightly reduces the risk of men being infected.

Many areas use needle exchange schemes, swapping used hypodermic needles for sterile ones. These aim to prevent the sharing of needles between intravenous drug users allowing users to inject themselves with clean needles.

Hypersensitivity (allergic and autoimmune) disorders

Hypersensitivity verses immunological tolerance

In health, the immune system exhibits immunological tolerance. This means the body does not generate immune and inflammatory reactions to any of the bodies own tissues or to outside substances such as latex, nuts or shellfish. However in hypersensitivity disorders, there is an exaggerated or inappropriate response to body tissues or outside agents which act as antigens. An antigen is anything the immune system recognises as being foreign. This means in people who suffer from hypersensitivity, there may be an immunological reaction to substances or body tissues which should be immunologically tolerated.

When the immune system recognises a substance as foreign, it usually mounts an inflammatory reaction. For example, when we have a viral throat infection, the redness and pain are caused by the bodies own inflammatory reaction, rather than by the virus itself. In hypersensitivity, the body is abnormally identifying substances as antigens which it should immunologically tolerate. This abnormal, immunologically generated inflammatory reaction, can lead to damage of body tissues. Clinically hypersensitivity gives rise to two categories of disorder. These are allergies and autoimmune disease.

Allergies

Allergy is the common term used to describe one group of harmful effects generated by hypersensitivity reactions. There is an exaggerated inflammatory response to an environmental compound. An antigen which generates such an allergic reaction is termed an allergen. Allergic disorders seen in regular clinical practice include urticaria, allergic asthma, atopic dermatitis, allergic rhinitis (hay fever) allergic conjunctivitis, allergies to food, drugs or insect stings and occasionally anaphylaxis.

Antibodies

Antibodies are immune proteins which are specifically synthesised to combat a particular antigen. Antibodies are made up of a class of protein molecules called immunoglobulins. There are 5 main classes of immunoglobulins, which play different roles in protecting the body against infection. Immunoglobulin is abbreviated to Ig, the classes are IgA, IgD, IgE, IgG and IgM. In an allergy, there is an abnormal antigen-antibody reaction which means the antibodies must be already present in the patient for the reaction to occur. This means the patient must have been previously exposed to the antigen, for the antibody synthesis to have been initiated. This process of antigen exposure followed by antibody synthesis is termed sensitisation. The patient becomes sensitive to the antigen which in future acts as an allergen.

Autoimmunity

As well as allergies, hypersensitivity may manifest as autoimmunity. In health, the immune system protects against invading infection by reacting against foreign proteins. The immune system should recognise body tissues as part of the 'self', and therefore not attack them. However, in autoimmune disease there is a breakdown in the self/non-self recognition system which results in the immune system attacking the bodies own proteins and tissues. In military terms this would be described as attack from 'friendly fire'. In autoimmunity the immune system reacts to some of the bodies own tissues as if they were invading infections agents which need to be eliminated. The immune system is making a mistake, and is attacking the very tissues it is supposed to defend. Autoimmune diseases you may come across include diabetes mellitus type 1, Graves' disease, Addison's disease, pernicious anaemia, rheumatoid arthritis and Hashimoto's thyroiditis.

Types of hypersensitivity reaction

The pathophysiology of allergy and autoimmunity are described under four types of hypersensitivity reaction, types I-IV. Allergic disorders are mostly caused by type I reactions. Autoimmune reactions are caused by types II, III and IV hypersensitivity reactions. Some autoimmune disorders are attributed to a specific type of reaction while others are caused by a more complex combination of types of hypersensitivity reaction.

Type I (immediate allergic) hypersensitivity reactions

Type I reactions typically develop rapidly (usually under 10 minutes) after exposure to the causative allergen. Common trigger allergens in type I reactions include moulds, animals, some foods, house dust mite, some drugs and pollens. Once antibodies have been produced, by the B lymphocytes, they attach to the cell membranes of mast cells. The antibodies formed in type I reactions are IgEs. When a patient is exposed to the antigen (which is now an allergen) on a subsequent occasion, the antigen binds onto the antibodies on the surface of the mast cells. This combination of the antibody and the antigen causes the mast cell to degranulate with release of histamine and other inflammatory mediators into the tissues and body fluids.

Clinical features in type I hypersensitivity reactions

In these disorders there may be localised or generalised (systemic) reactions caused by the release of inflammatory mediators. Local clinical manifestations depend on the site of antigen exposure and how sensitive the patient is. Reactions involving the skin often generate a wheal and flare. Reactions involving the upper respiratory tract and eyes cause nasal irritation, sneezing and conjunctivitis. This is the picture in 'hay fever' correctly termed allergic rhinitis. Angioneurotic oedema may develop with acute development of large, oedematous, painless, itchy lesions which may involve the mouth, lips, larynx, neck, chest, feet, hands and sometimes genitals. In severe cases, swelling of tissues around the upper airway may lead to asphyxiation. Systemic manifestations of type I reactions include bronchoconstriction, airway swelling with obstruction and hypotension, as seen in anaphylactic shock. Type I reactions may also trigger an episode of extrinsic asthma or urticaria.

Diagnosis

Type I disorders are recognised by the typical clinical history with features such as angioedema, urticaria and wheezing developing shortly (minutes) after exposure to an antigen. Skin prick tests are used to identify specific allergens. A droplet of dilute potential allergen is placed on the patient's forearm and a small prick is made in the skin. If the person is allergic to the allergen there will be a localised inflammatory reaction. This will allow the patient to clearly see what they are allergic to. These tests must be carried out in closely supervised conditions as there is a very slight risk of severe systemic reactions. It is also possible to check serum IgE levels for specific antigens. After a severe allergic reaction, blood can be tested for the presence of mast cell tryptase; if present this would indicate there has been a lot of mast cell degranulation, confirming a diagnosis of anaphylaxis.

Management principles

Patients with type I hypersensitivity should avoid exposure to the allergens they are sensitive to. Every time they are exposed to the allergen, there is the potential to stimulate even more IgE synthesis, making any future reactions more serious. One problem is that processed foods contain many ingredients so that something a person is allergic to may slip in unnoticed. Cross contamination is another problem. For example if a cook makes a chicken sandwich using a knife with some residue of peanut butter on it, this may cause anaphylaxis in a person with peanut allergy who eats the chicken sandwich.

Reactions may be treated with antihistamines or corticosteroids, both of which will act as anti-inflammatory agents. Inhaled bronchodilators may be useful for treating bronchoconstriction. More severe anaphylactic reactions should be treated with intramuscular epinephrine (adrenaline). Sodium cromoglycate will stabilise mast cell membranes and so prevent the release of histamine, an inhaled preparation is effective at preventing acute asthma and allergic rhinitis.

Atopy

Type I hypersensitivity reactions are more likely to occur in people who are atopic. Atopy describes a tendency to produce IgEs after exposure to everyday antigens. This is why people who suffer from one allergy are more likely to be allergic to something else, or have extrinsic asthma. The numbers of people who are atopic in the Western World is increasing and is currently about 15% of the population. Atopy is largely genetic but environmental factors are also involved in the pathogenesis. Conditions which damage the respiratory tract, such as viral infections or the inhalation of pollutants, may allow greater antigenic penetration and subsequent sensitization. Atopic conditions include allergic conjunctivitis and rhinitis, some cases of eczema (dermatitis), extrinsic asthma and allergies to foods, insect stings and other substances. Exposure to certain antigens in early life is another possible factor in the development of allergies. For example, mothers who eat peanuts while breast feeding secretes some nut antigen in their breast milk which may sensitise the child resulting in allergy in later life. The same effect has also been demonstrated in neonates who were massaged with oil containing peanut extracts. Similar effects have been seen with dairy products.

Healthy dirt

Despite these specific problems, early exposure to bacteria seems to increase the ability of the immune system to discriminate between antigens and therefore promotes immunological tolerance. Children who are reared in a very clean environment suffer more allergic problems than those who are exposed to 'normal' levels of bacteria as they grow up. Childhood exposure to soil bacteria seems particularly effective in promoting immunological tolerance. While over exposure to infectious agents may result in potentially dangerous conditions such as gastroenteritis there does seem to be a level of 'healthy dirt'.

Type II hypersensitivity

In these autoimmune reactions, antibodies act against antigens which are fixed in the cells or tissues of the body. Antibodies which act against 'self' targets are usually described as autoantibodies. As in type I and III hypersensitivity reactions the antibodies are produced by the B lymphocytes.

Pathophysiology

In type II hypersensitivity, the antibodies involved are IgG and IgM. Antibodies can attack 'self' cells and tissues in different ways. Sometimes antibodies attach to a particular self-antigen on a body cell. The presence of the antibodies targets the cell for phagocytosis, which clearly kills the body cell. In other cases, antibodies mimic the function of natural chemical transmitters. For example, in Graves' disease antibodies are formed which attach to, and stimulate, the thyroid stimulating hormone (TSH) receptors on thyroid producing cells in the thyroid gland. This leads to hyperthyroidism. In myasthenia gravis, antibodies occupy acetylcholine receptors on the motor end plates of muscles in the neuromuscular junctions. This blocks the binding of acetylcholine and so prevents normal stimulation of muscle contraction, leading to weakness or paralysis.

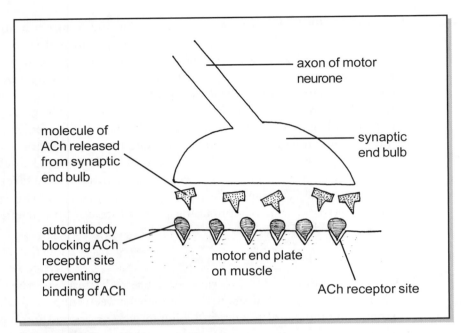

Diagram 3.2
In myasthenia gravis autoantibodies bind into and block the acetylcholine (ACh) receptors. This means ACh is not able to bind and cause muscle depolarization. As it is this depolarization which stimulates muscle contraction, paralysis results.

Disorders caused by hypersensitivity type II reactions

In some cases there may be single organ involvement. In others, many organs or body structures may be involved. These can be explained by an autoimmune reaction, attacking a particular form of tissue which is widely distributed throughout the body. Specific type II autoimmune conditions include Goodpasture's syndrome and thrombocytopenic purpura. ABO blood transfusion mis-matches are also a form of type II reaction. Treatments may be given to suppress inflammatory reactions generated by autoimmune reactions including local or systemic use of corticosteroids and immunosuppressant drugs.

Type III hypersensitivity (immune complex reactions)

These reactions are caused by the formation of immune complexes which lead to inflammatory changes. An immune complex is a combination of antigens and antibodies which form clumps. Antibodies, produced by the B lymphocytes, bind to specific sites on the surface of antigens called epitopes. In this way several antigens, for example bacteria or viral particles, can be clumped together in the process called agglutination. Once formed these immune complexes may become fixed in a particular tissue leading to localized reactions. Alternatively they may circulate leading to systemic effects.

Pathophysiology

Immune complexes can be detected in the plasma in many infections as antibodies agglutinate aetiological antigens; these do not usually cause any problems. Immune complexes are normally removed from the plasma by phagocytes located in the liver and spleen. However, some immune complexes are not readily removed and become persistent. These insoluble immune complexes can be deposited in body tissues or lead to inflammation in the blood vessel walls which they come into contact with. (Immune complex size and charge are other factors which determine pathogenesis.) Areas most commonly affected are the kidneys, blood vessels, joints, lungs and skin.

Immune complexes present in a tissue trigger the complement cascade. This can lead to the formation of membrane attack protein which can destroy local cells. Activated complement also acts as an inflammatory mediator. This leads to the vasodilation and increased capillary permeability typically seen in inflammation. Inflammatory mediators also attract neutrophils and monocytes to the area. These cells attempt to phagocytose the immune complexes which are lodged in the tissues. In doing so, the phagocytic cells also damage local cells and tissues, leading to further tissue injury and inflammation. In military terms this would be called 'collateral damage'.

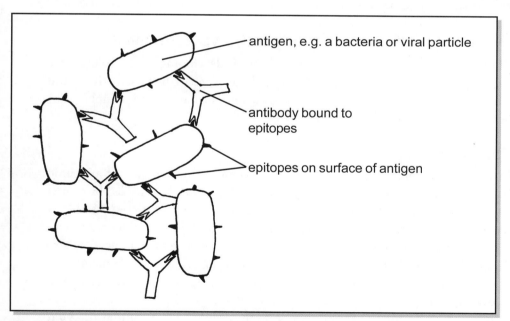

Diagram 3.3
Antibodies have agglutinated several antigenic particles to form an immune complex. The antibodies involved in type III reactions may be IgG IgM or IgA, (IgG antibodies are illustrated in this example). As antibodies have 2 arms they are able to 'grab' 2 antigens each. This means that several antibodies can 'clump' a group of antigens. This agglutination of antigens and antibodies forms an immune complex.

Clinical conditions associated with type III hypersensitivity reactions

Allergic alveolitis is a condition caused by the local development of antibodies. For example, in 'Farmer's lung' inhaled moulds act as antigens. This leads to the local synthesis of specific antibodies. Subsequent exposure to the mould leads to the formation of immune complexes, consisting of the mould antigen and the antibodies which have been synthesised by the immune system. These immune complexes in the alveoli lead to local inflammation and progressive lung fibrosis. Once a lung has been sensitised by the generation of antibodies it is important the person avoids further exposure to the antigen.

Systemic conditions caused by immune complexes include the vasculitis seen in rheumatoid arthritis. They also play a role in several connective tissue disorders including systemic lupus erythematosus (SLE). Type III inflammatory reactions are sometimes responsible for the kidney damage found in several forms of acute glomerulonephritis when immune complexes become fixed in the glomerular basement membrane. Serum sickness is another type III reaction; this is a self-limiting, acute disorder which presents 6-8 days after a person is injected with a foreign protein. It presents with an acute glomerulonephritis, fever, vasculitis and painful joints and was first identified after horse antisera were used for treating tetanus and diphtheria, (a treatment no longer used).

Type IV (T lymphocyte mediated) hypersensitivity

These reactions are often described as delayed, developing 24-72 hours after exposure to an antigen. Unlike the first three types of hypersensitivity, the reaction is not mediated by antibodies (which are produced by B lymphocytes) but by the T lymphocytes directly.

Physiology

In health, the ability of immune cells to recognise the presence of antigenic fragments is an important aspect of immunity. When a cell is invaded by a virus the infected cell is used to synthesise many more viral particles. As this is happening within the cell, antibodies in the tissue fluids are not able to interfere with the process of viral replication. However, the presence of viral biochemistry inside the cell, leads to some viral proteins appearing on the outside membrane of the infected cell. Immune cells such as cytotoxic T lymphocytes can recognise these viral antigenic fragments on the body cell surface. When these are recognised, the cytotoxic lymphocyte kills the whole cell, including the viral particles it contains. This prevents viral replication. Also immune cells are able to recognise some protein markers on outer cell membranes which indicate a cell has become malignant. This means cancer may be eradicated by the immune system when it only affects one or two cells. T cell mediated immunity is also essential in combating infections with fungi, protozoa and parasites.

Pathophysiology

The cells involved in type IV hypersensitivity are macrophages and T lymphocytes. First macrophages phagocytose an antigen (possibly a virus or bacterium). After the antigen has been digested and processed by the macrophage, parts of the antigen migrate to the outer cell membrane. Here, T cytotoxic and T helper lymphocytes recognise the antigen fragments, and are sensitised and activated. There will then be a proliferation of T cells which are sensitized to attack that particular antigen. These activated T lymphocytes then mistakenly recognise one of the bodies own proteins as an antigen. This may happen because one of the 'self' proteins has a similar shape to the infectious antigen the lymphocytes have been sensitised to.

Autoimmune activation of T cytotoxic lymphocytes will lead them to attack the bodies own tissues by depositing lethal chemicals onto the cells. T helper lymphocytes damage body tissues by releasing cytokines which activate macrophages which then attack the tissue cells. These immune cells can therefore kill body cells and damage tissues. As well as these immune cells, fibroblasts are attracted by the cytokines. Fibroblasts produce fibrous tissue resulting in fibrosis.

Clinical effects

Inflammation and direct cytotoxic effects caused by type IV reactions are the principle cause of several autoimmune conditions including diabetes mellitus type 1, Hashimoto's thyroiditis and primary biliary sclerosis. It is also very probably that T helper lymphocytes mediate the pathogenesis in the inflammatory bowel diseases, i.e. Crohn's and ulcerative colitis. At least part of the inflammation seen in multiple sclerosis is mediated by T lymphocytes penetrating the blood brain barrier and entering the CNS tissues. Cell mediated pathology is also involved in leprosy and causes the caseation and necrosis seen in tuberculosis.

T lymphocytes may also be activated against type II collagen which is a component of synovial joints. This is part of the pathogeneses in rheumatoid arthritis. It is also the main mechanism responsible for graft verses host disease, where the immune system seeks to 'reject' transplanted tissues. Another example is allergic contact dermatitis, this occurs when the skin is exposed to an antigen it has previously been sensitized to. Antigens causing contact dermatitis include cosmetics, topical drugs, metals, washing powders, poison ivy, oil and grease. Management in type III and IV hypersensitivity reactions include avoidance of allergens, corticosteroids and immunosuppressives.

CHAPTER 5

Disorders of Arteries

Physiology

Systemic circulation originates from the left ventricle, when this contracts blood is ejected into a single large artery called the aorta. From the aorta, numerous arteries branch off. These large arterial branches progressively divide into smaller branches which ultimately become arterioles and capillaries. An artery is essentially a tube or pipe through which blood may flow. A healthy artery has elastic walls and a patent lumen to allow smooth uninterrupted blood flow to all living tissues.

Pathophysiology

There are two common disorders of arteries, arteriosclerosis and atherosclerosis. Arteriosclerosis describes a thickening and hardening (sclerosis means hardening) of arterial walls which mostly affects the walls of the small arteries and arterioles. Arteriolosclerosis is a specific term which describes hardening of the arterioles. As the walls of a vessel thicken, the lumen becomes narrowed resulting in reduced perfusion of the tissues with blood. Hardening also causes the arterial walls to become inelastic. This reduces the ability of the vessel to expand and contract with the pulse which further reduces the efficiency of local perfusion, making the ischaemia worse.

Atherosclerosis

One of the most common disorders in Western countries is arterial atherosclerosis. Complications caused by atherosclerosis account for approximately half of the deaths in the developed world. Atherosclerosis affects large and medium sized arteries. In atherosclerosis there is accumulation of an abnormal material called atheroma under the inner layer of the arterial wall, (i.e. under the tunica intima). Atheroma is a fatty cholesterol based material which also contains inflammatory cells, smooth muscle and connective tissues such as collagen. As this atheroma accumulates it protrudes into the lumen of the vessel. A particular area of atheroma is described as a plaque. The presence of atheroma also affects the tunica media, (the middle muscular layer of the arterial wall) often resulting in thinning.

Causes of atheroma

Diseases caused by atherosclerosis are the most common cause of death in the Western World. Deaths occur primarily as a result of myocardial infarctions and strokes. Coronary heart disease is the most common single cause of death. In many developing countries the incidence of ischaemic heart disease and strokes is increasing as many adopt 'Western' life styles. The reason why an individual develops arterial disease however, is often difficult to identify. This is because the aetiology is multifactorial. In a multifactorial aetiology a number of factors contribute to the development of pathology, this means it is difficult to decide which factors are most important and how the factors interact. Despite this difficulty certain risk factors are now well accepted as aetiological and these will now be discussed.

Elevated plasma cholesterol

This problem is called hypercholesterolaemia. Cholesterol is a steroid based molecule which is fat soluble. Some cholesterol in the blood is derived from the diet but most is synthesised by the body in places such as the liver and intestines. Physiologically, cholesterol is an essential component of cell membranes and steroid based hormones such as hydrocortisone, aldosterone and testosterone. However, as plasma levels of cholesterol rise, the risk of death from coronary heart disease (CHD) also rises. The risk of developing CHD is four times greater with a cholesterol level of 8.6 mmol/litre than it is with a level of 4.8 mmol/litre.

High density and low density lipoprotein particles

As cholesterol is not water soluble, it must be transported in the plasma via specialised transporter particles called high-density lipoprotein (HDL) and low-density lipoprotein (LDL). The harmful effects of cholesterol on the arteries are modified by the opposing actions of this HDL and LDL cholesterol.

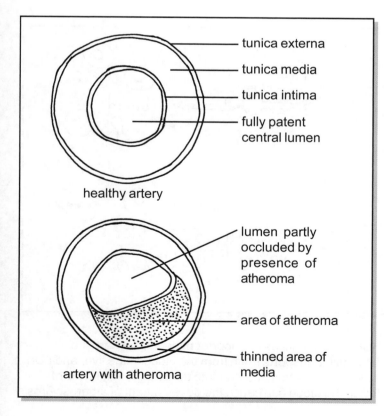

tunica externa

tunica media

tunica intima

fully patent
central lumen

healthy artery

lumen partly
occluded by
presence of
atheroma

area of atheroma

thinned area of
media

artery with atheroma

Diagram 5.1
Cross section of a healthy artery with a full patent lumen in comparison to an artery showing the presence of an atheromatous plaque.

HDL is protective against the development of atheroma so is sometimes called 'good cholesterol'. HDL takes cholesterol and fats from cell membranes in arterial walls and transports it, via the blood, to the liver. Once in the liver, cholesterol can be biochemically processed to make it less atherogenic, (i.e. less able to cause atheroma). Conversely, LDL particles transport cholesterol and fats from the liver, into the blood and so increase the proportion of cholesterol and other lipids in the blood, this is why LDL is often called 'bad cholesterol'. Once in the blood cholesterol comes into contact with the arterial lining so may contribute to the process of atheroma development.

From this it follows that factors which raise HDL or lower LDL will be protective against atheroma development. Conversely, factors which lower HDL or raise LDL will contribute to atheroma development. In addition to protecting against the development of atheroma HDL particles have effects on the functioning of platelets which help to prevent thrombus formation.

Population based studies have demonstrated a strong positive association between LDL cholesterol and the risk of developing coronary heart disease. Statins are drugs which lower the plasma levels of LDL and are know to reduce the likelihood of heart disease and stroke. While blood levels of cholesterol, LDL and HDL, are partly under genetic control they are also partly dependent on lifestyle factors.

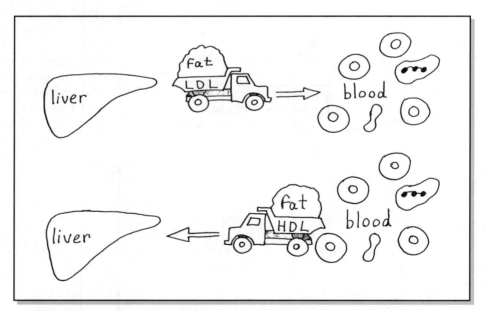

Diagram 5.2
In simple terms HDL and LDL act as transporter molecule for carrying cholesterol and fats. HDL transports them from the blood to the liver and LDL transports cholesterol and fats from the liver into the blood. High levels of cholesterol and fats in the blood can cause the development of atherosclerosis.

Harmful diets

Diets high in saturated fats increase the risk of developing arterial disease. These polysaturated fats increase the levels of harmful LDL cholesterol as well as increasing the total amount of fat in the blood. Foods derived from animal sources are often high in saturated fat, examples include, milk, cheese and fatty meat. Meat products such as pies and sausages are often particularly high in fat. This is why it is a good idea to grill meat products rather than to fry them. Grilling melts the fat and allows it to run out. In addition to animal sources there are a lot of saturated fats in many processed foods. When foods are processed the fat is often saturated by manufacturers, making vegetable fats as harmful as animal fats. Pastries, cakes and biscuits are examples of processed foods which contain a lot of saturated fat. Food manufacturers often describe fat as being 'hydrogenated' which means exactly the same thing as polysaturated.

In addition to eating harmful fats, diets which contain too many calories, are also harmful. In other words overeating is a risk factor. In western countries most people eat more than they need because high calorie foods are readily available.

Protective diets

Many dietary components are protective against the development of arterial atherosclerosis. Antioxidants such as beta-carotene, selenium, flavanoids and vitamins A, C and E are all found in foods, particularly fruit and vegetables. Flavanoids are naturally occurring compounds found in a variety of foods which act as antioxidants. This is one reason why people should be advised to eat at least 5 portions of fruit and vegetables per day. Tea is also a good source of flavanoids. Recent studies indicate that eating nuts is highly protective.

Normal metabolic processes in cells produce some oxygen molecules with an electron deficit. This form of oxygen is very reactive and is described as a free oxygen radical. These radicals have a tendency to take an electron from other compounds which may be in the area. Removal of an electron is a form of oxidation. Free oxygen radicals may therefore oxidise other molecules found in cells including DNA, the genetic material which controls all cellular processes. If such free radical damage occurs in the cells composing an arterial endothelial lining, atheroma may develop. Free radical damage may also lead to ageing and cancer. Dietary antioxidants have the ability to 'mop up' free oxygen radicals and therefore prevent them causing cellular damage. Therefore dietary antioxidants protect against free radical damage.

Oxidation of LDL and cholesterol in the blood by oxygen free radicals increases the capacity of cholesterol to cause the development of atherosclerosis. Again, it is believed that eating antioxidants prevents this oxidation of LDL and cholesterol so therefore reduces the development of atheroma.

Diets rich in water-soluble fibre from fruit, vegetables and oats have a slight cholesterol lowering effect. Some waste cholesterol from bile absorbs into water soluble fibre in the lumen of the gut and is subsequently passed out with the faeces. This means this waste cholesterol is not reabsorbed back into the blood. Evidence is also accumulating suggesting that adequate blood levels of vitamin D are protective against vascular disease. Vitamin D may be derived from the diet or by the action of sunlight on the skin. People with darker coloured skin need more time in the sun to produce vitamin D than people with light or white skin.

Alcohol

Some evidence exists that low doses of alcohol, probably 1-2 units per day, are protective. Alcohol slightly raises HDL levels and is a vasodilator. Despite these moderate benefits from low dose alcohol consumption, non-drinkers should not usually be advised to start, as some people find it hard to stop drinking once they start. Large doses of alcohol increase the risk of obesity, hypertension and arterial disease, as well as numerous other potential health and social problems.

Smoking

Tobacco smoking increases the risk of death from arterial disease. Smoking increases the adhesiveness of platelets, making thrombus formation more likely. Smoking increases heart rate, increases levels of adrenaline in the plasma and reduces the oxygen carrying capacity of blood. Smoking directly lowers the levels of protective HDL in the blood. The well known population based Framingham study found a direct relationship between smoking and risk of myocardial infarction, sudden cardiac death and overall CHD mortality in men and women. Smokers have a 2 to 3 times higher risk of cardiac related death when compared to non smokers. There is also clear evidence that smoking increases the risk of suffering a stroke.

The numbers of people in Western countries who smoke declined in the late 20th century and continues to do so in the 21st. This is partly because people know how harmful smoking is. What is so sad to see, is the increase in smoking in developing countries, sometimes as a result of high pressure sales and advertising campaigns by big tobacco companies. As professionals we need to protect our people from this danger by sound health education and example setting.

When smokers stop smoking, their risk of heart disease and stroke starts to fall within days. This reducing risk continues until after 2 to 3 years when the risk of an ex-smoker suffering a coronary event is comparable with someone who has never smoked, the risk of stroke takes longer to reduce, probably 5-10 years. This shows the importance of stopping as young as possible. We must help people not to start, or to stop.

Diabetes mellitus

It now seems clear that the risk of developing arterial disease in diabetes is dependent on the quality of diabetic control the individual is able to maintain. If blood sugar levels are kept low, arterial complications are less likely to occur. Overall, CHD is 2 to 4 times more common in diabetics when compared to non-diabetics. CHD contributes to death in 75-85% of diabetics. Diabetes is often associated with other risk factors such as obesity, dyslipidaemia and hypertension; these factors will increase risk synergistically. These risks illustrate why good patient education and management in diabetes is so important.

People may suffer from diabetes type 2 and be unaware of any problem. Despite being asymptomatic, damage to their arterial system will be progressing. This is why estimation of blood sugar level should, like blood pressure measurement, form a part of any routine examination.

Hypertension

High blood pressure damages the arteries directly and also contributes to the development of atheroma. Hypertension is a particularly important risk factor for strokes. The increase in risk of developing CHD is proportional to the level of high blood pressure. This means that the higher blood pressure is, the greater the risk of CHD. Population based studies of many people have found that with a diastolic blood pressure of 110 mmHg or higher, the risk of developing CHD is 10 to 12 times greater than people with a diastolic blood pressure of less than 79. Blood pressure measurement should be part of any routine examination, we have effective treatments for hypertension, but not for the arterial and organ damage high blood pressure can lead to. It is interesting to note that atheroma is found in blood vessels which are subject to relatively high blood pressures in the systemic circulation. Atheroma is not found in vessels which contain blood at low pressures such as the veins and pulmonary arterial system.

Physical activity

Increased levels of physical activity are associated with reduced risk of atheroma development while a sedentary lifestyle increases risk. Regular aerobic exercise helps to reduce blood pressure, reduce plasma LDL levels and increase HDL, combat obesity and lower blood sugar levels. Benefits from regular exercise have been claimed for low to moderate exercise for 20 minutes, 3 times per week. However as fitness increases, more vigorous exercise for longer, more regularly will have a greater beneficial effect. Regular teeth brushing also seems to be protective.

Gender

Population studies indicate that men have a greater chance of developing CHD in young to middle adult life, however rates of the disease in women 'catch up' with those of men in later life. This can partly be explained by the cardioprotective effect of high levels of oestrogen enjoyed by women before the menopause. Oestrogen lowers harmful LDL and raises protective HDL particles. This information might suggest that post menopausal hormone replacement therapy (HRT) would be cardioprotective however, trials have found no benefit from HRT in post menopausal women with established coronary artery disease.

Psychosocial factors

It has been suggested that emotions such as anger, cynicism and hostility adversely affect the cardiovascular system and may be risk factors for CHD and other arterial disorders. It may be that a calm personality, with good levels of social support is protective. Marriage is also probably protective and some studies indicate pets are helpful.

Age

The risk of developing arterial disease increases with increasing age. This can be explained simply in terms of more time allowing for risk factors to adversely affect the arteries.

Obesity

Obesity is a risk factor for development of atherosclerosis. Men who are 10% overweight have an overall 10% increased risk of death. For men who are 20% overweight the risk of death rises by 25%. Obesity is associated with increased blood pressure and plasma cholesterol levels. Weight loss should be encouraged because it is associated with reductions in blood pressure and cholesterol levels, as well as a decrease in overall mortality.

Risk factors are synergistic

We have seen that high cholesterol, hypertension and smoking are all independent risk factors for arterial disease. However if a person has high cholesterol and smokes, his or her chances of developing CHD increase to 8 times more than that of someone with normal cholesterol who does not smoke. In other words there is a multiplying effect if a person has more than one risk factor. A hypertensive, hypercholesterolaemic smoker has a 16 fold chance of developing CHD. Additional risk factors seem to enhance the damage done by plasma cholesterol, magnifying the harmful effect.

Complications of atheroma

Atherosclerosis has basically three complications. Firstly, because the lumen of the artery is narrowed, the volume of blood flow is reduced. This deprives areas of tissue past (i.e. distal to) the atheroma, of part of their normal blood supply. Reduction of blood supply to an area is termed ischaemia. Secondly, the presence of atheroma increases the risk that blood may clot within an arterial vessel forming a thrombus. If a vessel is thrombosed, the arterial lumen may be closed off completely, resulting in death of the area of tissue normally supplied. Such an area of dead tissue is called an infarct. Thirdly, atheroma can weaken the wall of an artery resulting in aneurysm formation. These may expand causing localised pressure effects or they may burst resulting in haemorrhage.

Ischaemia

Ischaemia means a reduced blood supply. If the lumen of an artery is partially obstructed by an area of atheroma, less blood can get through. This means that the blood supply to the tissues supplied by the artery is not cut off, as it is in infarction, but is reduced below normal physiological levels. Reduced volumes of blood perfusing a tissue will mean that there is a reduced amount of food molecules getting to the tissue cells; this will include the delivery of glucose, fatty and amino acids. These molecules are used as fuels in the process of metabolism which provide the energy essential for cell life. Reduced blood supply will also reduce the volumes of oxygen delivered. Like food molecules, oxygen is needed by the mitochondria in the cell cytoplasm to generate energy. Also reduced blood volumes passing through a tissue will allow the accumulation of chemical waste products which have been generated by metabolism. These wastes will therefore accumulate in the tissue.

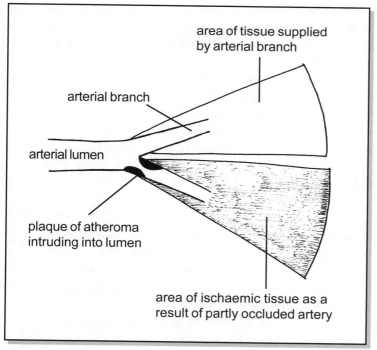

Diagram 5.3
Atheroma is partly occluding the arterial lumen resulting in a reduced blood supply to the distal tissues.

Diagram 5.4
A thrombus has developed over an atheromatous plaque; this has completely occluded the arterial lumen resulting in an area of infarction.

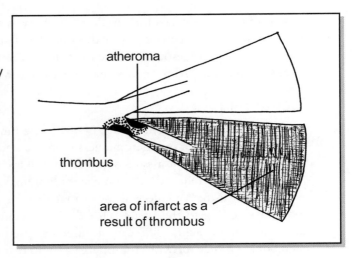

atheroma

thrombus

area of infarct as a result of thrombus

Aerobic and anaerobic metabolism

Lack of oxygen delivery causes a tissue to become hypoxic. This means there is not enough oxygen to generate the energy required for the living processes carried out by tissue cells. When this happens, metabolic processes still carry on and produce energy, so the tissue does not die immediately. What happens is that the form of metabolism changes, from aerobic to anaerobic. Aerobic metabolism refers to energy yielding metabolic reactions which occur in the presence of adequate supplies of oxygen. In contrast, anaerobic metabolism occurs in the absence of oxygen.

Anaerobic metabolism produces a waste product called lactic acid, which accumulates in the tissue. If the levels of lactic acid continue to rise, the tissue will eventually be poisoned and cease to function. This means anaerobic metabolism is an emergency measure which can only be maintained for a short period of time. Removal of lactic acid from a tissue will occur when the blood supply is able to wash the acid out into the systemic circulation. Lactic acid is also removed when fresh supplies of oxygen remove it by the process of oxidation.

In muscles, the accumulation of lactic acid, as a consequence of anaerobic metabolism, causes a pain we normally refer to as cramp. Cramps may occur in skeletal muscle as a result of muscle spasm but can normally be relieved by exercising the muscle concerned. Cramps may also occur, again as the result of lactic acid accumulation, in smooth muscles. This may occur in the smooth muscle walls of hollow structures such as the ureters, bile ducts, bowel or uterus. When this form of pain arises in a hollow structure it is called colic. The same principle applies to anaerobic metabolism in the myocardium. This will occur when the metabolic demands of the heart muscle exceed the delivery of oxygen by the blood passing through the coronary arteries. Lactic acid accumulation in the myocardium is associated with the pain referred to as angina.

The form of ischaemia caused by atheroma typically develops slowly and results in progressive deterioration of the affected tissue. Pathologically a tissue which has been subject to chronic ischaemia develops small, patchy areas of necrosis (tissue death) which may become fibrosed. However, in addition to being caused by atherosclerosis, ischaemia may also be caused by thrombosis and embolism. Ischaemia caused by these disorders often results in complete or near complete obstruction of the affected blood vessel and occur acutely.

Thrombosis

It is of course essential that blood is able to clot, without this mechanism we could bleed to death from a small wound, or even as a result of everyday rough and tumble. However, blood within the circulatory system is supposed to be liquid, if a clot forms within the lumen of a vessel this is abnormal. A thrombus is a pathological blood clot which occurs within the vascular system. This may be in the heart, arteries or veins. Thrombosis refers to the condition where a thrombus, or two or more thrombi exist.

Thrombus formation is promoted by the interacting effects of three factors; these are disease of blood vessel lining, reduced rates of blood flow and increased coagulability of the blood. These three factors are called Virchow's Triad, (named after the pioneering German pathologist, Rudolf Virchow, 1821-1902).

Disorders of vascular endothelium

The presence of atheroma under the lining of the arterial vascular endothelium greatly increases the risk of thrombus development. It is useful to think of two forms of atheromatous plaques, some are simple and stable while others are unstable and complicated. A stable plaque has an intact fibrous cap and a layer of vascular endothelium which separate the core of the plaque and the blood. This prevents platelets and other clotting factors in the blood from coming into contact with the core of the plaque. This is important as it is the core of the atheromatous plaque which is thrombogenic. In other words if blood comes into contact with the core of the plaque, the process of blood clotting and thrombus formation will be initiated. This means that as long as the fibrous cap is intact and stable, thrombus formation is very unlikely.

However, if an atheromatous plaque becomes unstable then thrombus formation becomes much more likely. Inflammatory processes can degrade the quality of the fibrous cap. This happens as inflammatory cells release enzymes which digest components of the fibrous cap. As the inflammatory processes thin the fibrous cap, fissures and ulcers may form which cause effective rupture of the cap. This plaque rupture means that the blood is no longer separated from the thrombogenic core. As blood comes into contact with components of the core, platelet aggregation will be triggered. This will lead to the formation of so called white thrombus, which can partly occlude the arterial lumen. The presence of white thrombus and continued exposure of the blood to the thrombogenic core can also lead the conversion of fibrinogen into the clotting protein fibrin. Once fibrin is formed red blood cells will stick to it forming a red blood clot. This red thrombus will completely occlude the arterial lumen and so completely cut off the blood supply to an area of tissue.

Sluggish or abnormal blood flow

Sluggish blood flow may result in thrombus formation in arteries or veins. When blood flow is sluggish, platelets and other clotting factors have time to accumulate, and may adhere to vessel walls, starting a clotting process. Sluggish venous blood flow may be caused by immobility and is a potential problem in deep veins where deep venous thrombosis (DVT) may develop. Abnormal or turbulent blood flow is also a risk factor in arteries where it may contribute to the rupture of unstable atheromatous plaques, as blood is forced to swirl around atheromatous intrusions into an arterial lumen. In atrial fibrillation (AF) the atria do not contract fully, potentially resulting in stagnant areas of blood. Blood clots which develop in the relatively stagnant areas of blood may be ejected from the heart as emboli.

Increased blood coagulability

Any condition, which increases the tendency of blood to clot, increases the probability of thrombus formation. When the proportion of cells to plasma is increased the blood becomes thicker and more likely to clot, this may occur in dehydration or at altitude, where more red cells are produced to improve the oxygen carrying capacity of blood. Smokers also produce more red blood cells to compensate for the proportion of their haemoglobin which is inactivated by the presence of carbon monoxide in the form of carboxyhaemoglobin. This means that despite smokers having a higher haematocrit than non-smokers, their blood has a reduced oxygen carrying capacity. (Haematocrit refers to the percentage of total blood volume made up by the red cells.)

Conditions which increase the viscosity or numbers of blood platelets, (correctly termed thrombocytes) also predispose to thrombosis. An increase in the number of platelets is called thrombocytosis. Platelets which are lost or broken down by the spleen are replaced by young platelets from the bone marrow. As a result of haemorrhage, caused by surgery, trauma or childbirth, lost platelets are replaced by new ones from the bone marrow. Young platelets are stickier than older ones, so if the proportion of young platelets is increased in this way, thrombus formation becomes more likely. This provides one reason why post operative patients should be mobilized as early as possible. Low dose aspirin has an antiplatelet action so reduces the likelihood of thrombosis and embolism. It is known that low dose aspirin reduces the incidence of myocardial infarction, stroke and mortality in high risk patients.

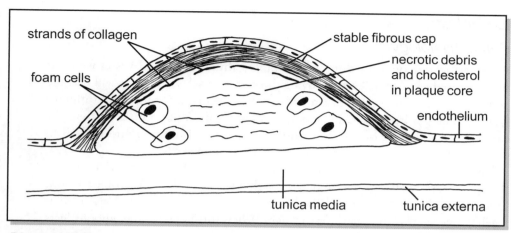

Diagram 5.5i

A stable plaque of atheroma. In a stable plaque, the trombogenic core and the blood are kept apart by the presence of a stable fibrous cap and an intact layer of normal vascular endothelial cells. Under the endothelial cells the fibrous cap is composed mostly of smooth muscle cells with some stabilising fibrous tissue. There are also some macrophages and lymphocytes. The central core contains foam cells, which are macrophages full of LDL cholesterol, necrotic cell debris and cholesterol crystals.

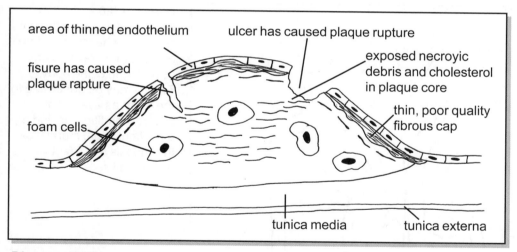

Diagram 5.5ii

An unstable (complicated) plaque of atheroma. In the unstable plaque inflammatory processes have thinned the fibrous cap and caused it to become unstable. This can result in plaque rupture. As a result blood can come into contact with thrombogenic collagen and a clotting factor produced by foam cells called tissue factor. It is therefore this plaque rupture which triggers off the process of clotting and thrombus formation. Interestingly, statin drugs have anti-inflammatory properties, as well as lowering LDL cholesterol. As a result statins prevent abnormal inflammatory processes thereby preventing inflammatory thinning of the fibrous caps. This will promote plaque stability and therefore make thrombosis less likely to develop.

Embolism

Pathophysiology

An embolus describes anything which moves through a blood vessel which is not supposed to be there. After moving through a vessel an embolus will become jammed, causing an occlusion. An embolus may be made of numerous different types of material including, air or gas, a piece of thrombus, a piece of tissue or tumour, or a globule of fat. The plural of embolus is emboli and embolism describes the pathological condition in which emboli exist.

Emboli formation is a possible complication of thrombosis. If part of a thrombus breaks off, this will move through a vessel in the normal blood flow. Once an embolus has formed, it will be carried in the blood flow, until it reaches a vessel it is too big to fit through. When this happens the embolus gets stuck and will block off the vessel.

Systemic emboli originate from the heart or systemic arteries. An embolus which originates from the left side of the heart may be carried by the systemic arterial blood flow to almost any part of the body and may lodge in the liver, spleen, gut, brain, kidneys or extremities, leading to infarction of the affected organ or limb.

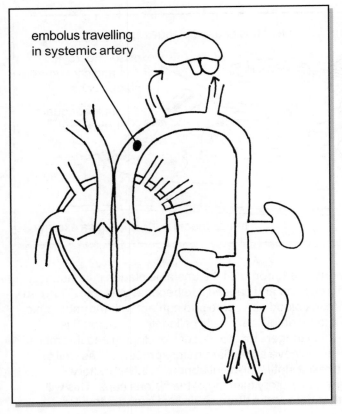

embolus travelling
in systemic artery

Diagram 5.6
Emboli arising from the left side of the heart or systemic arteries may travel to any other organ of the body. Emboli may be generated in the heart as a result of several conditions including atrial fibrillation, mural thrombosis and infective endocarditis.

Forms of emboli

In medical disorders the most common form of embolus is a piece of blood clot which has become detached from a thrombus. However several other forms may occur.

If any air is accidentally injected into the circulatory system it will travel through the blood vessels as an air embolus. Air embolus is a life threatening condition so we must ensure no air is ever inadvertently given intravenously. This is why we must always be careful to 'prime' all giving sets for intravenous infusions. During 'priming' air is excluded from the system by running through the intravenous fluid which is to be infused.

'Air' (actually nitrogen) emboli can form in the blood of deep-sea divers who ascend to the surface too quickly. At depth, the diver has to breathe air which is at the same increased pressure as the surrounding water. As this pressurised air contains more atoms of nitrogen than air at atmospheric pressure, more nitrogen enters the plasma in solution. If the diver ascends too quickly, this dissolved nitrogen will come out of solution in a gaseous form. These bubbles of nitrogen cause the condition called decompression sickness or 'diver's bends'.

Fat may also act as an embolus. After some fractures, fatty material from the bone marrow may leak out into the circulation leading to fat embolism. Fractures may also affect the way fat is chemically processed in the liver, contributing to the fat embolus. Fat embolism is most common after multiple fractures and fractures of the pelvis or long bones. The fat in the blood occludes numerous small capillaries in the lungs leading to dyspnoea, tachypnoea and possible hypoxaemia. There may also be neurological presentations and a petechial rash.

Septic emboli may occur as a complication of some infective conditions. Bacteria may spread around the body in this way, giving rise to metastatic areas of infection. Groups of cancer cells may break away from a tumour and lead to metastatic spread around the body.

A complication of labour may be that some amniotic fluid enters the maternal circulation; this may lead to the formation of multiple pulmonary emboli.

Aneurysm

The third complication of atheroma is aneurysm formation which describes a local enlargement of an artery. Accumulation of atheroma weakens and thins the arterial vessel wall which then undergoes expansion due to the pressure of the arterial blood. From this it can be seen that the two factors involved in aneurysm formation are vessel wall weakness and blood pressure. Sometimes, the entire arterial wall is weakened resulting in a generalised swelling of the vessel. On other occasions, only part of the wall is weakened giving rise to a one sided swelling. The presence of an aneurysm may give rise to local pressure effects, compressing surrounding tissues. Sometimes an aneurysm will burst causing haemorrhage. For example, if an aneurysm located in a cerebral artery bursts it will cause a haemorrhagic stroke.

Dissecting aneurysm

This form of aneurysm occurs in the aorta and usually affects the abdominal portion. The presence of atheroma on the aortic wall causes pressure effects on the inner layers of the artery which consequently become poorly nourished and so gradually deteriorate. As a result of this a tear may develop in the inner layer of the artery, (i.e. the tunica intima) allowing blood to penetrate into the weakened deeper layers of the wall. Blood then tracks between the middle and outer third of the arterial media, 'dissecting' the arterial wall.

Abdominal aortic aneurysm causes a pulsatile mass in the abdomen and may cause epigastric or back pain. Rupture of the aneurysm will cause pain radiating through to the back. If rupture does occur, the associated haemorrhage will be severe and usually fatal, unless there is emergency surgical intervention. Thoracic aneurysms may also occur and cause central chest pain radiating to the back. Pain may also radiate up to the neck and down the arms. This condition should be suspected in patients with chest pain who do not have the typical ECG cardiac presentation. Ultrasound scanning clearly demonstrates the presence of aortic aneurysm.

Berry aneurysms

These are so called because they look like fruit berries growing from the arterial wall. They most frequently occur on the circle of arteries at the base of the brain called the circle of Willis. Berry aneurysms are saccular in shape and are usually caused by a congenital weakness in the arterial wall rather than atheroma. Sometimes as these aneurysms grow they give rise to neurological symptoms as a result of pressure effects. However, they may burst with no previous warning signs. Berry aneurysms are the most common cause of subarachnoid haemorrhage and may present at any age. The patient suffers a very severe acute headache, often with vomiting and subsequent loss of consciousness.

Collateral circulation

Some areas of tissue are able to receive blood from two or more arterial vessels. This is referred to as collateral circulation. Some parts of the body have a good collateral blood supply while other areas do not. For example, the stomach has a good network of collateral vessels explaining why infarcts of the stomach are rare. Even if an occlusion develops in one arterial branch, gastric tissues may be perfused via an alternative vessel. However other important tissues such as the brain, heart and kidneys have a very poor collateral arrangement of vessels. This means that a thrombus or embolus in an artery supplying these organs will result in an infarction. Collateral circulation may however develop over time. If a vessel is partly obstructed by atheroma, other nearby vessels will dilate in an attempt to restore the reduced blood supply. This means that if ischaemia develops over time the body is, at least in part, able to compensate.

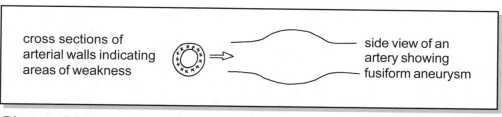

Diagram 5.7i
Atheroma has caused a circumferential weakness in the wall of an artery. (Crosses show weakened areas). Blood pressure has caused an area of expansion, resulting in the development of rounded distension. This is called a fusiform aneurysm.

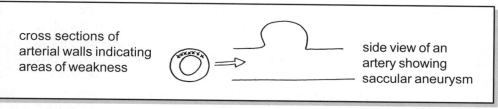

Diagram 5.7ii.
A localised weakness in the wall of an artery may occur in the area around the circle of Willis supplying blood to the brain. This congenital weakness may develop into a saccular (also called berry) aneurysm. Rupture will cause a subarachnoid haemorrhage.

Disorders caused by disrupted arterial circulation and inadequate tissue perfusion

Gangrene

Gangrene refers to tissue which has necrosed (necrotic means the tissue has died), usually as a result of being deprived of a blood supply. This may occur as a result of severe ischaemia, thrombosis or embolism. Gangrene may present as a complication of peripheral vascular disease where some toes or part of the foot dies and starts to decompose. Gangrene has a very unpleasant characteristic smell. In addition to progressive arterial disease, tissues may also be devascularised as a result of injury; this is a particular problem in high energy and crush wounds. Muscle, bone or other tissues may be involved. Some necrotising bacterial infections may also cause gangrene. Regardless of the cause, gangrenous tissue often needs to be surgically excised as infection is likely to develop in necrosed tissue.

Pressure sores

Causes

Pressure sores usually develop when tissue is compressed between an external surface and a bone. The external pressure is generated by the weight of the body. Pressure on a tissue will compress local blood vessels, depriving the area of a blood supply. As the blood supply to an area of tissue is reduced or occluded, an area of ischaemia or even infarction will be produced. Cells in the embarrassed area will become hypoxic, receive reduced supplies of nutrients and be unable to effectively remove waste products. Eventually this will result in death of the compressed tissue which will then break down to form a pressure sore or decubitus ulcer. In other words, prolonged pressure leads to tissue necrosis. Pressure also reduces the normal drainage of tissue fluid by compressing lymphatic vessels. In addition to the problems caused by pressure occluding blood and lymphatic circulation, some cells may burst as an effect of pressure on their external membranes.

Another risk factor for pressure sore development is shearing forces between the skin surface and deeper tissues. This form of force may be experienced when a patient is 'dragged' up a bed, using inappropriate moving and handling techniques. Moisture on the skin surface increases the levels of friction, and so increases the risk of shearing injury. Shearing can damage skin directly but may also damage the blood vessels which communicate between the skin and the deeper tissues. Consequent disturbance of blood supply will also lead to tissue ischaemia.

Prevention

All patients who have restricted mobility, for whatever reason, should have areas of pressure relieved regularly, before ischaemic tissue damage occurs. Normally this simply involves frequent changes of position, turning the patient from side to side and front to back. Once the pressure is relieved, blood will be able to perfuse the area as normal. Frequency of required turning will vary depending on the condition of the patient, forms of equipment being used and the hardness of the surface. In hospital beds, it has long been taught that a person should never remain in one position for more than 2 hours. However this time will vary depending on your assessment of the individual case. From the theory above on shearing and moisture, it naturally follows that part of pressure sore prevention should be good moving and handling techniques and removing excessive moisture from the skin surface. Good hydration and nutrition are also important. In the past it was thought that massage of pressure areas increased the circulation and so prevented tissue breakdown. However it is now realised that the tissue insult, caused by massage, contributes to pressure sore development.

Coronary heart and cerebrovascular disease

Thrombosis of the coronary arterial system is a leading cause of death in western countries. As the coronary arteries supply blood to the myocardium, an area of this muscle will be partly or completely deprived of a blood supply. The area which is cut off from a blood supply is called the area of infarct. This means that coronary artery thrombosis will cause myocardial infarction. Angina describes the pain caused by myocardial ischaemia. In this disorder there is ischaemia (reduced blood supply) to the myocardium. Accumulation of atheroma in the cerebral arteries may lead to transient ischaemic attacks (TIAs) and possible cerebrovascular accident (CVA or stroke).

Peripheral vascular disease (PVD)

In this disorder there is disease of the peripheral arterial system. The pathology involved is usually atherosclerosis.

Clinical features

As would be expected, this results in a reduced or absent blood supply to the legs and feet. The feet and lower areas of the leg often feel cold to the touch and there may be some cyanosis, caused by peripheral hypoxia. Poor blood supply leads to the skin appearing thin and shiny and there will be loss of hair. Poor wound healing is a feature of PVD and persistent arterial leg ulceration may be an ongoing painful problem. Severe cases may result in ischaemic gangrene.

Perhaps the best known feature of PVD is intermittent claudication, this usually presents over the age of 50 and is more common in smokers. Claudication refers to cramp like pains felt in the legs, often the calves. As a patient with reduced blood flow to the legs starts to walk, the oxygen demand of the muscles will increase. After a time the oxygen supply will be unable to support aerobic respiration and energy will be generated anaerobically. This will result in the accumulation of lactic acid, giving rise to the pain. Discomfort will initially cause the patient to limp, and then as the pain becomes more severe, to stop and rest. Rest reduces the oxygen demand of the muscle so the lactic acid will be washed away and oxidised. Removal of the lactic acid will also remove the pain, allowing the patient to carry on walking until the situation is repeated. The result is that the patient has intermittent pain and an intermittent limp. (Claudication is named after the Roman Emperor Claudius, 10 BC to 54 AD, who had a limp.)

Regular monitoring of the pulses in the groin and legs provides valuable information about the state and progress of the condition. In more serious disease the pulses will become progressively diminished. Pulses should be assessed in a warm room because cold causes vasoconstriction, which further reduces the pulse volume. In PVD the femoral, popliteal, posterior tibial and dorsalis pedis pulses should be assessed. It is useful to compare the volumes of the same pulse between the two legs. Ankle brachial pressure index should be measured.

Ankle : Brachial Pressure Index (ABPI)

Checking foot pulses is a quick test for the presence of PVD. However, as a result of reduced blood flow, the pulses may be very difficult to feel. In these cases, Doppler ultrasound can be used to generate an amplified sound which represents blood flow. Doppler ultrasound may be used to measure the ankle:brachial pressure index (ABPI). This is worked out by dividing the systolic blood pressure in the ankle by the systolic pressure in the brachial artery. If the pressures in the two ankles were different, as is common in PVD, a separate ABPI should be calculated for both legs. In a healthy person the pressures in the brachial artery, as compared to the ankle or foot should be about the same. However, if the leg is ischaemic, the pressure will be less in the leg than arm. This means the ABPI will be below 1.0. An ABPI of 0.8 or less is usually taken as an indicator of significant peripheral vascular disease. ABPI results should not be considered in isolation; other assessments of a limb such as temperature, colour and capillary refill should also be considered.

Treatment

All patients with PVD should have their risk factors for coronary heart disease assessed and when appropriate, modified according to current guidelines. This is because the factors which cause atherosclerosis in the peripheral arteries are essentially the same as those which cause arterial disease in other sites; patients should also be assessed for the presence of coronary and cerebral arterial disease. These patients should not smoke, and diabetes, hypertension, high cholesterol and obesity should all be treated. Supervised exercise will increase peripheral blood flow. Low dose aspirin and surgery may be considered.

Acute limb ischaemia

Acute presentation of peripheral ischaemia may occur as a result of thrombosis or embolism. Initial presentation of this disorder gives rise to the clinical features, sometimes described as the 6 Ps; pain, pallor, pulseless, paralysis (inability to wiggle toes), paraesthesia (abnormal sensation), perishing cold. This condition often requires emergency surgical intervention to remove the embolus or thrombus.

Raynaud's disease

Raynaud's disease affects about 5% of the population and is caused by excessive constriction of small arteries and arterioles. Most commonly it affects the fingers, but can also occur in toes. The condition is usually triggered by exposure to cold or emotional stress. Initially the fingers turn white, sometimes progressing to cyanosis, caused by the sluggish blood flow. An episode may last for several hours and is relieved by heat. Pain is often felt as an attack subsides when blood flow returns to the ischaemic fingers. Raynaud's disease is frequently seen in young women, the cause is unknown. A condition called Raynaud's phenomenon causes similar symptoms, but occurs secondary to an underlying disorder, often a connective tissue disease. Raynaud's phenomena has a progressive course and may eventually cause severe ischaemia and gangrene.

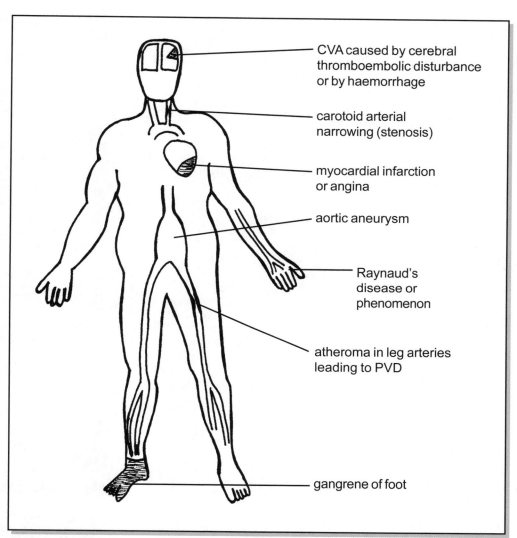

CVA caused by cerebral thromboembolic disturbance or by haemorrhage

carotoid arterial narrowing (stenosis)

myocardial infarction or angina

aortic aneurysm

Raynaud's disease or phenomenon

atheroma in leg arteries leading to PVD

gangrene of foot

Diagram 5.8
Review of disorders caused by arterial disease.

CHAPTER 6

Disorders of Veins

Introduction

A vein can usefully be defined as any vessel which carries blood towards the heart; this includes systemic veins draining blood back into the right atrium and pulmonary veins transporting blood into the left atrium. An essential area of knowledge for all health care workers is venothromboembolism (VTE). Despite being life threatening, VTE is common and in developed countries is the leading cause of preventable deaths in hospital patients. In VTE a thrombus forms in a vein and then embolises into the venous circulation. It is useful to consider this disorder under the headings of deep venous thrombosis and pulmonary embolism.

Deep venous thrombosis (DVT)

Development of a thrombus in a deep vein may occur as a result of interactions between the three factors of Virchow's triad i.e. changes in the vessel wall, changes in the rate of blood flow or changes in the tendency for blood to clot.

Physiology

Flow of blood through the venous system occurs by the operation of the normal mechanisms of venous return, the most powerful of which is contraction of skeletal muscles. Deep veins pass through skeletal muscles so are squeezed during muscle contraction. Squeezing deep veins between muscle layers causes a localized increase in venous blood pressure. Veins have an internal system of valves, directing blood flow from the periphery towards the centre of the body. As a skeletal muscle contracts, the increase in venous pressure will operate to close valves below or distal to the contraction while opening those above, or proximal. The effect of this is that blood moves from the peripheries towards the heart.

From this it can be seen that intravenous pressures generated by muscular contraction maintains efficient venous return. Lack of active skeletal muscle movement therefore reduces rates of venous return and leads to sluggish blood flow in deep veins. Such reduced rates of venous return will occur when patients are kept on bed rest, explaining why we encourage early mobilization of patients whenever possible. For example, post operative patients should be mobilized as soon as possible to reduce the risk of deep venous thrombosis.

Risk factors

In the hospital environment there is an increased risk of DVT after surgery, particularly of the abdomen, abdominal floor, knee and hip. DVT is typically a late complication of surgery with most developing about 10 days after the operation. Other risk factors include a history of chronic venous insufficiency, prolonged immobility, dehydration and obesity. As well as post operatively, it is common for DVT to complicate other disease processes such as coagulation disorders, heart failure, chronic airways disease, stroke and malignant conditions. Even otherwise apparently healthy people who are immobilised for prolonged periods of time are at risk. This is the so called 'economy class syndrome' and may occur as a result of long car or aeroplane journeys. Risk is also increased during pregnancy and the puerperium (the first 6 weeks after delivery). Use of oral contraception slightly increases risk.

Pathophysiology

The essential pathophysiology in DVT is the formation of a thrombus in a deep vein. If there is damage in a vessel wall, structural collagen can be exposed to the blood which may trigger off the process of platelet aggregation. Blood cells and fibrin then adhere to the aggregated platelets, forming a thrombus.

Reduced rates of venous blood flow occur during surgery as a result of immobility, use of muscle relaxants and in the case of orthopaedic surgery, unusual limb positioning. When muscle relaxant drugs are used there is a loss of skeletal muscle tone which further reduces venous return. Venous blood flow may remain low for some hours or days following surgery as a result of pain inhibiting mobility.

Other patients have factors which increase blood coagulability. Dehydration may be a factor so should always be prevented. Thrombophilia describes any condition where there is an increased tendency for thrombi to occur and may be caused by several inherited genetic traits.

Anatomy

Venous thrombosis is most common in calf veins but they may form or extend into veins higher up in the legs. DVTs can therefore be found in the popliteal veins behind the knee. Other possible sites include the femoral veins, iliac veins or even the inferior vena cava.

Clinical features

Some cases of DVT are described as being 'silent', this means the patient does not complain of any symptoms. In symptomatic patients the calf may be tender and warm on palpation. Oedema may be present with one leg swollen relative to the other. In some cases the first presentation of DVT may be a pulmonary embolism (PE).

Prevention of DVT

Several relatively simple management strategies can significantly reduce the risk of DVT. Early ambulation is important in all patients who have been immobilised. Patients who can not get out of bed should be encouraged to move their legs around in bed; it is particularly useful to flex the ankles regularly as this initiates compression of the deep veins in the calf muscles. Moving the ankles is such an efficient way of improving venous return that the mechanism is referred to as the 'calf pump'. If a patient is unable to do this actively themselves we can do it passively for them on a regular basis.

Compression bandages such as thromboembolic deterrent (TED) stockings reduce the pooling of blood in the legs. Correctly designed and fitted antiembolic stockings should give a graduated compression, being highest at the bottom and reducing as they fit up the leg. In other words the pressure will be greatest at the ankle and lowest at the thigh. Deep breathing exercises also promote venous return so should be encouraged. Sometimes drugs may be given as DVT prophylaxis. These may be aspirin or one of the heparin group of preparations. As these drugs are anticoagulant they reduce the tendency of the blood to clot so reduce the probability of thrombus formation.

Treatment principles

Rapid recognition and treatment of DVT can prevent extension of the thrombus, reduce the probability of pulmonary embolism and be life-saving. Normally low molecular weight heparin is given for at least 5 days with anticoagulation therapy being continued with oral warfarin. Low molecular weight heparin, given subcustaneously is just as effective as intravenous unfractionated heparin and is much easier to give. Warfarin therapy should be continued for at least 6 weeks and probably for 6 months in most patients. Some patients at high risk of recurrence may be anticoagulated for life. Patients should probably be kept on bed rest until anticoagulation is established as movement may cause emboli to break away from the thrombus. Analgesia should be given if pain is a significant feature.

Pulmonary embolism

Pathophysiology

If part of a DVT breaks away it will be carried along in the normal blood flow. This will carry an embolus up into the inferior vena cava and into the right atrium; it will then pass through the tricuspid valve into the right ventricle, through the pulmonary valve and into the pulmonary artery. What happens next depends on the size of the embolus. As emboli travel from a peripheral to a central vein, the lumen size of the vessels increases, so emboli may pass freely. Next, emboli are able to pass through the large chambers of the heart and on into the pulmonary vessels. After the heart, vessels of the pulmonary arterial system become progressively narrower, until ultimately they become pulmonary capillaries. This means an embolus will carry on in the pulmonary arterial circulation until it lodges in a pulmonary artery.

A very big embolus may completely occlude the main pulmonary artery; this is described as massive pulmonary embolism and will cause death from shock within minutes. Smaller emboli are able to fit through progressively finer pulmonary arteries before jamming in an arterial lumen. An embolus will occlude the lumen of the vessel preventing blood passing through the now blocked vessel; this will therefore result in a pulmonary infarct.

Emboli are most likely to detach from a thrombus which does not completely occlude the vein it formed in. When a thrombus is incomplete there will still be blood flowing past the partial occlusion before returning to the central veins and heart. Any bits which break away from a thrombus will be carried away in the blood flow as emboli. This means it is quite possible for a PE to arise from a DVT causing a partial obstruction which may present with no or only minor clinical features.

Clinical features

Small pulmonary emboli will impact in a terminal branch of the pulmonary arterial tree. These are lysed (i.e. broken down) fairly quickly so may give rise to minor or no symptoms. However, it is important to realise that small emboli may precede a large embolus if appropriate treatment is not started.

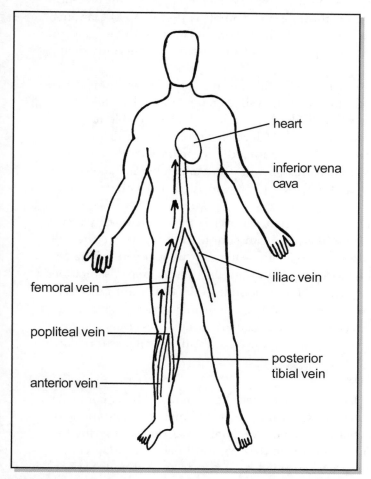

Diagram 6.1
The path of an embolus from the lower leg to the heart.

Larger emboli may give rise to a wide possible array of features. Rapid breathing (tachypnoea) is a common presentation and there may be feelings of dyspnoea (difficulty in breathing). Chest pain may present if there is involvement of the pleural membranes. Chest wall, shoulder and back pain should also arouse suspicion. Tachycardia, fever and sweating may present. If the chest is oscultated, crepitations (a sound of crackling or rattling) may be heard and the heart sounds may be altered. Haemoptysis (coughing up of blood) is a less common feature and may be delayed. On examination it may be possible to detect features of the original DVT.

Possible investigations include chest X-ray and arterial blood gases. X-rays are particularly useful in excluding other pathology such as pneumonia or pneumothorax. Blood gases typically show a reduced PaO_2 as might be expected from the reduced blood flow through the lungs. However, the tachypnoea will keep the $PaCO_2$ normal or below normal. The D-dimer test looks for the presence of degradation products from thrombi and emboli is useful. V/Q scanning uses radioactive isotopes to study V which is the ventilation of the lungs with air, and Q which describes the perfusion of blood through the pulmonary arteries.

Large pulmonary emboli will significantly obstruct blood flow through the lungs. This will have the effect of reducing venous return to the left side of the heart. As venous return is reduced, the heart will no longer be able to pump out normal volumes of blood, resulting in reduced left ventricular cardiac output. This will reduce the volumes of blood entering the coronary arteries to perfuse the myocardium. This reduced perfusion will cause anaerobic metabolism to occur, generating lactic acid and the severe chest pain associated with myocardial ischaemia.

Reduced cardiac output from the left ventricle will also reduce systemic blood pressure. This may cause the patient to faint or collapse. Heart rate will increase in an attempt to compensate giving rise to tachycardia. Severe respiratory distress and cyanosis will be accompanied by a reduction in oxygen saturation readings. As the pulmonary circulation is occluded, blood will not be able to drain freely from the systemic veins into the right atrium; this will give rise to the distended neck veins seen in raised jugular venous pressure. If a large pulmonary embolism affects the main pulmonary artery death will occur rapidly.

Management principles

Small and medium sized PEs should be managed the same as DVTs. For larger PEs, initial management measures will include giving high concentrations of oxygen, laying the patient flat to maximise cerebral blood flow and giving low molecular weight heparin. Thrombolytic therapy, to disolve the blood clot, is helpful in massive PE that is accompanied by shock. In unconscious patients external cardiac massage may break up large emboli, allowing the patients to be successfully resuscitated.

Diagram 6.2

A DVT has formed in association with a venous valve in a deep vein. The presence of the thrombus in the deep vein may cause venous backlog leading to damage of other venous valves. This will increase the risk of chronic venous insufficiency in the future. In the short term, part of the thrombus may detach and become an embolus. From the deep vein the embolus travels through the venous circulation to the heart and is then pumped into the pulmonary arteries where it forms a pulmonary embolism.

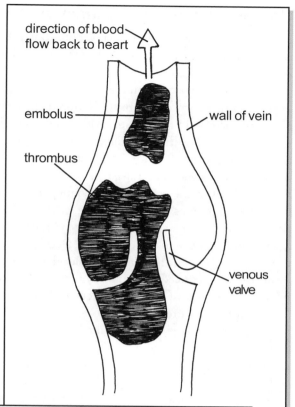

Diagram 6.3

From the heart an embolus will pass into the pulmonary arterial tree and become lodged in a branch of pulmonary artery. Arrows indicate the path emboli travel; up the inferior vena cava, into the right atrium, through the tricuspid valve, into the right ventricle, through the pulmonary valve, into the pulmonary artery and in this case the embolus has lodged in the lower right lobar artery.

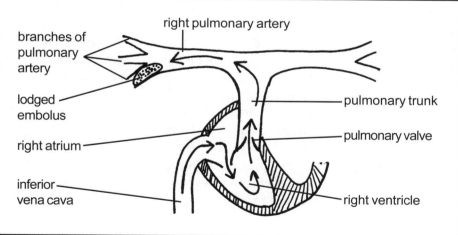

Chronic venous insufficiency and hypertension

Any condition obstructing normal venous drainage will lead to a backlog of blood which will increase the pressure within the veins. This increased pressure will damage the venous valves which do not have good powers of recovery. As a result an episode of acute venous hypertension may result in a permanent reduction in the efficiency of the venous return mechanisms. Reduced efficiency of venous return will lead to a chronic increase in the pressure within the effected peripheral veins. These factors explain why DVT is the most important pathogenic mechanism in the causation of chronic venous insufficiency. This insufficiency can contribute to the development of varicose veins and venous leg ulcers.

As a result of the venous insufficiency there is a chronic backlog of blood in the peripheral veins. As the volume of blood in these veins increases so does the pressure. Increased hydrostatic pressure in the veins in turn increases hydrostatic pressure in the capillaries. Backlog of blood in the capillaries reduces the rate of circulation as arterial blood is not able to enter efficiently. As a result there is reduced delivery of nutrients and oxygen to the tissues as well as inhibited removal of waste products such as carbon dioxide and nitrates.

Increased pressure in the venous ends of capillaries also reduces the rate of reabsorption of tissue fluid; this increases the volume of tissue fluid resulting in oedema. Oedema in tissues increases the volume of fluid through which nutrients must diffuse in order to pass from capillary blood into the tissue cells. Also oedematous swelling increases the diffusional distance from blood to tissue cells. This reduces the efficiency of transporting oxygen and nutrients to cells and removing carbon dioxide and other metabolic waste products. Both of these effects will reduce the viability of tissue cells in the presence of oedema.

Increased pressure in a capillary will also lead to dilation of the vessel. This will stretch the capillary walls and so widen the gaps (or pores) between individual cells which compose the endothelial wall. Increased capillary pore size allows larger molecules such as proteins to migrate from blood into the tissue spaces. One of the plasma proteins is fibrinogen which can pass through the enlarged pores. Once in the tissues fibrinogen is converted into the clotting protein fibrin. Fibrin is composed of long sticky strands which may form a cuff around a dilated capillary. It may be that the presence of such a 'fibrin cuff' further reduces the interchange of oxygen, nutrients and waste products between capillary blood and tissue fluids and so further reduces tissue viability.

Varicose veins

This common condition results in tortuous dilated veins which engorge with venous blood. Varicose veins are usually thought of as occurring in the legs but they may also present in the rectum and oesophagus. If the problem occurs in the rectum this is usually referred to as piles or haemorrhoids, in the oesophagus they are called oesophageal varices.

Physiology

In the legs there are deep veins and superficial veins. Deep veins run in the muscle bundles of the leg, under muscle fascia. Superficial veins are found under skin and subcutaneous tissue, above the muscle fascia. When leg muscles contract this has the effect of rapidly increasing the pressure of blood in the deep veins, resulting in rapid return of blood to the centre of the body. As blood has now been returned to the large central veins, the pressure in the deep veins drops, allowing more blood to flow from the superficial veins into the deep system, prior to the next muscular contraction. Blood is able to pass from the superficial to the deep venous system via short veins called communicating veins. These communicating veins are sometimes referred to as perforating veins because they perforate the muscle fascia.

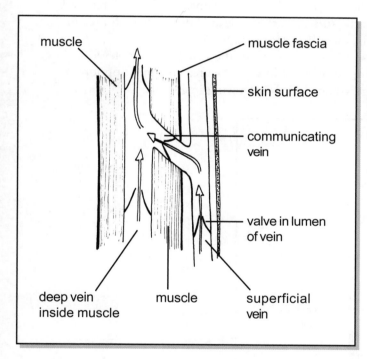

Diagram 6.4
In normal physiology one-way blood flow is ensured by the action of valves located within the lumen of the veins. (Arrows indicate normal direction of blood flow.)

Causes of varicose veins

Varicose veins have a hereditary factor which may cause weakness in the vein walls or valves. Weak valves may easily become incompetent; this means they lose their ability to prevent backflow of blood. Another factor in the aetiology is increased pressure in the abdomen which may occur as a result of multiple pregnancies, obesity or abdominal tumours. If the pressure in the abdomen is increased this will compress the inferior vena cava, reducing the rate of venous drainage from the legs. This will increase intravenous pressure in the legs leading to pressure on vein walls and valves.

Any complete or partial occlusions in the deep veins will also lead to an increase in peripheral venous pressure; this may be caused by a DVT or thrombophlebitis. If there is obstruction to deep venous drainage, muscle contraction will still dramatically increase deep intravenous pressure. However as the normal anatomical route back to the inferior vena cava is obstructed, blood will be forced from the deep to superficial venous systems. This is a reverse of the normal physiological direction and will rapidly damage the valves in the communicator veins.

Complications of varicose veins

Haemorrhage is well known complication of varicose veins. Dilated veins have stretched thin walls which are not as resistant to trauma as their healthy counterparts. In addition, if the wall of the vein is damaged there is a relatively large volume of blood near the surface of the body at abnormally high pressure. These factors explain why bleeding from varicose veins can be profuse. Haemorrhage from varicose veins is arrested in the usual way, by elevation of the bleeding limb and the application of direct pressure. Treatment options for varicose veins include surgery and directly sclerosing injections.

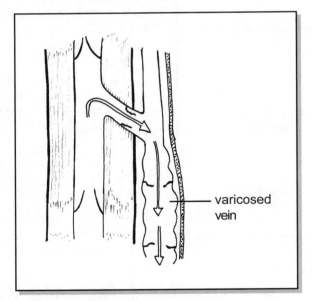

varicosed
vein

Diagram 6.5
If the valves in the communicator veins fail,
venous reflux can increase the pressure on
valves in the superficial veins, this will lead to
further valve failures and increased pressure in
the superficial veins. Increased pressure will
cause a dilated tortuous superficial vein. (Arrows
indicate direction of abnormal blood reflux.)

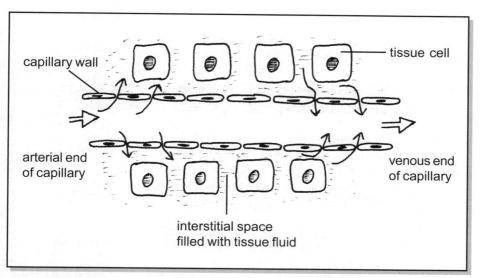

Diagram 6.6

In normal physiology, tissue fluid is formed at the arterial end of a capillary and reabsorbed at the venous end. (White arrows represent direction of blood flow and dark arrows tissue fluid.)

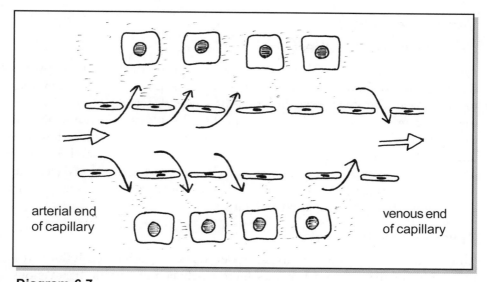

Diagram 6.7

Venous hypertension increases the pressure at the venous end of the capillary therefore reducing tissue fluid reabsorption. In this diagram more tissue fluid is being formed than absorbed. As a result fluids accumulate in the tissues causing oedema, this in turn increases the diffusional distance between blood and cells reducing the viability of tissue cells. (This capillary is also somewhat distended, again due to increased pressure of blood caused by the venous backlog.)

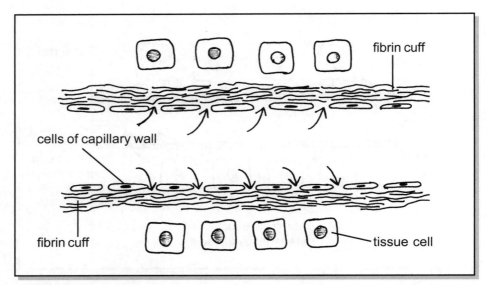

Diagram 6.8
The fibrin cuff hypothesis. Soluble fibrinogen leaks out of the enlarged pores in the capillary wall and is converted into long sticky strands of fibrin which form a cuff around the capillary. Arrows indicate direction of fibrinogen escape.

Venous leg ulcers

Classification of leg ulcers

Leg ulcers are usually defined as wounds which occur on the leg or foot, involve skin loss and take more than 6 weeks to heal; they are usually classified according to their cause. Chronic venous hypertension caused by venous insufficiency is the most common cause, so these are termed venous ulcers. Ulcers may also be caused by the chronic ischaemia seen in peripheral vascular disease, these are termed arterial ulcers. Leg ulcers are also seen as a long term complication of diabetes mellitus; such lesions are therefore classified as diabetic ulcers. Diabetic ulcers may be primarily ischaemic or neuropathic. Rheumatic ulcers may occur as a complication of rheumatoid vasculitis.

Aetiology of venous ulcers

This often chronic condition affects about 1.5 to 3 people per 1000 of the population of the UK and becomes increasingly common with age. Venous ulcers occur secondary to venous disease. Poor or obstructed venous drainage leads to a chronic venous hypertension in an affected leg. This will reduce the viability of leg tissues by reducing the efficiency of the circulation of blood. Venous hypertension also causes oedema and fibrin cuff formation. Several factors can lead to chronic venous insufficiency; these include DVT, venous congenital disorders, degenerative changes with age, pregnancy, ankle joint fixation and congestive cardiac failure.

Clinical features

Venous hypertension causes dilation of capillaries which allows red blood cells to escape into the tissues through dilated capillary walls. Over time this leads to a characteristic brown staining caused by the presence of haemosiderin, a breakdown product of haemoglobin. Venous ulcers are typically described as 'wet' wounds as tissue fluid oozes onto the wound bed. The ulcers are usually shallow with diffuse edges and oedema is often present in the whole limb. Venous ulcers are usually painful. It is important to decide if a given ulcer is venous or arterial. If an ulcer is purely venous then the arterial blood supply will be normal. Quality of the arterial supply should be assessed by determination of the ankle brachial pressure index (ABPI). This assessment is vital as arterial ulcers must not receive compression therapy. In a purely venous ulcer the ABPI will be greater than 0.8. In practice some patients have venous and arterial insufficiency in a leg; this can give rise to a mixture of venous and arterial ulcer features. Such ulcers are described as being of mixed aetiology.

Treatments

It is known that compression using four layer bandaging or other techniques improves healing rates of venous ulcers. Leg compression progressively compresses leg veins and so improves venous return. If the venous return is improved the adverse effects of chronic venous hypertension are relieved. In addition to aiding healing, compression also significantly reduces the risk of recurrence of venous ulcers. Administration of oral flavanoids further increases the proportion of ulcers healed. It may be that flavanoids are helpful because of their antioxidant effect on harmful free radicals inside cells. Other helpful treatments include the use of cultured skin replacement and oral pentoxifylline.

Oesophageal varices

Oesophageal varices are varicose veins which occur in the wall of the oesophagus. The most common cause of this disorder is fibrosis of the liver seen in hepatic cirrhosis. Abnormal fibrous tissue present in the liver obstructs the entry of venous blood from the hepatic portal vein. This portal vein is formed by a union of the veins which drain the lower third of the oesophagus, spleen, pancreas, gall bladder and most of the gastrointestinal tract.

As blood entry into the liver is partly obstructed in cirrhosis, a backlog of blood in the portal venous system develops which gives rise to a portal venous hypertension. This increased blood pressure in the portal vein eventually leads to varicosity in the veins of the lower oesophagus. Varicose veins in the oesophagus are easily traumatised and may rupture leading to potentially life threatening haemorrhage. Bleeding takes place into the lumen of the oesophagus and blood usually collects in the stomach. Patients with bleeding oesophageal varices may present with the clinical features of shock. Haematemesis may result in the vomiting of large volumes of blood which may often appear fresh and frank. Management principles include fluid resuscitation, endoscopic variceal band ligation or baloon tamponade.

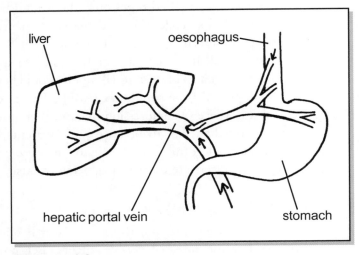

Diagram 6.9
Obstruction of blood flow from the hepatic portal vein into the liver causes portal hypertension. Normal portal venous pressure is about 5 to 8 mmHg. In portal hypertension this may rise above 12 mmHg. Chronic pressure rise in the veins of the oesophagus leads to varicosity. Rupture of oesophageal varices may lead to torrential blood loss.

Haemorrhoids

Haemorrhoids (also called piles) are varicose veins which occur in the rectum. They may be internal, occurring in the rectum, or external haemorrhoids, which may protrude from the rectum.

Aetiology

Haemorrhoids occur as a result of phenomena which increase rectal intravenous pressure leading to venous distension. Causes of increased venous pressure in this area include prolonged sitting, pregnancy and obesity. Another important factor is straining at defecation. Straining to pass a stool will lead to an increased pressure in the veins in the rectum. Risk of varicosity formation increases with duration and frequency of straining. Most commonly, straining is caused by constipation which should be prevented by exercise and diet with plenty of fibre and fluids.

Clinical features

Clinically there may be itching and feelings of discomfort, although often there will be no pain associated with the condition. Bleeding from haemorrhoids is the most common cause of rectal haemorrhage producing fresh blood which may be seen on the stools or toilet paper. External haemorrhoids will be obvious on examination of the anus. Internal haemorrhoids can be seen using proctoscopy.

If haemorrhoids prolapse they will need to be reduced. Straining to pass stools may also result in rectal prolapse. Prolapses may be reduced using a water soluble lubricant and direct pressure to push the rectum or haemorrhoids back in.

Treatments

Treatment involves avoidance of factors which may increase intravenous pressure in rectal veins. Local anaesthetic and anti-inflammatory preparations may help to reduce symptoms and swelling. Surgical options include freezing, ligation and haemorrhoidectomy.

CHAPTER 7

Shock

Introduction

Shock is a much misused term that is frequently applied to mean a fright or used to describe the psychological effects of trauma. This is not the correct clinical use of the term and health care professionals should use the word shock in a strict sense. Shock describes a state of circulatory failure when the circulation of blood around the body is reduced to such an extent that body tissues are embarrassed or damaged as a result. Tissue embarrassment is caused by factors which may compromise normal function, the principle ones being reduced delivery of oxygen and nutrients and the accumulation of waste products of metabolism. A possible definition of shock is 'a state with significant reduction in systemic tissue perfusion, resulting in decreased delivery of oxygen and reduced removal of metabolic waste products, leading to tissue injury'.

In shock the blood supply and so the oxygen delivery to the tissues of the body are insufficient to meet the metabolic demands of the tissues. In all forms of shock low blood pressure will develop in time. However, this is a sinister development in the progression of shock and the organs and tissues of the body may be seriously hypoperfused before blood pressure starts to fall. This means that the development of shock should be recognised at an early stage, preferably before blood pressure starts to fall. Shock is not a specific disease but can complicate many conditions caused by trauma or disease.

Factors affecting blood pressure

Blood pressure is needed to push blood through the arterial system and to perfuse the capillaries in all body tissues. Blood pressure is a combination of the pressure generated by contraction of the ventricle and the resistance to this blood flow as it passes through the arterial system. The relationship is summed up in the following equation:

Blood pressure	=	Cardiac output	x	Peripheral resistance

All forms of shock can be explained using this one equation. This means that if there is a reduction in cardiac output or peripheral resistance, blood pressure will drop and shock may ensue. Peripheral resistance is often described as systemic vascular resistance (SVR). It is also useful to note that cardiac output is determined by the volume of blood pumped out per ventricular contraction (i.e. stroke volume) and heart rate. Heart rate is the number of cardiac contractions per minute. This relationship is defined as follows:

Cardiac output	=	Heart rate	x	Stroke volume

A normal cardiac output at rest is about 5.6 litres per minute in a fit young man, but the average for all adults, including women and the elderly is about 5 litres per minute. Women generally have a cardiac output about 10% lower than men because cardiac output is correlated with body surface area.

Venous return

Venous return describes the volume of blood returning to the heart via the venous system. While venous return is not a term in the blood pressure equation, it is essential to maintain cardiac output. If we decide we would like to spend some money, we cannot do so if there is no money in our purse, in the same way the heart cannot pump out blood that has not been returned to it by the veins.

Cardiac output is therefore dependent on, and indeed largely determined by, venous return. This aspect of physiology is described by Starling's law of the heart. Starling (1866-1927) identified that increased volumes of venous return cause increased stretching of the myocardium, as the ventricles fill with blood. This increased stretching in turn causes a stronger contraction of the myocardium to eject the increased blood volume. In the same way, if venous return is reduced, the force of myocardial contraction will be reduced and stroke volume will fall.

Physiological response when blood pressure falls

Neurological response

Blood pressure in the systemic arterial system is monitored by specialised nerve endings located in the walls of the aorta and carotid arteries. These pressure receptors are referred to as baroreceptors. At the start of the internal carotid artery is a widened area referred to as the carotid sinus which is where most baroreceptors are located.

Increased blood pressure in the carotid sinus will stretch the arterial walls in the area of the baroreceptors. This will stretch the baroreceptors causing them to produce nerve impulses, the greater the degree of stretching the more nerve impulses are produced. Baroreceptors respond very rapidly to a change in blood pressure, in fact their firing rate changes during systole and decreases with diastole.

Sensory nerves travel from the baroreceptors to the medulla oblongata of the brain stem. Here they influence the activity of the vasomotor and cardiac centres. These centres control the activity of the circulatory system by controlling the tone of arteries and veins and the level of cardiac output. Impulses from the baroreceptors inhibit the sympathetic outflow from these centres. Sympathetic outflow causes an increase in blood pressure by generating vasoconstriction and increasing cardiac output.

When blood pressure falls there is a reduced firing rate from the baroreceptors which in turn reduces the number of nerve impulses travelling to the medulla oblongata. Reduced baroreceptor impulses arriving in the medulla oblongata reduces their inhibitory effect on the sympathetic outflow from the vasomotor and cardiac centres. This results in increased sympathetic outflow from the medulla oblongata which will cause vasoconstriction and attempt to increase cardiac output. These physiological changes will work to compensate for the drop in blood pressure.

When blood pressure rises, the converse is true. Increased baroreceptor firing inhibits the sympathetic outflow from the medulla oblongata and so leads to vasodilatation and a reduced cardiac output, both of which will lower blood pressure.

Endocrine system response

A fall in blood pressure will cause more adrenaline and noradrenaline (i.e. the catecholamines) to be secreted by the adrenal medulla. These will cause vasoconstriction and so increase peripheral resistance directly. The result of this vasoconstriction is that the diastolic blood pressure can be maintained for a period of time. This explains why the first blood pressure reading to fall as shock progresses is the systolic. The combination of a lowered systolic and maintained diastolic pressure results in a lowered pulse pressure. The pulse pressure describes the difference between the systolic and diastolic blood pressures.

Another endocrine response is that increased sympathetic outflow from the medulla oblongata stimulates the kidneys to secrete more renin which will stimulate the renin-angiotensin-aldosterone system. Renin release is also directly stimulated by any reduction in the pressure of blood perfusing the kidneys. Angiotensin II has a powerful constricting effect on the arterioles, so increases blood pressure. It also promotes the release of aldosterone which leads to the conservation of salt and water by the kidneys, both of which preserve or increase plasma volume. Falling blood pressure also causes the release of antidiuretic hormone, (ADH also called vasopressin). This conserves water in the plasma and is also a vasoconstrictor. Increased amounts of ADH in the blood explain why urine volumes will decrease in hypovolaemia.

Another mechanism which also plays a role in compensating for a drop in blood pressure is the increased absorption of fluids from the gastrointestinal tract and interstitial fluid. This water movement has the effect of increasing intravascular volume. Intravascular relates to the volume of blood in all of the blood vessels.

Clinical features of shock

The classical features of shock are particularly seen in hypovolaemia, cardiogenic and obstructive shock. As we have seen, when blood pressure starts to fall this is detected by the baroreceptors which then initiate powerful sympathetic reflexes

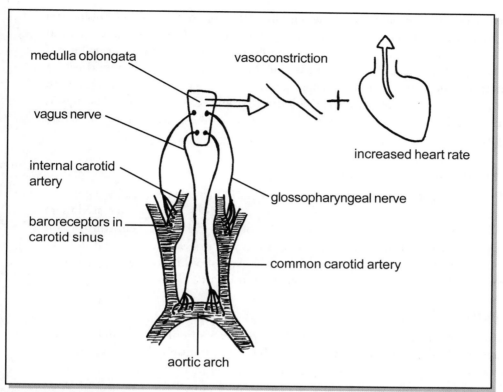

Diagram 7.1
The common carotid arteries derive from the arch of the aorta. In the upper part of the neck these divide into the internal and external carotid arteries. The internal carotids supply blood into the cranial cavity to perfuse the brain. Sensory fibres of the vagus nerve carry impulses from baroreceptors in the arch of the aorta into the medulla oblongata. Sensory fibres of the glossopharyngeal nerve carry impulses from the carotid sinus into the medulla oblongata.

intended to increase blood pressure. This increased sympathetic activity will stimulate heart rate and cause widespread arterial and venous constriction. These changes, combined with the release of catecholamines, explain most of the clinical features seen in classical shock.

Arterial vasoconstriction

Sympathetic stimulation of the arterial system causes constriction, particularly at the level of the arterioles. Vasoconstriction reduces the overall lumen of the arterial system so has the effect of increasing peripheral vascular resistance. This is a useful compensatory response as an increase in peripheral resistance will increase blood pressure, as blood pressure is equal to cardiac output multiplied by peripheral resistance. Arterial constriction will reduce the volumes of blood perfusing the peripheries so reducing blood flow to the hands and lower parts of the legs generating the clinical features of cold peripheries. Arterial vasoconstriction near the surface of the body will reduce the volumes of red blood perfusing capillary beds near the skin surface. This will give rise to a characteristic pale appearance called pallor. This is easy to see in people with white skin but harder in darker coloured people. Observation of the lips is particularly helpful in all races as these will demonstrate pallor if they are hypoperfused.

Venous vasoconstriction

Widespread constriction of the venous system will increase venous blood pressure and help to maintain essential venous return. If venous return is increased there will be a proportionate increase in cardiac output. Clinically, venoconstriction can make it very difficult to site a venous cannula in a shocked patient. Ideally, any patient who is at risk of becoming shocked should have two intravenous lines sited before significant venoconstriction occurs.

Tachycardia

Heart rate will increase as a result of sympathetic stimulation giving rise to a tachycardia. As cardiac output is equal to heart rate multiplied by stroke volume, a low stroke volume may be compensated for by an increase in rate. This means that a near normal cardiac output may be maintained for a period of time. Tachycardia will present before blood pressure starts to fall.

Clammy

As well as being pale, a drop in blood pressure causes the person to be clammy. This is caused by a cold sweat, that is a sweat which occurs in the absence of an increase in body temperature. This happens because sweat is produced in response to sympathetic stimulation. In this sense the sweating is a side effect of the sympathetic compensatory mechanisms.

Thirst

Shocked patients are thirsty; in hypovolaemia thirst may be extreme. Thirst is stimulated in dehydration because a reduction in the volume of water in the blood increases its concentration. This has the effect of increasing osmolarity which in turn leads to intracellular dehydration of neurones in the thirst centre of the hypothalamus. If the water content of these thirst centre neurones falls, thirst is greatly stimulated. Thirst will be present in other forms of shock as the thirst centre is also stimulated by a reduction in blood volume or drop in blood pressure. In addition the increased sympathetic activity will lead to a dry mouth. This is because saliva is physiologically produced as a result of parasympathetic stimulation.

Respiratory effects

The presence of anaerobic metabolism in ischaemic tissues leads to an accumulation of carbon dioxide and lactic acid, both of which stimulate respiratory effort. In addition the presence of hypoxia will also stimulate respiratory rates. Despite a rapid ventilatory rate the respirations are often shallow. This shows the importance of accurately monitoring respiratory rate in any ill or potentially deteriorating patient.

Coronary and cerebral circulation

It is vital that perfusion of the myocardium and brain continue as failure of either one will rapidly lead to death. The sympathetic response to a drop in blood pressure described above does not cause significant vasoconstriction in the coronary and cerebral blood vessels. This means that blood flow is shunted away from areas which can survive for a time with a restricted supply, but maintained in vital areas. Significant hypoperfusion of the brain and myocardium does not occur until systolic blood pressure drops significantly, probably to about 70 mmHg. When it does occur, reduced perfusion of the brain can lead to clinical features such as anxiety, drowsiness, confusion, irritability and reduced levels of consciousness.

Effects on other body tissues

There is however a price to pay for this maintenance of cerebral and myocardial circulation. As shock develops there will be vasoconstriction of the vessels supplying the peripheries, skeletal muscles, kidneys and gastrointestinal tract. As the volumes of blood perfusing a tissue are reduced there is a corresponding reduction in oxygen delivery. This will lead to widespread hypoxic damage to cells and tissues partly explaining why shock can be associated with multi-organ failure.

Ischaemia of the bowel and other tissues causes a change from aerobic to anaerobic metabolism, with consequent production of lactic acid. This can lead to the development of a systemic acidosis. Bowel ischaemia also predisposes the patient to endotoxic complications and peptic ulceration. The liver is also at risk if the volumes of perfusing blood are reduced. As in other tissues, patchy areas of necrosis develop. In the liver necrosis develops first near the centre of the liver lobules, as these are furthest away from the arterial blood supply. The longer and more severe the shock, the more cells will die, enlarging the areas of necrosis.

Renal effects

Reduced blood supply to the kidneys, and the effects of ADH, explains why urine volumes will drop and the patient will develop oliguria and eventually anuria. Renal hypoperfusion will reduce rates of ultrafiltration from the glomerular capillaries into the nephrons as this process is dependent on an adequate blood perfusion pressure. If glomerular filtration pressures are significantly reduced there will be a corresponding reduction in glomerular filtration rate. This will lead to acute renal failure and then to the development of acute tubular necrosis. Increased levels of ADH work by increasing tubular reabsorption.

Oliguria is often diagnosed when urine volumes fall below 30 mls per hour in an adult. More specifically, a urine output of less than 0.5 mls per hour per Kg of body weight indicates reduced perfusion of the kidneys. In children the minimum required urine output is 1 ml per hour per Kg.

Stages of shock

It is useful to discuss the development and classification of shock under the headings of compensated, progressive or irreversible.

Compensated shock

Compensated shock is sometimes described as nonprogressive. In this situation the sympathetic and endocrine responses discussed above are able to maintain blood pressure at reasonable levels by the use of compensatory mechanisms. While these compensations prevent the development of hypotension, the vasoconstriction will significantly reduce the blood supply to most body tissues and organs meaning that some hypoxic damage may already be starting to develop. However, if shock, and the pathology causing the disorder, can be successfully identified and corrected at the compensated stage the shock will not progress. Ideally, all cases of shock should be recognised and corrected at the compensated stage to prevent the onset of the progressive phase.

Progressive shock

Progressive shock is also referred to as decompensated shock and can develop, regardless of the initial cause of the shock. During this stage, despite the presence of the compensatory mechanisms, the condition deteriorates and the blood pressure will progressively fall. There will be developing hypoxic damage to all of the body cells and tissues. Once the circulation of blood has decreased to a particular point, the integrity of the circulatory system is compromised. For example, if the myocardium is hypoperfused, cardiac output will drop, resulting in more severe myocardial hypoperfusion. This means that once shock reaches a certain level of severity, a vicious downward spiral is set up which, without active treatment, will result in death.

Another factor which contributes to progressive shock is reduced blood circulation to the gut causing many gram-negative bacteria in the gastrointestinal lumen to die and break up. Some components of the bacterial cell walls are therefore released into the gut lumen. These bacterial components act as endotoxins, which are toxic to the heart muscle. If endotoxins are absorbed into the blood they will further depress the activity of the myocardium.

Eventually there will be hypoperfusion of the vasomotor centre in the medulla; this will mean it can no longer initiate the required sympathetic responses, which compensated in the early stages of shock. If there is no longer sympathetically induced vasoconstriction and cardiac stimulation the blood pressure can drop rapidly. When a person is in progressive shock it is essential to treat the condition before the shock becomes irreversible. The progressive phase is the last window of opportunity for curative treatment.

Irreversible shock

A person in irreversible shock is still alive, but will shortly go on to die from shock. After shock reaches a particular stage it will cause widespread damage to numerous essential body tissues which can not be reversed. There will be permanent damage to the circulatory system and other body tissues such as the brain. Active treatment may increase cardiac output and blood pressure for a period of time, but the person will still go on to die from shock in the following minutes or hours. It is therefore vital to treat shock before this stage is reached.

The Golden Hour

The rationale behind the concept of 'The Golden Hour' is that shock is the principle cause of mortality after trauma. Poor tissue perfusion leads on to irreversible chemical changes and tissue damage in the body – but these take one hour to develop. Patients who have experienced significant shock for more than one hour are likely to die. This means they have crossed the line between progressive and irreversible shock. In cases of trauma, most patients could be saved if we could stop the bleeding, treat injuries and restore blood pressure within one hour. If significant shock is prolonged for more than one hour death becomes much more likely, even if extensive treatment is subsequently given. This critical period is the Golden Hour, an hour of 'golden' opportunity. Clearly this means patients in shock must receive prompt treatment. The Golden Hour of course begins at the time of trauma, not from the time when the patient enters our care.

Clinical forms of shock

Shock has traditionally been categorised according to the cause. All causes can be explained in terms of the blood pressure equation. That is the cause of a particular case of shock can be reduced cardiac output, reduced cardiac output caused by reduced venous return or decreased peripheral resistance.

Cardiogenic shock

Cardiac pertains to the heart and genic to beginning. In cardiogenic shock blood pressure is reduced as a result of decreased cardiac output. Cardiogenic shock can be described as 'pump failure shock'. Causes include reduction in the heart rate, or a reduction in the amount of blood ejected per cardiac cycle, i.e. reduced stroke volume. Specific causes of cardiogenic shock include myocardial infarction, severe valve dysfunction, cardiomyopathy and abnormal heart rhythms.

Myocardial infarction

Cardiogenic shock is a possible complication after myocardial infarction. An infarcted area of heart muscle will die as it is deprived of the normal blood supply. In other words there will be an area of dead, necrotic muscle in the myocardium which will not be contractile. As a result, the overall pumping efficiency of the myocardium will be reduced. If the compromise of myocardial contraction is such that cardiac output cannot be maintained, then blood pressure will drop. This would be expected from the blood pressure equation as blood pressure is dependent on cardiac output. If blood pressure drops to the extent that there is reduced tissue perfusion and oxygenation then the person will be shocked.

Early thrombolysis (clot busting) or other reperfusion therapies are the key to preventing cardiogenic shock after infarction. If a blood clot occluding a coronary artery can be removed, the infarcted area of myocardium can be reperfused before necrosis has developed. This means the infarcted area of myocardium will not die and so will remain actively contractile. If the myocardium remains contractile it is able to function as a pump and to generate cardiac output.

Severe heart valve dysfunction

The four valves in the heart are essential to ensure one way flow of blood through the heart. For example when the left ventricle contracts the bicuspid atrioventricular valve is closed and the aortic valve is opened. If there is failure of the bicuspid (also called mitral) valve, blood will be pumped from the left ventricle, back into the left atrium. This will reduce the volume of blood ejected into the aorta, and so lower cardiac output. Valve replacement surgery can sometimes be carried out to treat this condition.

Cardiomyopathy

'Myo' pertains to muscle and 'path' means disease of. Cardiomyopathy is therefore disease affecting the heart muscle fibres. Cardiomyopathy is a possible cause of sudden cardiac death. The most common cause of infective cardiomyopathy is viral infection, although other infectious agents can be aetiological. Hypertrophic cardiomyopathy has a genetic cause. Alcohol abuse may also damage the heart muscle. If no particular aetiological factor is identified, the condition is then referred to as primary or idiopathic.

Dysrhythmias

If normal sinus rhythm is altered, the heart will work less efficiently. If the reduction in cardiac efficiency is sufficient to reduce cardiac output then cardiogenic shock may ensue. Abnormal heart rhythms can often be treated with drugs, cardiac pacing and sometimes by direct current (DC) electrical shock, as long as the patient is anaesthetised or unconscious.

Hypovolaemic shock

As the name implies this form of shock is caused by a low blood volume. This reduces intravascular volume and so reduces venous return. Causes include haemorrhage, burns, significant oedema and dehydration.

Haemorrhage

If blood is lost from the circulatory volume venous return will fall, which will lower cardiac output and blood pressure. Haemorrhage is the most common cause of shock in trauma patients. For example, 750 mls of blood can be lost into the tissues from a fractured tibia or humerus. Up to 1.5 litres of blood may be lost from a fractured femur and more than 2 litres can be lost from a significant pelvic fracture.

Burns

Fluid and electrolytes are lost through a burned area as a result of increased rates of evaporation from exposed tissue fluids. Large volumes of inflammatory exudates are also produced; the fluid exuded from the capillaries is therefore lost from the circulating volume. The result of this is that large volumes of fluid can be lost, particularly in the first 12 hours after the injury before a coagulum forms over the burn. Children with burns affecting 10% or more of body surface, and adults with 15% or more, need intravenous fluid replacement. Fluids should be aggressively replaced as soon a possible to prevent the development of hypovolaemia. In cases where the area of burn is less than these figures, oral fluid replacement will normally be adequate. A ready way to estimate percentage surface area involved is to use the area of the flat of the patient's hand, including the palm and fingers which approximates to 0.8% of body surface area.

Fluids should be titrated carefully with the patient's condition and individual requirements. Observations must include hourly urine volumes, pulse and respiration rate, blood pressure and core temperature. The following Parkland formula is commonly used in the UK to estimate the total additional volume of fluid replacement required over the first 24 hours after a burn injury.

Fluid volume required = 4 mls x weight (KG) x % burnt area

As most fluid is lost in the first hours after the burn has been sustained, half of the volume calculated by the Parkland formula should be given over the first 8 hours and the other half over the next 16 hours. In addition to these volumes, an adult requires 3 litres of fluid per day to meet fluid maintenance requirements. Ringer's lactate (Hartmann's solution) is probably the best fluid for the first 24 hours. After the first 24 hours colloidal fluids will also normally be given. Other injuries leading to loss of substantial areas of the skin can also cause extensive fluid loss.

Oedema

After soft tissue injury, inflammatory mediators will cause localised vasodilatation and increased permeability of the capillaries. This can lead to the accumulation of significant volumes of fluid in injured soft tissues. The volumes of fluid lost from the intravascular compartment will be proportional to the extent of the soft tissue injury.

Dehydration

Perhaps the most common cause of dehydration and electrolyte loss is infection of the gastrointestinal system. Diarrhoea and vomiting are useful defence mechanisms to eject infection from the gut, but if prolonged may lead to dehydration. This problem may develop fairly rapidly in children who have relatively low blood and fluid volumes in their bodies compared to adults. In global terms, dehydration which is secondary to gastroenteritis is still the most common cause of death in young children.

Another cause of dehydration induced shock is intestinal obstruction. In this condition there is dilation of the gut with fluids. As these fluids derive from the blood there will be reduced volumes left in the plasma. In peritonitis large volumes of fluid may accumulate in the peritoneal cavity, also depleting fluid levels in the blood. These gut pathologies will also prevent absorption of fluids in the normal way, leading to further dehydration, electrolyte deficiency and hypovolaemia.

When fluids collect in potential spaces such as the peritoneal sac, or within the lumen of the gut, the condition is described as fluid 'third spacing'. In this context the first and second fluid spaces are the intracellular and extracellular fluid compartments. If fluids accumulate anywhere else they are in a third space and are clearly not available to the component of extracellular fluid which comprises the circulating blood volume. Dehydration may also have a medical cause such as osmotic diuresis seen in diabetic ketoacidosis and hyperglycaemia. It may also develop during the diuretic phase of resolving acute renal failure.

Tachycardia and hypovolaemia

When blood volumes are low, the heart beats more rapidly. This decreases the circulation time of the blood and so increases delivery of oxygen and nutrients to tissues. In other words, increased heart rate attempts to compensate for reduced blood volume. This is referred to as a compensatory tachycardia. In the early stages of fluid or blood loss, this mechanism may be able to maintain blood pressure for a time.

When blood volumes are low, venous return of blood to the heart will be correspondingly reduced. This means that volumes of blood entering the heart will be low, resulting in a low stroke volume. Low stroke volume is explained by the fact that the heart can only pump out the volumes of blood it receives in venous return. When stroke volume is reduced, the volume of the pulse will also be reduced. This explains why the pulse feels weak and thready in hypovolaemic shock, despite being rapid.

Management principles in hypovolaemia

Basically, the treatment for hypovolaemia is to treat the underlying cause, for example in haemorrhage definitive control of bleeding must be established. Next blood and fluid volumes need to be restored. This often means giving intravenous infusions of crystalloid fluids and blood transfusions if needed. In all situations of fluid loss it is essential to think of the electrolyte values as well as fluid levels. Electrolytes are often lost with fluid and will need to be monitored and appropriately replaced. Sodium, potassium, chloride, calcium and magnesium are very important as these dissolve in body fluids as ions where they act as electrolytes. The correct balance of electrolytes is essential as nerve and muscle cells work by generating an electrical potential difference (i.e. voltages) across their cell membranes by controlling the relative concentration of ions.

Oral rehydration therapy

In dehydration caused by gastroenteritis, intravenous therapy may be indicated, but for the majority of cases oral rehydration salts (ORS) are remarkably effective. ORS at its most simple is made up from water, sugar, salt and preferably some potassium as well. In the home situation fruit juice or mashed banana are good sources of potassium. ORS works by replacing lost water and salts.

ORS is rapidly absorbed from the gut into the blood because glucose is actively absorbed using a process called active transport. This uses energy to transport glucose from the lumen of the gut into the lining mucosa. Once the glucose has been rapidly absorbed by this active process, water will passively follow by osmosis. After being absorbed the water will rapidly enter the capillaries and so increase intravascular volume. ORS therapy is particularly appropriate for children with diarrhoea and vomiting. If parents all over the world could be taught how to use this simple treatment, potentially millions of children could be saved every year. In addition to replacing water and electrolytes, ORS also supplies sugar. This is good as hypoglycaemia is a further complication of gastroenteritis in children.

Intravenous fluid replacement

Intravenous fluids may be crystalloid or colloidal. Crystalline fluids contain small molecules which will crystallise if removed from the water they are dissolved in. Examples include normal saline, dextrose saline and Hartmann's solution. The small molecules in crystalloid fluids may pass out of the capillaries into the interstitial fluids, and into the intracellular fluid compartment. This means they are useful to increase the total volume of fluid in the body. Pure water is not given intravenously (except in small volumes as a vehicle for some drugs) as it has a low osmolarity, in other words pure water is hypotonic. Hypotonic fluids would cause water to diffuse into red blood cells by the process of osmosis. This would cause the cells to swell, leading to haemolysis – the breaking up of blood cells.

Colloidal fluids contain large molecules which may be protein or carbohydrate based. As the molecules are large, they are not able to readily leave capillaries to enter the tissue fluids. As a result these large molecules stay in the intravascular fluid compartment. Large molecules are osmotic and so retain water in the blood, increasing plasma volumes. This is why colloids are sometimes referred to as plasma expanders. If a colloid increases intravascular volume it will increase venous return, which will increase cardiac output and blood pressure.

Any patient with shock, or who is at risk of developing shock, should have two large caliber peripheral venous catheters inserted. These will allow for rapid infusion of fluids as required. If these are impossible to insert, a central line should be considered. Intraosseous infusions, running fluids directly into a bone such as the tibia, may also be used in emergency situations. After shock and haemorrhage intravenous fluids should be warmed to 39°C before they are given. This is to prevent the patient becoming hypothermic. Any drop in blood temperature will reduce the efficiency of the enzyme based blood clotting mechanisms.

After significant haemorrhage isotonic crystalline solutions should be given for initial fluid resuscitation. If more that 1500 mls of blood are lost in an adult a blood transfusion should be considered. As a general principle the '3 for 1' rule should be used after significant acute haemorrhage. This says that a patient should receive 3 mls of crystalloid fluid for every 1 ml of blood lost. However, fluid replacement must always be tailored to individual patient response.

Obstructive shock

This may occur secondary to a blockage in the circulatory system, often affecting venous return to the heart. For example, if a patient has a large pulmonary embolism, this will obstruct blood flow through the lungs. Blood pumped out by the pulmonary artery will not be able to get through to the pulmonary veins to return to the left atrium. This will lower venous return and therefore cardiac output. These patients are usually started on heparin as an anticoagulant and thrombolysis should be considered.

Another possible obstructive cause is a tension pneumothorax which will push the heart and major blood vessels to one side; this will tend to flatten the large blood vessels, effectively obstructing the circulatory system. The treatment is to relieve the pressure in the pneumothorax as an emergency.

Cardiac tamponade may be caused by blood collecting within the pericardial sac. This will compress the heart and prevent normal venous return from filling the chambers of the heart which will again obstruct the normal circulation of the blood. This will normally be managed by removing blood from the pericardial sac using the process of pericardiocentesis.

Uncomplicated sepsis, severe sepsis and septic shock

Uncomplicated sepsis, severe sepsis and septic shock represent differing levels of severity of infection. These three descriptions represent a continuum of increasing severity, with the potential for uncomplicated sepsis to become severe sepsis, and for severe sepsis to develop into septic shock.

Uncomplicated sepsis

This describes the clinical situation of any person with a systemic infection, most commonly bacterial or viral. These infections are very common and normally resolve with no treatment, or simple home care treatments. Common causes of uncomplicated sepsis include chest and urinary tract infections and influenza. The person feels generally unwell and will have some of the following clinical features. A pyrexia above 38°C (or below 36°C), a resting heart rate of over 90 beats per minute, a respiratory rate of over 20 breaths per minute and a raised white cell count of over 12,000 (or less than 4000). An increased body temperature (pyrexia) and white cell count (leucocytosis) are by far the most common responses to infection, but occasionally the temperature or white cell count may be lower than normal. There may also be an altered mental state. Blood glucose levels may be raised, in the absence of diabetes, as part of a generalized stress reaction. Plasma C-reactive protein (an inflammatory marker) levels may be raised. There may also be evidence to indicate the site of infection, such as a soft tissue infection, dysuria or a cough.

Uncomplicated sepsis caused by viral infection will normally resolve as the body develops specific immunity. Some cases of uncomplicated sepsis caused by bacterial infection may resolve more rapidly if antibiotics are given. These common, almost routine, infections are still classified as sepsis because they are caused by infecting agents which live in body tissues and fluids during the acute phase of the illness. However, this sepsis is uncomplicated as it does not affect organ function or cause hypotension.

Severe sepsis

In severe sepsis the systemic infection is more serious. In addition to the clinical features which can be present in uncomplicated sepsis the condition will be complicated by organ dysfunction or tissue hypoperfusion. A severe infection will lead to the release of cytokines and inflammatory mediators. Cytokines are signal molecules released from cells, in this case particularly from macrophages and polymorphonuclear cells such as neutrophils. These white blood cells will release cytokines when they come into contact with bacterial derived components. Together with toxins released by infecting bacteria, these cytokines and mediators can adversely affect many tissues and organs.

All of the major organs can potentially be affected in severe sepsis. As tissues become hypoperfused they will change from aerobic to anaerobic metabolism with the consequent production of lactic acid. This waste product will accumulate in the blood giving rise to raised lactate levels. Renal involvement can lead to reduced urine volumes (acute oliguria) and the consequent retention of water and waste products. Acute lung injury, caused by infective toxins and the body's own inflammatory response can lead to reduced pulmonary function with consequent hypoxaemia. Cardiac and blood vessel involvement can lead to hypotension. Normal blood coagulation may be impaired resulting in an increased international normalised ratio (INR). Liver involvement may reduce normal liver function test results and involvement of the GI tract lead to bowel stasis (ileus).

As most cases of severe sepsis are caused by bacterial infection, early identification of the causative bacteria is essential, but intravenous antibiotic therapy must not be delayed. (In the past severe sepsis and septic shock have been referred to as blood poisoning and septicaemia, but these terms should not be used in current clinical practice)

Septic shock

This is described by the international Surviving Sepsis Campaign (SSC) as severe sepsis plus hypotension which is not reversed with fluid resuscitation. Septic shock develops as a complication of severe sepsis and does not resolve after giving intravenous fluids.

Vasodilation as part of the problem

In the first three classifications of shock we have considered, i.e. cardiogenic, hypovolaemic and obstructive, peripheral vasoconstriction occurs as part of the physiological attempted compensation. However, in septic, allergic and neurogenic shock vasodilation is part of the underlying, causative pathophysiology. In these three classifications of shock there is pathological vasodilation which will reduce peripheral resistance. As peripheral resistance is lowered, blood pressure will also be lowered as blood pressure is partly determined by peripheral resistance. This vasodilation explains why these forms of shock are usually associated with warm peripheries (sometimes referred to as 'hot shock') and full or bounding pulses. This is in clear contrast to the vasoconstriction induced cold peripheries normally seen in the cardiogenic, hypovolaemic and obstructive forms.

Vasodilation also increases the size of the gaps in capillary walls, increasing permeability. Increased volumes of tissue fluid exude from these dilated capillaries. This leads to the development of oedema and reduced plasma volumes, possibly leading to hypovolaemia. If plasma volumes are reduced, venous return will also be reduced. This reduction in venous return will reduce cardiac output which will further reduce blood pressure. Toxins and inflammatory mediators may also depress the function of the myocardium, resulting in a cardiogenic component, further exacerbating the vasodilation and hypovolaemia.

Management principles in severe sepsis and septic shock

As in all forms of shock, treatment should be started as soon as possible. Ideally infection should be managed before severe sepsis or septic shock has time to develop. Blood cultures should be taken to ascertain the bacterial species present in the blood. Once bacterial sensitivities are known the treatment can be modified and refined. This identification of the nature of an infection, using culture and sensitivity testing, allows for specific antibacterial treatments to be given. However, intravenous antibiotic treatment should be started as soon as possible, before specific culture results are available. If there is any delay in giving antibiotics mortality increases. For example if a patient is suspected to be suffering from meningococcal septicaemia they should immediately be given high doses of intravenous benzylpenicillin.

If possible the anatomical source of the infection should be identified. It may be that specific treatments are then indicated. For example an infected wound can be debrided, with the removal of necrotic and infected tissue. A leaking gastrointestinal perforation causing peritonitis could be surgically closed. Abscesses can be drained, cleaned and packed. Potentially infecting foreign bodies or devices, such as intravenous cannula, can be removed.

Fluid resuscitation with intravenous crystalloid or colloidal fluids should be given. Fairly large volumes may be needed to maintain central venous pressure, especially in the first 24 hours of management. Vasopressive drugs such as norepinephrine or dopamine will cause vasoconstriction in order to maintain blood pressure and consequent tissue perfusion. Blood pressure may also be helped by giving inotropes. These drugs, such as dobutamine, increase the force of cardiac contraction. Attention should also be paid to hameoglobin levels, respiratory support, sedation, blood glucose control, renal function and the prevention of deep venous thrombosis and stress ulcers.

From this it is seen that it is essential to treat the underlying precipitating cause and the accompanying organ and circulatory failure. If these are both well managed in the early stages of the condition the prognosis is good. However, if the condition is allowed to deteriorate then organ function will decline, leading to eventual multiple organ failure (MOF) which is associated with a high mortality.

Anaphylactic shock

Anaphylactic (allergic) shock is also referred to as anaphylaxis. As the clinical features present within a few minutes of exposure to an antigen it is classified as a severe form of type 1 hypersensitivity reaction. It is an extreme abnormal allergic reaction to a drug or other substance introduced into the body. Reactions usually present suddenly, within seconds to a few minutes after exposure to the antigenic substance. However, reactions delayed by up to half an hour may occur.

When a person is first exposed to a substance to which they are hypersensitive, the B lymphocytes will produce antibodies. These antibodies become attached to mast cells. On subsequent exposure to the antigenic substance the antigen will combine with these antibodies causing the mast cells to release large amounts of histamine and other inflammatory and vasodilatory substances into the blood and tissue fluids.

Histamine is a powerful vasodilator and bronchoconstrictor. Arteriole vasodilation reduces the peripheral resistance and therefore blood pressure. In addition to this the capillaries become more permeable so fluid leaks from the blood into the tissues, leading to oedema and hypovolaemia. Pulmonary oedema may also develop. Heart rate will usually increase in an attempt to compensate for the hypotension.

Clinical features

Often the first indication of a developing reaction is patient anxiety and unease. This has been described as a feeling of impending doom. The severity of reactions may vary considerably from skin irritation and a feeling of unease to complete collapse. Indeed in young children the collapse has been of such severity that the child becomes completely flaccid, so called 'rag doll' syndrome. In addition to the hypotension and bronchospasm already described, angioedema may develop. This may affect the face, tongue and larynx resulting in progressive occlusion of the upper airway, compounding the respiratory embarrassment caused by the bronchospasm. These respiratory problems will lead to wheezing, distress, stridor and cyanosis.

Because pathological vasodilation is caused by histamine and other substances, anaphylaxis often causes patchy or global redness of the skin. In addition to redness, intensely itchy urticarial wheals may develop. Sneezing and other irritation of the respiratory tract may be a feature.

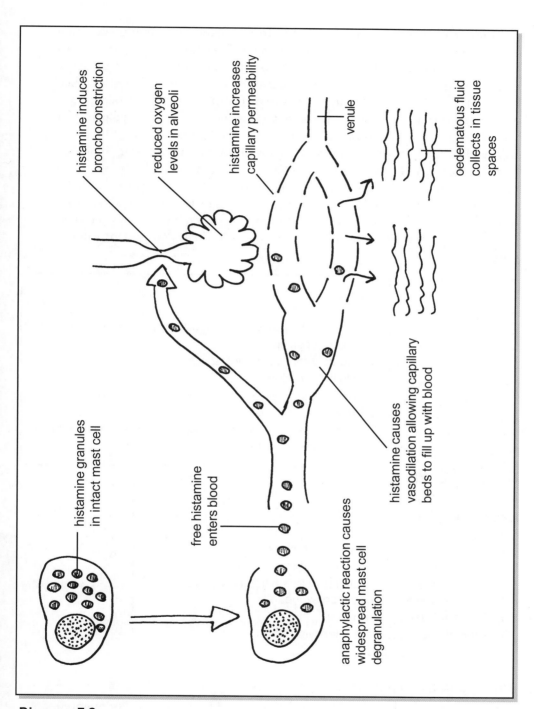

Diagram 7.2
In anaphylaxis mast cell degranulation leads to a sudden increase in circulating histamine. This causes bronchoconstriction and dilates blood vessels and capillaries. Vasodilatory effects lead to reduced peripheral resistance and oedema.

Young children rarely, if ever, faint after a medical procedure such as a vaccination, so any case of collapse in children will be organic in nature. Adults however frequently faint, and so this is the most likely cause of acute unconsciousness. In a faint the patient regains consciousness very quickly when lying flat and there is no redness or wheals on the skin. A central pulse is maintained during a faint or convulsion. Central pulses should be palpated for 5 to 10 seconds as there is often a bradycardia during a faint.

Anaphylactic reactions are more common in people with a history of allergy or previous reactions; there may also be a history of asthma. There is often a history of previous localized allergic reactions to the offending antigen. Gaining information about an individual's allergies and any previous abnormal reactions is therefore a vital part of a patient assessment. However, almost any agent may cause anaphylaxis in idiosyncratically sensitive individuals and present without warning.

FAINTING

Clinical features

- Full carotid pulse persists, but may be bradycardic
- Respiration continues
- No upper airway oedema
- No bronchospasm
- No itching
- Pallor
- Patient regains consciousness rapidly when lying down
- Young children do not faint

ANAPHYLAXIS

Clinical features

- Usually sinus tachycardia
- Hypotension
- Possible apnoea, especially in children
- Upper airway oedema, sneezing may occur
- Bronchospasm, possible retrosternal tightness, dyspnoea, may be an audible expiratory wheeze
- Urticarial lesions, erythema
- Patient does not revive when lying down

Management principles in anaphylaxis

The causative agent should be identified and if possible discontinued or removed. Airway patency must be established and high concentrations of oxygen should be given if available. The patient should lie flat to maximize cerebral circulation. Intravenous fluids may be needed to improve blood pressure. If there is no

---

AGENTS WHICH MAY CAUSE AN ANAPHYLACTIC REACTION

- Antibiotics
- Blood and blood products
- Vaccines
- Muscle relaxants
- Morphine and codeine based preparations
- Latex, natural rubber, (e.g. in clinical gloves)
- Some foods, e.g. shell fish, nuts, bananas, eggs, mangoes, chocolate
- Nonsteroidal anti-inflammatory drugs
- Colloidal intravenous infusions
- Insect stings
- X Ray contrast mediums

---

cardiac output the situation may present as a cardiac arrest and then should be treated as such. Epinephrine (adrenaline) should be given promptly via deep intramuscular injection, normally an initial dose of 0.5mg for an adult with a corresponding reduced dose for children. This dose may be repeated after 5 to 10 minutes if indicated. Epinephrine is a potent bronchodilator and vasoconstrictor; it is therefore capable of reversing the principle effects of histamine. (Inadvertent intravenous injection of a bolus dose of epinephrine may well lead to ventricular fibrillation so is one to avoid.) Chlorpheniramine (piriton), hydrocortisone and salbutamol may also play a role in management.

All patients who have had an anaphylactic reaction should be automatically admitted to hospital for review by a physician. Once the causative agent is identified patients must be instructed to avoid it in future. Patients should also be issued with self-injectible epinephrine and they and their relatives should be taught how and when to administer this. MedicAlert bracelets should be worn. Alert stickers should be placed on patients' notes and prescription charts.

Neurogenic shock

Neurogenic shock begins with a problem in the nervous system. In this form of shock there is a reduction in sympathetic or an increase in parasympathetic outflow from the central nervous system. These effects will reduce peripheral resistance and reduce cardiac output.

As it is sympathetic stimulation which provides vasomotor tone leading to constriction, a loss of this stimulation allows vasodilation of the arterial system. This will reduce peripheral resistance and so lower blood pressure. Loss of sympathetic tone also allows venodilation. This allows blood to pool in the peripheral veins resulting in a lowered central venous pressure which in turn lowers venous return to the heart. As cardiac output is dependent on venous return this will be correspondingly reduced.

Cardiac output will be directly reduced if there is a reduction in sympathetic innervation of the heart. Increased vagal parasympathetic stimulation will also slow heart rate and reduce stroke volume. Spinal shock and neurogenic syncope are both forms of neurogenic shock.

Spinal shock

Normally sympathetic nerves leave the spinal cord from level T1-L2 (Thoracic 1 to Lumbar 2). If this sympathetic outflow is disrupted, as in a spinal cord injury or high spinal anesthesia, the stimulation of the vagus parasympathetic nerve is unopposed. As the vagus nerve is a cranial nerve it is not affected by the spinal cord injury. Spinal shock may last from a few hours to a few weeks and resolves as spinal reflexes recover after acute injury. If the blood pressure, heart rate or urine output are too low, the patient will need physiological support for a period of time. Atropine may be used as an occasional treatment or an infusion of dopamine used for longer term support.

Vasovagal (neurogenic) syncope

Common faint was previously termed vasovagal syncope but is now also described as neuroregulatory or neurogenic syncope. Syncope describes an acute loss of consciousness caused by reduced perfusion of the brain. Strong parasympathetic stimulation, via the vagus nerve, slows down the heart and therefore pulse rate. Reduced heart rate reduces cardiac output which in turn lowers blood pressure. There is also reduced sympathetic stimulation of the peripheral blood vessels, resulting in peripheral vasodilation. This lowers the peripheral resistance further contributing to a lowering of blood pressure. If blood pressure drops significantly there will be a consequent reduced perfusion of the brain with blood. If the hypotension generates a slightly reduced cerebral perfusion this will cause temporary dizziness and is described as presyncope. A more serious reduction in cerebral perfusion and oxygenation will lead to an acute, but usually brief, loss of consciousness (syncope).

Most people probably faint at some point in their lives; it is more common during youth and pregnancy. It is more likely to occur if a person is forced to stand for a period of time as this leads to pooling of blood in the legs and reduced venous return. Dehydration is another risk factor as this will lower blood volume. Heat makes fainting more likely as the blood pressure will be reduced as a result of peripheral vasodilation.

Pain is another possible cause of vasovagal syncope. A person in pain will often complain of feeling dizzy and need to lie down. In this situation it is important to remove the cause of the pain and/or to give analgesics. For example a patient with a lower arm fracture will often feel much better after an analgesic and when the fracture has been immobilized in a back slab to promote stability and reduce pain.

Syncope may occur for emotional reasons as a result of clinical procedures such as giving injections or taking blood. If such fainting is a possibility, the procedure should be carried out with the patient lying down, as fainting almost never occurs in this position.

Students (and sometimes qualified staff) sometimes feel faint when watching some clinical procedures. This is common, and can be considered a normal part of learning to adapt to new situations. If you feel faint, it is important to admit it, and to lie down for a little while. Perhaps the key is not to worry too much about it. Fainting is in no way a sign of personal weakness. This form of fainting seems to be most common in situations we are not used to. Once we have seen, or assisted in, a procedure a few times we start to feel much more comfortable.

If a person faints when they are standing up they may injure themselves as they fall. However once they are lying flat on the ground, the blood is able to perfuse the brain without fighting against gravity. As a result the person comes round quickly, usually within a few seconds. Laying the person flat is a simple but essential aspect of management. These patients should be laid flat with no pillow. The legs may also be elevated to increase venous return from the bottom half of the body. If a person faints, but remains propped in an upright position, they may start to fit as a result of worsening cerebral hypoxia, (reduced oxygen supply to the brain).

Shock and children

In children all the fluid volumes in the body are less, simply because children are smaller than adults. Blood and fluid loss should therefore be viewed in percentage terms, rather than in simple volumes. Total child blood volume can be estimated as 80mls per Kg of body weight. For example a child of 6 months has an approximate blood volume of 500 mls, rising to 750 mls at one year and one litre at age 2 years. Even at age 10 years most children will only have a total of 2 litres of blood, as opposed to 5 litres in an adult of average size.

If children do lose blood they do not show the progressive development of tachycardia and hypotension seen in older adults. Children are able to compensate extensively. This means that as they lose blood the blood pressure is well maintained for a period of time. However, once blood volumes drop to a certain level they will decompensate very rapidly and will collapse. In this situation the child's life is in imminent danger. This is why it is important to estimate volumes of blood lost by children and to treat accordingly before the decompensation point is reached. Young adults are also good compensators. This again means that they may maintain blood pressure for a period of time but then deteriorate rapidly.

CHAPTER 8

Haemorrhage

Damage to blood vessels

As blood is only supposed to be found within the circulatory system, that is within the heart and blood vessels, it follows that haemorrhage is caused by damage to blood vessels. This damage allows blood to leak out causing bleeding. Haemorrhage is just another word for bleeding.

Arterial haemorrhage

As the pressure of blood in arteries is high, a cut artery may lose blood rapidly. Initially there will be loss of pulsating, bright red blood. Pulsation means the blood comes out in spurts, with the normal arterial pulses. Fortunately, a cut artery will undergo reflex constriction to reduce blood loss. This may give rise to the presence of bright red oxygenated arterial blood in a wound without obvious pulsation.

Venous haemorrhage

This gives rise to a steady stream of dark red blood. The loss is steady as venous blood does not undergo the pressure changes found in arteries. Venous blood is relatively deoxygenated so is dark red.

Capillary haemorrhage

This often takes the form of oozing from a wound surface. Another presentation of capillary haemorrhage is a bruise (correctly termed a contusion). These develop when there is an accumulation of blood in the tissue spaces. Contusions often result from capillary haemorrhage caused by blunt trauma.

Forms of haemorrhage

Primary haemorrhage

Primary haemorrhage describes bleeding which occurs at the time of injury. For example primary haemorrhage occurs at the time of operation when a surgeon makes an incision or when we cut ourselves with a kitchen knife.

Management principles in primary haemorrhage

Use of pressure

The mainstay in the initial management of external haemorrhage is to apply direct pressure. Even significant haemorrhage from an artery can be arrested with very firm direct pressure over the damaged area of vessel wall. Firm direct pressure may be applied for long periods while waiting for surgical help. If there is a foreign body in a wound, which we would not want to press into undamaged tissue, we can apply pressure around the site. This will provide ring pressure which compress vessels which are carrying blood to the bleeding site. If a limb is bleeding it may be also elevated while still applying direct pressure. This will reduce venous pressure within the limb and so reduce venous bleeding.

Indirect pressure, over arteries which supply a bleeding area, is not usually recommended in first aid, but is sometimes useful in clinical practice as a short term measure. In accident and emergency situations obvious or large bleeding vessels should be visualized then ligated. Ligation describes the surgical process in which a string (i.e. a ligature) is placed tightly around a tissue and tied. Bleeding arteries or veins are normally clipped off using artery forceps, and then ligated. In serious injuries, such as traumatic amputations, early ligation of bleeding vessels can be life-saving.

Tourniquets

Use of tourniquets in first aid situations is not routinely recommended but merits discussion. A tourniquet will occlude venous return and so increase the pressure of blood within the veins. You can easily demonstrate this by applying a tourniquet to your own arm for a short period and notice how the veins fill up with blood. Such localised increase in intravenous pressure is therefore likely to increase venous haemorrhage. There can also be problems if a tourniquet is left on for too long. Healthy tissues in the limb will lose their blood and oxygen supply, this will result in tissues distal to the tourniquet converting from aerobic to anaerobic metabolism. As a result of this localised hypoxia there will be accumulation of lactic acid and other metabolic waste products which are unable to leave via the now occluded venous drainage. Then, when the tourniquet is finally released these toxins will enter the systemic circulation as a 'bolus'. If the heart is already embarrassed as a result of blood loss, this metabolic insult could be life threatening. Despite these considerations judicious use of a tourniquet can be very helpful in such situations as transferring a patient with a traumatic amputation.

Prevent hypothermia

Patients suffering from haemorrhage must not be allowed to become hypothermic because blood clotting requires the activity of enzymes in the blood. Physiological enzyme activity works most efficiently at 37°C therefore as blood temperature falls so will the efficiency of the enzymes which activate essential clotting factors. Therefore, if an injured patient is hypothermic, they will bleed more due to reduced blood clotting. If there is a reduced ability of the blood to clot this is described as a coagulopathy. This enzyme based physiology explains why traumatized patients should be kept warm and intravenous fluids should be warmed to 39°C prior to administration. Despite the need to avoid hypothermia in emergency situations, patients should not be too hot. If someone is hot, this will encourage peripheral vasodilation which will increase blood loss. Superficial cold will also induce peripheral vasoconstriction which can help to reduce haemorrhage. Alcohol is contraindicated in haemorrhage as it is also a vasodilator. Hot drinks can have the same vasodilatory effect so should be avoided.

Patient position

If blood loss is significant the patient should lie flat and the legs may be raised. These measures will prevent pooling of blood in lower parts of the body, and so help to maintain venous return to the heart. Lying flat will also remove the constraint of gravity from cerebral arterial circulation which will help to maintain perfusion of the brain.

Reactionary haemorrhage

Reactionary haemorrhage describes bleeding which occurs as a reaction to increase in blood pressure. Primary haemorrhage may cause a drop in blood pressure, leaving the patient temporarily hypotensive. During this time blood clots will form over the ends of ruptured arterial vessels. These blood clots may arrest the haemorrhage resulting in haemostasis. (Haemostasis means there is no bleeding.) However as the person recovers and the blood pressure increases to return to normal, the blood clot may be 'blown' off resulting in renewed, or reactionary haemorrhage.

Reactionary haemorrhage may also occur after surgery. During an operation the blood pressure may be relatively low, as a result of bleeding or as an effect of the anaesthetic. When the patient returns to the ward, probably on an intravenous infusion, the blood pressure rises back to normal. This may dislodge a clot or surgical ligature, which was able to maintain haemostasis at the lower blood pressure, but not at the higher. In post operative reactionary haemorrhage it may be necessary to return a patient to theatre.

Another cause of reactionary haemorrhage is over zealous fluid replacement. This was a problem in the Vietnam War where severely wounded soldiers were given large volumes of intravenous fluids, at an early stage, while being transferred to a surgical facility. The aim of these infusions was to restore blood pressure after haemorrhage. While it is essential to prevent shock, it can be argued that a degree of hypotension after injury is a normal response which protects against excessive haemorrhage. Rapidly increasing blood pressure can dislodge blood clots sealing damaged blood vessels. While it is possible to maintain blood pressure by giving even more fluids, these will lack the oxygen carrying capacity of blood, resulting in potentially life threatening hypoxia. Once haemostasis has been definitively established, for example by tying off bleeding vessels, then it would become appropriate to give more rapid fluid replacement.

Secondary haemorrhage

This occurs as a result of infection complicating a wound. The presence of wound infection can compromise the integrity of blood vessels resulting in renewed haemorrhage. This was relatively common in the era before antibiotics and modern wound management. We still see the problem in infected, friable granulation tissue. Wound cleaning procedures and antibiotics will be indicated to treat the infection.

Presentations of haemorrhage

External haemorrhage

This is bleeding which occurs from the surface of the body so is usually fairly obvious and easy to diagnose. However, even external haemorrhage can be underestimated or missed. It is important to get a good history from Paramedics who transfer a casualty from the scene, if there was a lot of blood on the floor; this has clearly been lost from the patient. Also if a person is bleeding from the back, blood may pool under the body or be missed under clothes, covers or bandages. This is why, after any significant trauma, the whole surface of the body should be inspected, (E for exposure).

It is also important to note where bleeding is occurring. For example bleeding from the ear, (i.e. from the external auditory meatus), after trauma may indicate a basal skull fracture. Bleeding from the nose may also be an indicator of basal skull fracture but is more likely to be caused by trauma to the nose. Leakage of clear fluid from the nose or ears may indicate loss of cerebrospinal fluid (CSF) and can also occur after basal skull fracture.

Internal haemorrhage

Clearly internal bleeding cannot be seen on the surface of the body. However, internal haemorrhage should be suspected after some forms of trauma or surgery as well as in some medical conditions. If haemorrhage takes place into the abdominal cavity or pleural space it will not be seen without aspiration or some form of scanning. After certain injuries, such as blunt abdominal or pelvic trauma a high index of suspicion for internal haemorrhage should be maintained. For example this form of trauma may be associated with lacerations to the kidneys or liver or rupture of the spleen. There will also be haemorrhage from the broken ends of fractured bones. In the days after internal haemorrhage has occurred, bruising may be seen over the local area of body surface, as blood diffuses from the haemorrhage site.

This thinking guides the principle in trauma that blood can be lost 'onto the floor and four more'. So after injury blood loss may be external, i.e. onto the floor. The four likely sites for internal blood loss are into the chest, abdomen, pelvis or into the limbs from fractured bones.

If significant amounts of blood are lost this may be detected by recognition of systemic manifestations such as peripheral vasoconstriction generating pallor and cold hands and feet. There will also be an increase in heart rate, (the pulse becomes fast, weak and thready) and eventually a reduction in blood pressure. Other forms of internal bleeding may become revealed in vomit, faeces, urine or sputum as discussed below.

Management principles in internal haemorrhage

Patients should be kept as still as possible as movement may dislodge blood clots which have formed over ruptured internal vessels. Hypothermia must be prevented to keep the enzymes responsible for blood clotting working at physiological temperatures. Very often the clinical management in this situation involves emergency preoperative care. If there is significant internal bleeding it will probably be necessary to identify the location of the bleed and to arrest the haemorrhage surgically. Intravenous fluid or blood replacement will usually be started.

Blood in vomit

Blood which is vomited is called haematemesis; this indicates a bleed into the lumen of the upper gastrointestinal (GI) tract which may suggest such disorders as peptic ulceration, oesophageal varices or gastric malignancy. Haematemesis may have the appearance of fresh blood, if it is vomited shortly after the haemorrhage occurred. Blood, which looks like blood is often described as frank, a term which means that something is obvious or blatant. However, if blood remains in the stomach for a period of time, it is altered by digestive processes. In this case the blood often has the classical 'coffee grounds' appearance. (This altered blood looks like the used grounds left in the pot after making percolated coffee.) In practice vomited blood often has an appearance inbetween these two classical presentations of frank and coffee grounds. If we are unsure if blood is present in vomit we should test it using a urine dipstick.

Blood in faeces

Blood may also be noted in faeces. As was the case with haematemesis, blood in the faeces may be fresh and frank, or it may be altered as it spends time in the lumen of the gut. Fresh blood in the faeces often indicates a bleed low down in the GI tract, while this may indicate colitis or cancer the most common cause is haemorrhoids (piles), these are varicose veins in the rectum which are prone to bleeding.

If there is bleeding into the upper gastrointestinal tract, which is not vomited, the lost blood is subsequently altered by digestive processes. When this blood is passed in the stools it has a characteristic dark 'tarry' appearance, this is called melaena. There is also a characteristic very unpleasant smell. These observations should lead us to check definitively for the presence of blood with a laboratory based diagnostic test. Any blood in faeces is abnormal and should always be explained.

Sometimes it is not possible to see blood in a stool by direct observation, but if the faeces is tested the blood can be detected. This hidden blood is called occult, (occult means hidden); again this is abnormal and should be explained. We should test for occult blood whenever we suspect it might be present. Faecal occult blood may be an early indicator of cancer of the colon.

Blood in urine

Haematuria (blood in urine) is always significant and may indicate malignancy, calculi, infection or obstruction of part of the urinary tract. (A calculus is an abnormal stone or other aggregate of solid material in the urinary or biliary tract.) Other possible causes include trauma to the bladder, pelvis or kidneys. Blood from menstruation often contaminates urine samples in women. If blood is detected in urine from a woman who is menstruating, the test should be repeated after the period has finished. Haematuria is expected after urinary tract or prostatic surgery and needs to be managed to prevent clots causing urinary retention.

Blood in sputum

Coughing up of blood is described as haemoptysis. This may occur after penetrating lung injuries or as a sign of lung cancer or tuberculosis. Sometimes blood in the sputum takes on a rust coloured appearance which is a sign of pneumococcal pneumonia. If pink, frothy sputum is observed this is a clear sign of pulmonary oedema, a potentially very serious disorder. Blood in the sputum, like blood in vomit, faeces or urine is always abnormal and should be explained.

Bleeding from bony injury

Bones have a copious blood supply. This means that when a bone is fractured, the blood vessels it contains will be torn. This is why fractures cause bleeding from the broken ends of bone. Larger volumes of blood are lost from larger bones, for example 1.5 litres of blood may be lost from a fractured shaft of femur. Unstable fractures of the pelvis are also associated with massive haemorrhage, possibly a life threatening 2 litres or more. Fractures in smaller bones are associated with smaller volumes of blood loss, but if there are several fractures, possibly in combination with other injuries these may all add up to a dangerous blood loss.

Site of haemorrhage

Haematoma

Internal blood loss which accumulates locally within a tissue is referred to as a haematoma. Such a collection of blood in a tissue space will clot and form a semisolid mass. Some haematomas can be left and will be broken down by enzymic systems and absorbed by phagocytes over time. As a general principle, a haematoma should be removed if it is easy to do so. This is because the mass of clotted blood will separate living tissues and so retard healing. As a haematoma provides substrate (food) and habitat for any bacteria there is an infection risk. Also as a haematoma takes up space it causes compression of surrounding tissues. Risk associated with internal haemorrhage depends on place (i.e. site) and volume of blood lost. Some internal haemorrhages may exert pressure on vital structures.

Thyroid related haematoma

There is a risk that there may be bleeding from the thyroid gland, or surrounding tissues after thyroid surgery. A haematoma in this area may exert pressure on the trachea causing compromise of the airway.

Intracranial haematoma

Bleeding into the vault of the skull will increase intracranial pressure (ICP) which will reduce the level of consciousness. Raised ICP may also lead to reduced or absent pupillary reflexes and may ultimately cause death by compromise of the vital structures in the brain stem.

Pressure on a nerve

If a haematoma causes compression of a peripheral nerve there may be loss or alteration of motor and/or sensory function distal to the site of pressure. If nervous compression is continued over time there may be permanent nerve damage.

Cardiac tamponade

If there is bleeding or an accumulation of fluid in the pericardial sac, which is between the parietal and visceral pericardium, there will be compression of the heart chambers. This problem is referred to as cardiac tamponade. External pressure reduces venous filling, and so reduces blood flow through the heart. If the compression is severe there will be an acute life threatening reduction in cardiac output. Emergency aspiration of the blood or fluid from the pericardial sac is usually indicated.

Effects of haemorrhage

Blood volumes

In an average 70Kg man the blood volume is about 7% of body weight. This would mean the total blood volume would be about 5 litres. If a person is obese, their blood volume should be calculated on what their ideal weight would be for their height. This is because adipose tissue does not have an extensive blood supply. In children the blood volume is about 8 to 9% of body weight, in other words about 80-90mls per Kg of body weight.

Acute haemorrhage

In acute haemorrhage there is a sudden loss of circulating blood volume and it is useful to assess this blood loss using a classification of 1 to 4. The following figures are based on a 70Kg man.

Class I haemorrhage

In this class of haemorrhage the blood loss is less than 750mls, or up to 15% of total blood volume. The patients pulse might be slightly faster than normal, but blood pressure will be maintained at normal levels. All other physiological parameters should also be normal, but the patient may feel a little anxious for a period of time. Normally fluid can be replaced by giving drinks, but if needed crystalloid intravenous fluids could be given.

Class II haemorrhage

This classification represents blood losses of 750-1500mls or 15-30% of total blood volume. This will typically result in a compensatory tachycardia of 100-120 beats per minute. Respiratory rate will be increased with a tachypnoea of 20-30 breaths per minute. Despite a decreased pulse pressure, the blood pressure is usually maintained at normal or near normal levels. The patient may feel anxious. Intravenous crystalloid fluids are indicated.

Class III haemorrhage

This involves blood losses of 1500-2000mls or 30-40% of total blood volume. Tachycardia will usually be in the 120-140 range. Tachypnoea will be about 30-40 breaths per minute. Pulse pressure will be reduced and blood pressure will be low giving rise to hypotension. The patient will feel anxious and may be confused and the other clinical indicators of shock will be present. It is vital to identify and treat the cause of the haemorrhage. Crystalloid infusions will be needed and a blood transfusion may also be indicated.

Class IV haemorrhage

If more than 2000mls of blood are lost, representing over 40% of total volume, the patient is in class IV haemorrhage and their lives are in immediate danger. Pulse rate will be above 140 beats per minute. Respiratory rate over 35 breaths per minute. The patient will be profoundly hypotensive and in a shocked state with cold clammy skin. Mentally the patient is likely to be confused, lethargic or unconscious. Without rapid infusion of crystalloid fluids and definitive haemorrhage control the patient will die within minutes. Blood transfusion will also be needed.

Chronic haemorrhage

Chronic haemorrhage may occur in a number of conditions such as uterine fibroids, ulcerative colitis, some cancers and peptic ulceration. If small volumes of blood are lost over time, the fluid component can be replaced, therefore maintaining normal blood volumes. However, if the loss of red blood cells exceeds the ability of red bone marrow to replace them, the number of red cells in circulation will progressively decline. This will result in a reduced oxygen carrying capacity of the blood causing anaemia. Chronic haemorrhage may therefore present with insidious symptoms such as tiredness, faintness, blackouts and dizziness.

Discussion of treatment principles in haemorrhage

In principle management of haemorrhage is simple, fix the leak, and replace fluid loss. We have already mentioned strategies for the establishment of haemostasis. The method chosen for restoration of fluid loss depends on the degree of blood loss. For small losses oral fluids can replace the lost water and reserves of blood from the spleen may be rapidly mobilised to replace lost red cells.

In dehydration, especially if caused by gastrointestinal disturbance, oral rehydration solutions may be given. In patients who are unable to drink it may be worth considering using a nasogastric tube to give fluids. Subcutaneous crystalloid infusions are also used to maintain hydration in some patients. Per rectum infusions are not used in hospitals, but may be of value in some situations where the necessary equipment and skills for intravenous therapy may not be available.

More severe haemorrhage of course requires intravenous fluid infusions. For more severe blood loss, the only fluid known to science which will transport oxygen efficiently around the body is blood. This is why blood transfusions are often essential. Blood transfusions save many lives. With correct screening, storage and administration the risks from blood transfusions are slight. Administration of all intravenous fluids should be given in the context of blood pressure, pulse, vasotone, cardiac function and if possible, central venous pressure measurements.

In the medium term urine output is monitored on an hourly basis. This provides accurate information on the hydration status of the patient. If a patient is dehydrated or hypovolaemic, urine output will be reduced. We therefore need to treat hypovolaemia and dehydration until good hourly volumes of urine are passed.

In the days and weeks after blood loss patients should eat enough protein to allow for the production of new red blood cells. Sufficient energy giving foods such as fats and carbohydrates are also necessary. Substances which are essential for the formation of new haemoglobin and red blood cells include, iron, folic acid and vitamin B_{12}. These essential nutrients are sometimes called haematinics.

Restoration of blood volume following haemorrhage

Background physiology

The mean arterial pressure in the aorta will normally be about 100 mmHg. This will drop to a mean of around 90 mmHg in smaller arteries and will represent the pressure at the start of an arteriole. By the time blood has passed through the arterioles and enters capillaries, the pressure will have dropped to about 32 mmHg. As blood passes from the arterial to venous end of a capillary, the pressure continues to drop to about 12 mmHg. The blood pressure in the arterial ends of the capillaries is essential for the formation of tissue fluid and the reduced pressure at the venous end of the capillaries allows for the reabsorption of tissue fluid. Reabsorption is facilitated by a plasma osmotic pressure of about 25 mmHg, principally generated by plasma proteins.

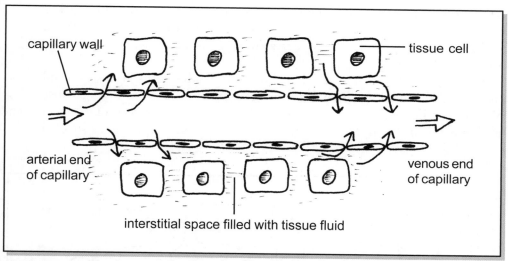

Diagram 8.1
Tissue fluid is formed at the arterial end of a systemic capillary as the blood (hydrostatic) pressure is greater than the osmotic pressure. Tissue fluid is reabsorbed at the venous end of a capillary because osmotic suction pressure is greater than blood hydrostatic pressure.

Physiological compensations after haemorrhage

Haemorrhage will start to cause a reduction in systemic arterial blood pressure. This is detected by the arterial baroreceptors which cause the medulla oblongata of the brain stem to increase sympathetic outflow. This increased sympathetic activity will cause a widespread vasoconstriction of the systemic arterioles. As it is the arterioles which provide most of the peripheral resistance, this vasoconstriction will increase blood pressure. This vasoconstriction is therefore a compensatory mechanism which attempts to maintain systemic blood pressure.

However, vasoconstriction of the arterioles will reduce the diameter of their lumen. This will reduce the volumes of blood which are able to pass through into the systemic capillaries. As there is now less blood in the capillaries, the blood pressure in the capillaries will be correspondingly lower. This means that after vasoconstriction induced by haemorrhage, the pressure of the blood entering the capillaries may drop from 32 to about 20 mmHg. As blood passes through a capillary the pressure continues to drop from 20 mmHg to as low as 5 mmHg at the venous end. (These figures are only approximate as they will vary depending on the degree of vasoconstriction.)

This means that after a significant haemorrhage, the blood pressure along the whole length of a capillary will be less than the osmotic pressure of the plasma. At the arterial end of the capillary, osmotic pressure will exceed blood pressure by about 5 mmHg and at the venous end the difference will be 20 mmHg. The result of these pressure changes is that tissue fluid will not be extruded from plasma into the interstitial spaces but tissue fluid will be sucked into the blood along the capillary length. As tissue fluid moves into the blood, total intravascular volume will be increased which will increase blood pressure back towards normal.

This response to haemorrhage has clear survival advantages. It means blood pressure can be increased, even if external sources of fluid are not immediately available. As this mechanism increases blood pressure, the person becomes much more functional and is able to instigate future behaviour to enhance survival probability.

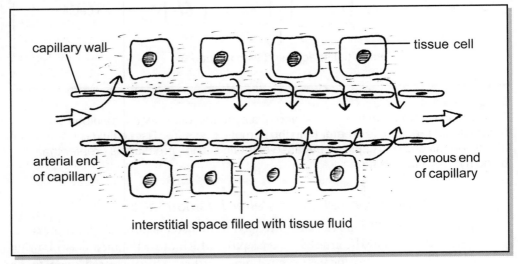

Diagram 8.2
After haemorrhage there is movement of water from tissue fluid into the blood, this is good as restoration of blood volume will help to restore blood pressure.

Haemorrhage, haematocrit and haemoglobin concentrations

Haemorrhage results in the loss of whole blood. This means that immediately after a haemorrhage, the proportions of blood constituents, in the blood which is left, will be the same as they were before haemorrhage took place. This will be true for haematocrit, red cell count, haemoglobin content and the concentration of proteins in plasma. It is the presence of normal levels of plasma proteins, generating osmotic potential, which allows for the shift in fluid into the intravascular compartment, described above. This means that if blood is tested shortly after haemorrhage the results will be normal, it will not be possible to tell, just from the blood, that haemorrhage has taken place. However over the next few hours, as the remaining blood is diluted by water from tissue fluid, haematocrit, red cell count and haemoglobin concentrations will drop. Drinking water or giving intravenous crystalloid fluids will have a similar diluting effect.

Red blood cell replacement after haemorrhage

As haemorrhage will reduce the total number of red blood cells in the circulatory system, the oxygen carrying capacity of the blood will be reduced. Initially, the red cells stored in the spleen will be released into the circulating blood, these are probably equivalent to about a unit of packed cells. If more blood is lost the reduced levels of oxygen will be detected by the kidneys which respond by releasing more erythropoietin (EPO). EPO will circulate to the red bone marrow where it will stimulate increased red cell production to replace those which have been lost. Some of the newly formed red cells enter the bloodstream before they are mature. These slightly immature cells are called reticulocytes, and are characterized by the presence of residual ribosomal material in their cytoplasm. Reticulocytes normally make up about 1% of the total RBC count, but this will be increased when compensating for anaemia or haemorrhage. An increase in the proportion of reticulocytes is termed a reticulocytosis.

Disorders of blood clotting

If normal blood clotting is inhibited, there may be haemorrhagic complications. Wounds will keep bleeding for longer than normal. There will be a susceptibility to bruise, even in the absence of trauma. Bleeding may also occur from the nose, eyes, gastrointestinal tract and into joints. In addition to hypothermia, reduced blood clotting may occur in genetic disorders such as haemophilia or Christmas disease. As platelets (thrombocytes) are needed for blood clotting, haemorrhage may occur whenever there is a thrombocytopenia (low levels of platelets in the blood), regardless of the cause. Excess anticoagulation may occur iatrogenically as a result of giving too much heparin or warfarin. Aspirin will also lead to longer clotting times. Viper venom also acts as an anticoagulant leading to haemorrhage.

CHAPTER 9

Cardiac Disorders

The electrocardiogram (ECG)

The muscular heart wall.

An ECG may be recorded by detecting and amplifying the electrical activity generated by the myocardium, as detected on the surface of the body. In order for muscle to contract it must depolarize. After contraction the muscle will repolarize, prior to the next depolarization. P waves are generated by atrial depolarization and so represent atrial contraction, QRS complexes are generated by ventricular myocardial depolarization so represent ventricular contraction. T waves are generated by ventricular myocardial *Repolarization* repolarization and so do not represent active muscular contraction. As each QRS complex represents ventricular contraction, each is associated with one arterial pulsation. A three lead ECG is commonly used to monitor the heart rhythm. However, if a 12 lead ECG is used the heart may be 'viewed' from 12 different positions. This allows any pathology in the myocardium to be localised.

Diagram 9.1i
The ECG records the electrical activity of the myocardium, as detected on the surface of the body. A normal ECG has a PQRST in the right order, and is regular with a rate of 60–100 complexes per minute; this is a sinus rhythm.

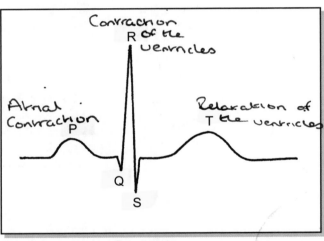

Contraction of the ventricles R

Atrial Contraction P

Relaxation of the ventricles T

Q

S

Coronary heart disease (CHD)

Reduction of blood flow to the heart.

CHD is caused by pathology in the coronary arteries. This results in myocardial ischaemia which is why the term ischaemic heart disease (IHD) is also used. Right and left coronary arteries carry blood directly from the aorta to the myocardium, the muscle of the heart. CHD most commonly occurs as a result of the deposition of atheroma within the lumen of the coronary arteries. This *Fatty deposits in the arteries* disease process is termed atherosclerosis. CHD is the most common form of heart disease and is the leading single cause of death in western countries. Heart disease caused by atherosclerosis is less common in developing countries, although if these areas adopt western life styles, the incidence increases. CHD may lead to stable angina pectoris, unstable angina, myocardial infarction, heart failure, dysrhythmias and possible sudden death. Under the age of 65 CHD is less common in women, probably due to the protective effects of oestrogen.

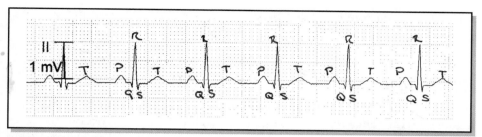

Diagram 9.1ii
This strip shows a short run of normal sinus rhythm.

Slow Rate below 60bpm – Relaxation or sleep?
Bradycardia

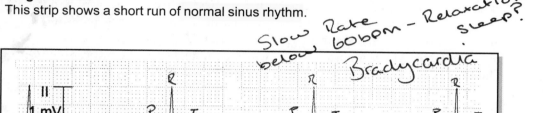

Diagram 9.1iii
If there is a PQRS and T wave, in the right order and the rhythm is regular with a rate below 60 per minute this is described as a sinus bradycardia. This rhythm is normal in fit individuals and may present during relaxation or sleep.

Tachycardia BPM – greater than 100.

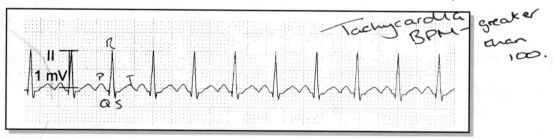

Diagram 9.1iv
When the normal rhythm rises above 100 it is described as a sinus tachycardia, physiologically this occurs during exercise, excitement or in emergencies.

Latin for chest.

Stable angina pectoris

(See CHD)

Stable angina is a relatively common disorder and describes the pain generated as a result of myocardial ischaemia. (Pectoris refers to the Latin word pectus meaning chest, so only partly describes the distribution of the pain.) Pain will be generated whenever the metabolic demands of the myocardium exceed the ability of the blood supply to transport nutrients and oxygen to the muscle cells. This form of angina is described as stable because there is reduced coronary arterial perfusion as a result of fixed or stable areas of atheroma within the coronary arteries. Also the severity of the condition may remain relatively stable over long periods of time.

Pathophysiology

blocked.

Low O₂ levels

Patients usually only complain of stable angina when the coronary arteries are 75% occluded by atheroma. In this sense angina is a clinical feature of reasonably advanced CHD. Coronary arterial narrowing reduces blood flow and so reduces oxygen delivery, which leads to myocardial hypoxia. If oxygen delivery is not adequate to meet myocardial work load at a particular time the metabolism of the myocardial cells changes from aerobic to anaerobic. Anaerobic metabolism generates lactic acid as a waste product which accumulates in the myocardium. The presence of lactic acid is associated with pain. — *Anaerobic!*

Blood test
liver on admission
identify anaerobic bacteria.

Angina is not associated with any pathological changes in the myocardium unless the ischaemic episodes are long enough to lead to myocardial injury. Although coronary arterial atherosclerosis is by far the most common cause of stable angina the pain may also be caused by other conditions such as aortic valve disease, disorders of the aorta or hypertrophic cardiomyopathy (enlargement of the myocardium).

Clinical features

Upper central region of the abdomen.

The common presentation is pain as a result of exercise or other forms of stress. This means the onset of pain is often predictable. Pain is usually felt in the centre of the chest and may radiate up into the neck, lower jaw, left arm or down into the epigastrium. It is therefore important to realise that pain in any of these areas should be treated with suspicion. For example, the most common cause of epigastric pain is probably simple indigestion, but it is not always safe to assume this. Angina pain is usually described as being tight, heavy or vice like. Some patients just complain of a general feeling of 'heaviness' in the chest. Severity of the pain can vary from mild to very severe. This common, stable form of angina is sometimes described as exertional angina, with pain developing during exercise and passing off with rest. Most patients will be pain free after resting for five minutes. Exertional angina is more likely to present in cold weather and after large meals. Many patients also complain of pain caused by walking into the wind. Breathlessness is a common feature during an episode of pain. Some patients complain of pain when they start walking but become pain free with continued effort, this is termed 'warm-up angina'.

Between attacks of stable angina pectoris the ECG is usually normal. However, during an attack there are often reversible ST changes, usually depression. If a patient complains of angina an ECG performed during an attack can be very helpful in diagnosing the disorder. Another common investigation is a stress or exercise test. This records the ECG while the patient exercises on a tread mill; if angina is induced, the ST changes can usually be seen. Extensive ST depression

Threaded in through the wrist either or femoral artery).

Also an echo can show atheroma.

is an indication of more severe coronary arterial narrowing. Using a 12 lead ECG will also help to decide which part of the heart is most affected. More precise information about the position and extent of coronary arterial atheroma can be gained using coronary angiography. As well as providing an absolute diagnosis, essential information is provided to inform future percutaneous coronary interventions or coronary bypass grafting.

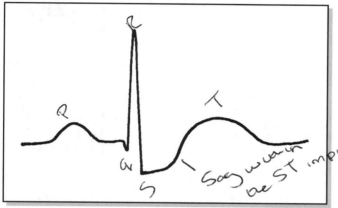

Sag within the ST impulse , this is mostly very clear on an ECG

Diagram 9.2
During an episode of angina there is usually ST depression (also sometimes called ST sag).

Treatment principles

GTN Spray).

Patients who experience exertional angina should rest; this usually results in the pain passing off fairly quickly, usually within minutes. Sometimes they may need to rest for more than five minutes (even up to 15 minutes) for the pain to pass off completely. The other standard treatment is to give sublingual (under the tongue) glyceryl trinitrate. This usually gives immediate benefit. Some patients will take sublingual nitrate before undertaking an activity they know is likely to induce pain. *1-2 sprays under tongue.*

Various drug treatments may be given to control angina such as longer acting nitrates, calcium channel blockers or beta-blockers. Another approach to treatment is revascularization therapy. This involves invasive procedures to increase the volumes of blood which reach the myocardium. Percutaneous coronary intervention (PCI) involves coronary angioplasty where a catheter is passed into a coronary artery and a balloon is inflated at the point of obstruction. This can widen the lumen of the artery and improve blood supply. A coated metallic coronary stent can then be placed in the narrowed section of coronary artery to increase the diameter of the lumen. Alternatively, open surgical procedures may be used involving coronary artery bypass grafting. A blood vessel is harvested from the patient, and used to bypass an occluded coronary artery. This allows blood to reach the ischaemic area of myocardium via the bypass vessel.

e.g Amlodopine

e.g. Atenolol (most oral (oral))

CABG

c cabg, done in major heart centres. outbanzation of blocked vessels.

Overall the prognosis in angina is fairly good with a mortality of less than 2% per year. Patients should be assessed to see if they have any risk factors which may need to be corrected, e.g. diabetes, hypertension, hypercholesterolaemia, obesity or hypothyroidism. Patients must not smoke and should take regular exercise. A healthy diet should be taken. As angina is a consequence of coronary arterial disease, patients are at risk of further coronary events. This is why patients with proven coronary arterial disease should be given antiplatelet therapy. This will reduce the risk of platelet activation and blood clot formation within the coronary arteries. This explains why low dose aspirin (75-150 mg daily) reduces the risk of adverse events such as myocardial infarction. Individuals who have side effects from aspirin can take clopidogrel (75 mg daily) as an equally effective alternative.

Uncommon forms of angina
Variant angina

Variant (also called Prinzmetal's) angina typically occurs when the patient is at rest, as a result of coronary arterial spasm. As a section of a coronary artery goes into spasm the lumen is greatly reduced leading to an acute hypoperfusion of an area of myocardium. Typically during an episode of variant angina pain, there is ST elevation, in contrast to the more usual ST depression. Variant angina usually occurs in atherosclerotic arteries but may occasionally present in patients with otherwise healthy arteries.

Syndrome X

A minority of patients complain of stable angina on exertion but are found not to have coronary arterial atheroma. Often, when investigated by stress testing these patients are found to have definite myocardial ischaemia. It appears that these individuals suffer from a microvascular (small vessel) dysfunction. Normally, when a healthy person exercises and cardiac workload increases, the small coronary arterial vessels dilate to increase the blood supply to match metabolic demand. However, if this mechanism fails and the blood supply to the actively contracting myocardium is not increased, ischaemia will result. This condition is associated with a good prognosis and is often referred to as syndrome X

Acute coronary syndrome (ACS)

Acute coronary syndromes are caused by acute obstruction of a coronary artery resulting in a reduced or occluded blood supply to an area of myocardium. Consequences of the arterial blockage depend on the degree and location of obstruction. Low grade, partial obstructions will cause low risk unstable angina, with a greater degree of obstruction causing high risk unstable angina. Still more severe obstruction will cause a non-ST elevation myocardial infarction (NSTEMI) and complete arterial obstruction will cause ST elevation myocardial infarction (STEMI). Sudden cardiac death is another complication of acute coronary syndrome, usually resulting from a ventricular dysrhythmia such as ventricular fibrillation.

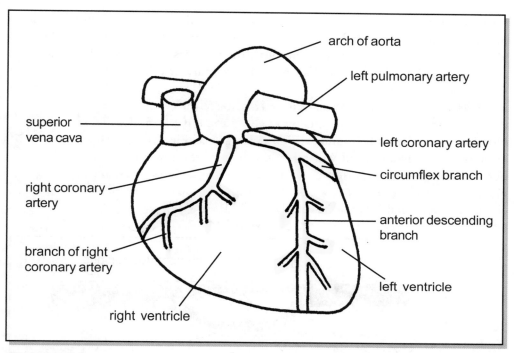

Diagram 9.3
Normal arrangement of coronary arteries. The left artery divides into two branches; the circumflex branch carries on around the left side of the heart to the posterior surface. The coronary arteries are the first to leave the aorta and their anatomy can be used to describe the three most common presentations of MI.

Pathophysiology in acute coronary syndrome

In all forms of acute coronary syndrome there will be varying degrees of myocardial ischaemia. The immediate cause of almost all cases of ACS is rupture of an atherosclerotic plaque. Atherosclerotic plaques develop within the coronary arteries over many years and may be stable or unstable. In a stable plaque the area of atheroma will be covered by the usual lining layer of endothelial intimal cells under which there is a fibrous cap. This fibrous cap is composed largely of collagen and there will be associated smooth muscle cells which promote repair and stabilization of the plaque. However, if the roof of the plaque is disrupted it may fissure or rupture. When this happens the plaque is described as unstable. This will mean that blood is able to come into contact with constituents of the plaque core. These contents may include lipids, collagen, smooth muscle and fat containing macrophages described as foam cells. Contact between these core constituents and the blood leads to platelet aggregation and adhesion to the vessel walls. The aggregation of platelets leads to the development of white thrombus which will partly occlude the lumen of the coronary artery. Unstable angina and NSTEMI are usually caused by this form of white, partly occlusive platelet rich thrombus. Because the white thrombus only partly occludes the lumen of the artery, some blood is still able to perfuse the distal myocardium, although the volumes will be reduced. The presence of the thrombus may also provoke coronary arterial spasm, making the ischaemia worse.

Platelet activation and aggregation may stimulate the coagulation cascade in the blood leading to the development of red thrombus (i.e. a blood clot). Red blood clot contains fibrin and will completely occlude the arterial branch. *– MI!!* This means no blood at all will reach the part of the myocardium normally perfused by the thrombosed coronary artery. In other words the area of myocardium will be infarcted. This will give rise to the classical picture of ST elevation myocardial infarction seen in a STEMI. *tha Shown with ST elevation on an ECG*

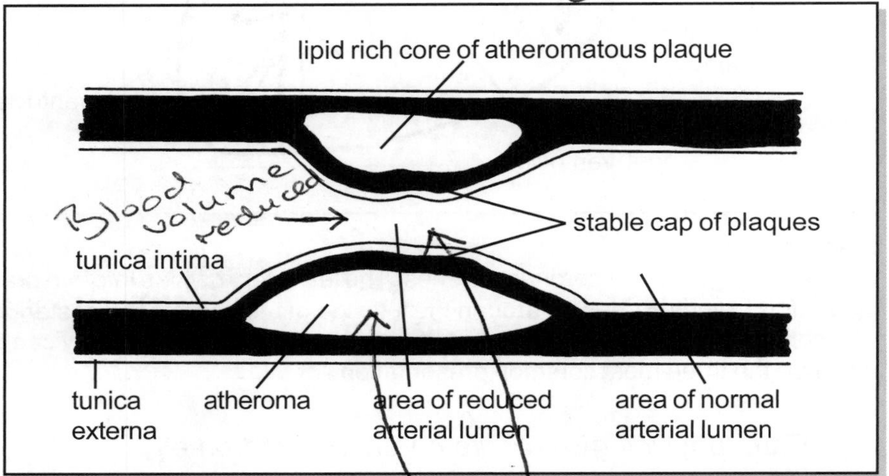

Diagram 9.4i
This is a length of a coronary artery in an individual who suffers from stable angina pectoris of effort. There is a fixed area of stenosis (abnormal narrowing) as a result of the presence of stable plaques of atheroma. Clearly, this reduces the volumes of blood which may pass through the artery in a given time. This pathology generates myocardial ischaemia which explains the predictable clinical features associated with exertion.

Unstable angina

This condition may present in a patient who already suffers from stable angina, or as a new clinical condition. The platelet rich white thrombus leads to an acute coronary insufficiency and myocardial ischaemia which generates the clinical features.

Clinically unstable angina pain may come on while the patient is at rest or during exercise. Pain is usually felt in the centre of the chest and referred to the usual areas where anginal pain is experienced. Patients may present with pain which is of new onset or is getting worse (crescendo angina), despite the patient *oral or IV*

If central chest pain continues for longer than 20 for mins, check ECG or drop to see if MI or unstable angina.

paracetamol codeine morphine

resting. If angina pain persists for more that 20 minutes it is likely to be caused by unstable angina or MI as opposed to stable angina. The patient will usually be short of breath and clammy. In low risk unstable angina there should be no release of troponin from the myocardium. Patients should be admitted and given bed rest and analgesia, oxygen should be given if oxygen saturations are low. In order to reduce the probability of further thrombi formation, aspirin, clopidogrel and heparin are given. Beta blockers are also often used. If low risk unstable angina is not treated it may develop into high risk unstable angina. The presentation and management of high risk unstable angina is essentially the same as the low risk form. However, in high risk unstable angina there are increasing levels of troponin detectable in the blood. These are released from damaged myocardium and increasing levels in the blood indicate more myocardial damage and increasing risk of the condition developing into myocardial infarction. So if this condition is not treated it may go on to develop into, NSTEMI or STEMI.

'enoxaparin'

Less than 94% consider

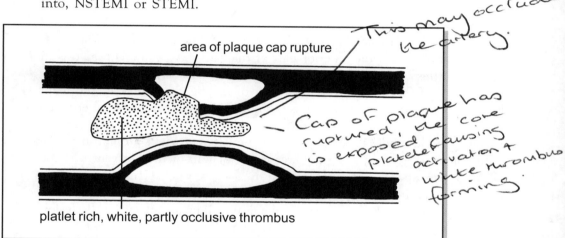

This may occlude the artery.

area of plaque cap rupture

Cap of plaque has ruptured, the core is exposed causing platelet activation + white thrombus forming.

platlet rich, white, partly occlusive thrombus

Diagram 9.4ii
This diagram illustrates an atheromatous plaque where the cap has ruptured. This allows platelets to come into contact with the core of the plaque which causes platelet activation and subsequent white thrombus formation. White thrombus is platelet rich and may occlude the artery to various degrees. A certain degree of thrombotic occlusion will cause unstable angina and a greater degree of occlusion will lead to a NSTEMI. This is a dynamic stenosis causing unpredictable symptoms which may present at rest.

Myocardial infarction (MI)

— Heart attack Then visit to CCU to check heart
— A+E admission

This is a common and serious condition with a high mortality. In the days and weeks before an acute event many patients experience prodromal symptoms such as crescendo angina, fatigue and shortness of breath. The clinical features in NSTEMI and STEMI are the same. However, as the names imply, there will be ST elevation in STEMI which is not present in NSTEMI.

Can be caught early.

"Sense of impending doom"

Just in non st elevation MI

Red thrombus   White thrombus
linked to   caused by opening
Stemi   of plaque
*   build ups.*

Pathophysiology

MI is almost always caused by the development of a thrombus in a coronary artery. NSTEMI is caused by white thrombus and STEMI by red, blood clot, thrombus. In other words coronary thrombosis causes myocardial infarction. Rupture of an atheromatous plaque causes activation of clotting mechanisms leading to thrombus formation. After the thrombus has occluded an arterial lumen the affected area will be deprived of a blood supply and irreversible cellular necrosis will start to develop 20-40 minutes after infarction. An infarct may be transmural; this means the full thickness of the ventricular wall is affected, involving the endocardium, myocardium and epicardium. Conversely, subendocardial infarcts involve only the inner third to half of the ventricular wall. Over time any necrosed area of myocardium is replaced by fibrous scar tissue which lacks the elasticity of normal myocardium and has no powers of contraction.

Tired easier

Lesser heart function

Peripheral chilling

The region of the heart affected by infarction is determined by the branch of the coronary arterial system which is occluded by the thrombus. Thrombosis in the left anterior descending branch leads to infarction in the anterior wall of the left ventricle and the anterior part of the cardiac septum. Thrombosis in the circumflex branch of the left coronary artery leads to infarction in the lateral wall of the left ventricle and part of the right ventricle. If the main branch of the left coronary artery is occluded this will prevent blood entering the anterior descending and circumflex branches. This will therefore result in a massive anterior and lateral infarction of the left ventricle. Thrombosis in the right coronary artery affects the lower posterior wall of the left ventricle, the posterior part of the septum and part of the right ventricle. This is because the right coronary artery curls around the back of the heart to supply blood to these areas. Because the lower areas of the myocardium are affected by occlusion of the right coronary artery the infarct is often described as an inferior MI.

Clinical features

Acute myocardial infarction (AMI) typically presents with the sudden onset of severe chest pain which may also be felt in the usual myocardial referred sites as illustrated below. Pain in AMI is often described using the following words; crushing, tight, constricting, heavy, 'like a weight on the chest'. AMI pain is not relieved by GTN and does not pass off with rest, as it does with stable angina pain. AMI causes very severe pain and should be treated with intravenous diamorphine or morphine as an emergency. Pain and anxiety stimulate the sympathetic nervous system leading to peripheral vasoconstriction and sweating. This is why these patients are usually pale, cold and clammy. Sympathetic stimulation can also give rise to tachycardia. Nausea, vomiting and breathlessness are other features. Anxiety is often severe, with a feeling of 'impending doom'. Impaired myocardial function may give rise to hypotension and shock may develop. In the days after MI a low grade fever often occurs as a result of pyrogens

ST elevation

being released from necrotic myocardial tissue. STEMI is diagnosed using three criteria; the clinical presentation discussed above, presence of evolving ECG changes and the detection of cardiac markers in the blood. *No symptoms shown*

Despite the above typical severe clinical features, a minority of myocardial infarcts are described as being 'clinically silent' and are not reported by the patient. These infarcts are only identified later by an ECG, blood tests for cardiac markers or at post mortem. Such silent infarcts are more common in the elderly and diabetics where there may be some sensory neuropathy. Also after cardiac transplantation the heart is not connected to the nervous system of the recipient. This means the patient cannot feel pain from the donated heart should an infarct develop. — *Post transplant - no pain felt in heart as nerves not connected.*

(handwritten left margin: biomarkers used to assess heart function: also called cardiac enzymes.)

(handwritten right margin: if infarct sensory nervous system.)

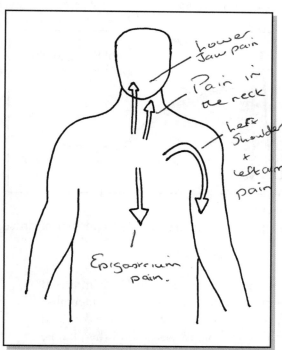

(handwritten diagram labels: Lower Jaw pain; Pain in the neck; Left Shoulder + Left arm pain; Epigastrium pain.)

Diagram 9.5
Myocardial pain caused by angina or infarction has frequently seen patterns of distribution. Pain is reported in the neck, lower jaw and even lower teeth. It may go down to the epigastrium or into the left shoulder and arm; it is rare for pain to be referred to the right shoulder or arm. Most patients suffer some chest pain, but pain is often felt at one or more of these referred sites. Sometimes pain is only felt at one of the referred sites. Pain in any of these areas should arouse suspicion. If in doubt, perform a 12 lead ECG; this is a safe non-invasive procedure. This myocardial distribution of pain is the same for angina and infarction, however in myocardial infarction the pain does not pass off with rest as in exertional angina.

(handwritten: Perform if one. Site of pain is identified.)

ECG changes in STEMI

After an ST elevation myocardial infarction, the ECG changes progressively over a few days. After a few minutes there is ST segment elevation which persists for a day or so. ST elevation occurs as a result of the occluded blood supply and the myocardial injury present in the acute stages of an STEMI and is usually fairly pronounced. Also in a full-thickness transmural infarct, the Q waves will widen and deepen. These changes are most useful for diagnostic purposes and are usually obvious by the time a patient is admitted to hospital. Infarcts that occurred months or years before can often be recognized by the presence of abnormal Q waves which persist after the ST changes have returned to normal.

(handwritten right margin: Widening of the Q wave. Q wave.)

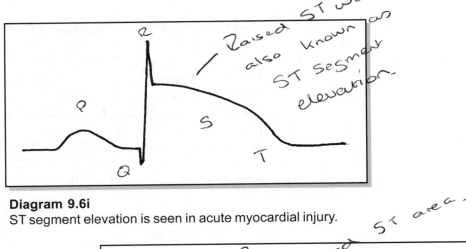

Diagram 9.6i
ST segment elevation is seen in acute myocardial injury.

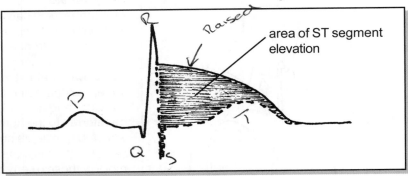

area of ST segment
elevation

Diagram 9.6ii
The same area of ST segment elevation compared to the normal trace.

Cardiac markers

As myocardial cells become progressively hypoxic or necrosed in an infarcted area, their surrounding cell membranes are no longer able to compartmentalise the cytoplasm. This means that chemicals such as enzymes, which were confined inside the cells when the cells were healthy, are able to escape into the plasma. If blood is analysed for increased levels of these markers, then myocardial cell injury and necrosis can be deduced. ⎯Troponins tested by blood test.

Chemicals called troponins are released from damaged myocardium and may be detected in the blood 4-6 hours (or sooner with sophisticated equipment) after high risk unstable angina or AMI. Raised levels of troponins may persist for up to 2 weeks. Cardiac specific troponins are only released by damaged myocardium which makes this test useful and accurate. The most common form of troponin measured clinically is troponin type T, but type I may also be used. Increasing levels of troponin will be released in high risk unstable angina, NSTEMI and STEMI. As higher levels of serum troponin are released by greater volumes of damaged myocardium, increasing levels are a marker for increasing severity of the condition.

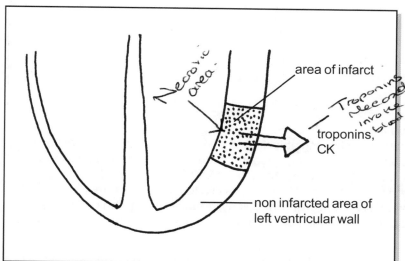

area of infarct

Necrotic area.

Troponins leecond invoke blood

troponins, CK

non infarcted area of left ventricular wall

Diagram 9.7
CK (creatine kinase) and cardiac specific troponins are released into the circulation from a necrotic area of myocardium. These act as 'markers' for myocardial damage.

Complications following MI

Aaure Myocardial Infarction

Dysrhythmias

AMI may lead to dysrhythmias. These are abnormalities of the normal cardiac rhythm which occur as a result of myocardial damage. Dying and dead myocardial cells are no longer able to generate normal electrical activity and so will not function normally. Any changes in heart rhythm can be readily seen using continuous ECG monitoring. As some dysrhythmias are immediately life threatening early detection is vital. For example, ventricular fibrillation is most likely to occur in the immediate time after an MI has occurred, with the first hour being the most dangerous time. About 10-50% of patients who suffer AMI may suffer from VF in the first few hours after infarction. If ventricular fibrillation is not treated with defibrillation, death will follow in a few minutes. Early professional help with full resuscitation facilities therefore improves the prognosis significantly. Another relatively common dysrhythmia is atrial fibrillation (AF). This is caused by an abnormal electrical focus in the atria which may have been caused by infarction, ischaemia or pericarditis. AF significantly increases the probability of thrombus formation in the atria. Other possible dysrhythmias after MI include ventricular tachycardia, sinus bradycardia and heart block.

Conduction disorders

The electrical stimulus for cardiac contraction originates in the sinoatrial (SA) node (or pacemaker). From here, specialised conducting tissues spread the impulse through the atria, atrioventricular (AV) node, bundle of His (also called the AV bundle), right and left bundle branches and Purkinje fibres. If any part of this pathway is infarcted the electrical stimulus will be blocked as an impulse

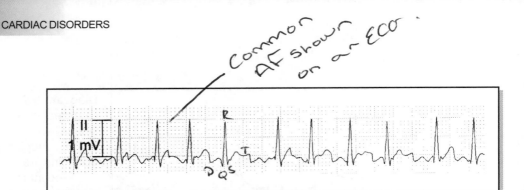

Common AF shown on an ECG

Diagram 9.8

A three lead ECG showing atrial fibrillation. The rate of atrial contraction is high resulting in a completely uncoordinated twitching of the atria. Some impulses are able to descend through the atrioventricular node to the ventricles, but most do not. This results in a totally irregular response by the ventricular myocardium giving irregularly irregular contractions and QRS complexes. The pulse will have a corresponding irregular rate and volume.

cannot be transmitted through dead tissue. Clinically this pathology gives rise to heart block. Varying severities of heart block are recognised and they may be of long or short duration. More serious cases may require an electrical pacemaker to be fitted on a temporary or permanent basis.

Acute left ventricular failure

This is a serious complication that usually indicates a significant part of the left ventricular myocardium has been devitalised. As the left ventricle is not working properly it is not able to pump out blood efficiently. This means blood is left in the heart after contraction which in turn prevents blood draining freely into the heart from the 4 large pulmonary veins. This leads to pulmonary venous congestion, which dams back into the capillaries, leading to increased hydrostatic pressure. This increased hydrostatic pressure in the pulmonary capillaries prevents tissue fluid reabsorption, leaving more free fluid in the lung tissue. In other words LVF causes pulmonary oedema. Patients complain of shortness of breath, especially when lying down and in severe cases there may be pink frothy sputum. Patients should be managed sitting up to reduce pulmonary congestion. LVF should be treated by improving ventricular function as much as possible. Diuretics will usually be given to reduce the total volume of water in the body. Oxygen should be given at high concentrations and CPAP (continuous positive airway pressure) may be helpful.

Cardiogenic shock

In this severe complication the heart is unable to generate enough force to maintain blood pressure. This results in reduced tissue perfusion and oxygenation. Cardiogenic shock is a form of severe heart failure and is associated with a high mortality. This complication tends to develop soon after infarction and indicates that 40% or more of the left ventricle has been lost.

Pericarditis

A transmural infarct involving the epicardium may also lead to inflammation of the pericardium; the inflamed pericardium causes chest pain which is often sharp and made worse with respiration. Pericardial pain often responds well to paracetamol rather than opioids.

Ventricular rupture

Death of myocardial tissue that extends from the endocardium to the epicardium as a result of a myocardial infarction

This complication is most likely to occur between the first and fourth day after a transmural infarct, at the time when the damaged ventricular wall is weakest. During this time the infarct is composed of soft, necrotic tissue which may give way, resulting in massive haemorrhage through the ventricular wall. Haemorrhage through the ventricular wall will cause blood to accumulate in the pericardial sac. This will compress the heart causing the condition of pericardial tamponade and may lead to death. It is still possible that ventricular rupture may occur at any time in the first 3 weeks after AMI, however after this time the necrotic tissue will have been replaced by collagen rich fibrous tissue which acts as a 'patch', making rupture less likely. Rupture may also occur through the intraventricular septum causing a ventral septal defect. This will allow a communication between the left and right ventricles leading to combined ventricular failure.

Ventricular aneurysm

CHF

Left ventricular aneurysm may present as a later complication after transmural infarcts. The weakened wall of the ventricle bulges out with every cardiac contraction. As part of the ventricular wall bulges (or balloons) out with every contraction there is reduced efficiency of cardiac contraction and output causing chronic heart failure. Electrical abnormalities associated with the weakened area also make ventricular tachycardia more probable. This condition gives rise to persistent ST elevation and is usually obvious using echocardiography. Mural thrombosis is also associated with ventricular aneurysm.

Mural thrombosis

A mural thrombus is a blood clot which forms overlying an infarcted area of endocardium within the ventricle. After infarction, inflammation of the endocardium promotes platelet deposition and clot formation. Emboli may detach from a mural thrombosis and enter the systemic circulation. Such emboli may cause strokes, MI and infarcts of other organs such as the gastrointestinal tract or kidneys. The lower limbs may also be affected causing acute lower limb ischaemia. Prevention of mural thrombosis is one reason why antiplatelet medication such as aspirin should be taken after MI.

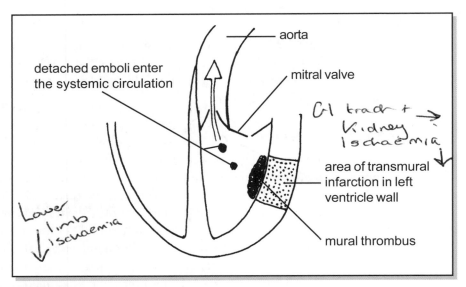

Diagram 9.9 labels: aorta; detached emboli enter the systemic circulation; mitral valve; GI tract + Kidney ischaemia; area of transmural infarction in left ventricle wall; mural thrombus; Lower limb ischaemia

Diagram 9.9
A mural thrombus has developed overlying an infarcted area of myocardium and endocardium. Emboli from a mural thrombus can break off, and be carried in the flow of blood as it passes through the left ventricle and out of the aorta. From here the emboli may lead to occlusion of a systemic artery, e.g. if emboli lodge in a cerebral artery a stroke will be caused.

Infarct of a papillary muscle

An infarct affecting a papillary muscle will cause death of part of that muscle. This dead muscle will eventually snap, leading to rupture of the papillary muscle. In normal physiology, contraction of papillary muscles causes tight closure of the atrioventricular valves. As the left side of the heart is most commonly involved in MI, rupture of a left ventricular papillary muscle will lead to sudden onset of mitral incompetence. This will mean that when the left ventricle contracts, blood will be pumped back through the incompetent mitral valve, causing acute mitral regurgitation. This will greatly reduce the efficiency of the left ventricle and will present with acute heart failure and pulmonary oedema; this may be severe and lead to a rapid death.

Management principles in MI

Patients who are suspected of suffering AMI should be given 300 mg of aspirin to chew. If the aspirin is left in the mouth it will be absorbed more rapidly than if the drug is swallowed. This is because the absorbed aspirin does not need to pass through the hepatic portal circulation and liver before reaching the systemic circulation. Aspirin has some independent benefit and also increases the effectiveness of subsequent thrombolysis. Adequate oxygen saturations should be maintained to maximize oxygenation of the myocardium. Intravenous access must be established for analgesia and any other drugs which may need to be given. Bloods are taken for cardiac markers.

Cardiac Troponins and Enzymes

A 12 lead ECG should be carried out immediately. If this shows ST elevation then primary percutaneous coronary intervention (PCI) should be immediately considered if available. PCI carries a good prognosis after AMI as it removes the blockage within the coronary artery and restores blood flow to the previously infarcted area of myocardium. If PCI is not available or appropriate the patient should be screened to see if they have any contraindications to thrombolysis. If there are no contraindications this should be given intravenously as soon as safely possible. Thrombolysis is the process of lysing or breaking down the thrombus. Patients receiving thrombolysis must be monitored very closely for signs of hypotension, allergic reactions, haemorrhage and stroke.

Both of these reperfusion therapies allow restoration of the blood supply to a previously infarcted area of myocardium. Removing or dissolving the thrombus means that a coronary thrombosis causes much less myocardial damage than would be the case without treatment. In both forms of reperfusion therapy time is of the essence. Giving reperfusion therapy as soon after diagnosis as possible is more important than the form of therapy used. *1/2mg via IV*

Adequate analgesia must be given; intravenous diamorphine or morphine are used combined with a suitable antiemetic such as metoclopramide. Other drugs such as beta-blockers and nitrates may also be indicated. During the first *Constant* 48 hours after AMI there is a risk of cardiac arrest, most of which are caused by *monitors* ventricular fibrillation. This is why patients should be monitored on a coronary care unit for this time period with defibrillation facilities to hand. Most centres start gradual mobilisation on the second day. Advice should be given on treatment and management of arterial disease risk factors, preferably by a specialised cardiac rehabilitation nurse; this will include management of diabetes, hypertension, diet, smoking cessation and the benefits of early mobilisation. Patients must also be taught the importance of good compliance with taking prescribed drugs such as aspirin and statins.

Cardiac failure

This is a common and serious condition which becomes more prevalent with increasing age. *heart working some Faster causes issues*

Aetiology

In Western countries the most common causes of heart failure are hypertension and coronary heart disease. Hypertension may cause heart failure as the heart must work harder in order to discharge blood into the pressurised arterial circulation. Angina or infarction will decrease the pumping efficiency of the myocardium leading to reduced cardiac output. Disorders of the heart valves may also lead to a reduced pumping efficiency of the heart. The normal function of valves is to ensure a one way flow of blood around the heart, therefore failure of any valve will lead to some blood flowing in the reverse direction.

Disease of the heart muscle [handwritten annotation]

Blood flowing in the reverse direction within the heart due too valve weakness. [handwritten annotation]

This abnormal situation is called valvular regurgitation. Other possible aetiological factors in heart failure include excessive alcohol consumption, cardiomyopathy, dysrhythmias such as atrial fibrillation, narrowing (stenosis) of the aorta and constrictive pericarditis. In addition to these factors right heart failure may also be caused by acute or chronic lung diseases or pulmonary embolism.

inflammation of the pericardium [handwritten annotation]

Pathophysiology

In cardiac failure the heart is unable to maintain an adequate cardiac output despite there being sufficient venous return. In patients without valvular disease the primary pathology in cardiac failure is in the ventricular myocardium. Myocytes (myocardial cells) initially enlarge in the process of hypertrophy but eventually there will be progressive myocyte death with areas of focal myocardial necrosis. This leads to reduced contractility of the ventricles and a fall in cardiac output.

ischaemia [handwritten annotation]

In the early stages of heart failure, compensation mechanisms are able to maintain cardiac output and tissue perfusion. Increase in heart rate can maintain cardiac output for some time despite reduced stroke volumes. This is because cardiac output is determined by heart rate multiplied by stroke volume. However, as the condition develops, this mechanism is no longer able to compensate and cardiac output drops.

Starling's law of the heart (sometimes called the Frank-Starling reflex) also maintains cardiac output for a time. Starling's law states that the degree of myocardial contraction during systole is determined by the degree of myocardial stretching during diastole. In health, this law means that cardiac output is always equal to venous return. As cardiac failure develops the volume of blood pumped out per contraction is reduced, leaving larger residual volumes of blood in the ventricle than normal. This residual blood contributes to myocardial stretching, which therefore generates increased myocardial contraction, an effect which will increase stroke volume and so cardiac output. However, as cardiac failure progresses, the failing myocardium is no longer able to obey Starling's law and stroke volume will drop.

In order to maintain tissue perfusion in cardiac failure there is a reactionary peripheral vasoconstriction. This mechanism increases blood pressure and so maintains tissue perfusion. This is explained by the fact that blood pressure equals cardiac output multiplied by peripheral resistance. However, peripheral vasoconstriction increases the outflow resistance (or afterload) the heart must work against, increasing ventricular workload. Over time this increased workload contributes to ventricular hypertrophy and the development of cardiac failure. As cardiac output falls there will be reduced perfusion of the kidneys. This causes activation of the renin-angiotensin mechanism, leading to the formation of angiotensin II which will also cause constriction of the systemic arterioles, also increasing afterload, ventricular workload and blood pressure.

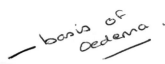
— basis of
oedema.

Fluid overload in the venous system is made worse by the activation of the renin-angiotensin-aldosterone mechanism. This leads to the retention of more salt and water which increases blood volume and venous return (or cardiac preload), which in turn increases cardiac workload, as the myocardium attempts to obey Starling's law.

Over time these effects lead to myocardial cell (myocyte) damage, failure and decreased cardiac output. As in the other mechanisms discussed in this section, this leads to a vicious circle of progressive cardiac failure.

Left and right ventricular failure

In practice, cardiac failure usually presents with involvement of the right and the left ventricles. This can partly be explained by the underlying causative pathology. For example, coronary arterial disease may lead to ischaemia of the right and left ventricular areas of the myocardium. Also LVF will lead to RVF and vice versa. For example, LVF will cause a damming back of blood into the lungs which will reduce the volume of blood which can pass through the lungs. This will lead to less blood being able to enter the lungs and so increase pulmonary arterial pressure and right ventricular workload. Chronic increase in right ventricular workload will lead to hypertrophy and RVF.

Clinical features of LVF

Patients often complain of tiredness, listlessness and fatigue. Fatigue can be explained by the reduced perfusion of skeletal muscles with oxygen and nutrient carrying blood. Feelings of tiredness can result from reduced perfusion of the brain. Exercise tolerance is also reduced, with patients becoming short of breath on exercise, (also described as exertional dyspnoea). Even if a patient with cardiac failure is not short of breath at rest, the heart has little or no ability to increase output during exercise. This will greatly reduce the ability of the circulatory system to supply oxygen and remove carbon dioxide from the tissues. As a result exercise will cause CO_2 levels to rise and O_2 levels to fall rapidly.

As the failing left ventricle is no longer able to pump out blood efficiently, the volumes of blood returning to the left atrium via the pulmonary veins can no longer pass through the heart efficiently. This results in damming back of blood into the pulmonary veins which increases the pressure within the pulmonary capillaries. This reduces the reabsorption of tissue fluid from the lungs, leading to pulmonary oedema and subsequent dyspnoea. This difficulty in breathing is worse when lying down, a feature referred to as orthopnoea. When a patient with cardiac failure is lying down, the pulmonary oedema is able to spread throughout the lung fields. Clearly if there is fluid in the alveoli, air will not be able to enter and dyspnoea will result. However, when the patient is managed sitting up or leaning forward on a bed table, the oedematous fluid will fall by gravity to the bases of the lungs, allowing effective air entry and

175

Orthopnic position

therefore relieving dyspnoea. Fluid overload also leads to a moderate increase in the jugular venous pressure (JVP) and to some leg and ankle oedema.

On a chest X-ray the heart can be seen to be enlarged as a result of the ventricular hypertrophy, a condition termed cardiomegaly. Pulmonary blood vessels can be seen to be dilated and in more advanced cases basal pulmonary oedema can be seen as hazy white areas.

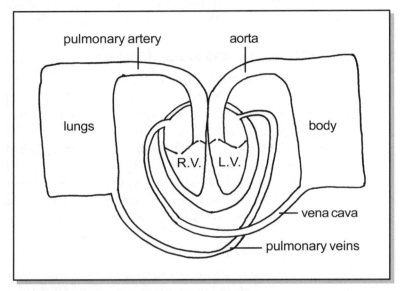

Diagram 9.10

LVF will initially lead to congestion of the pulmonary circulation with blood, resulting in pulmonary oedema. RVF will initially lead to congestion of the systemic venous circulation leading to congestion of the organs and limbs with blood. This is why cardiac failure is sometimes referred to as congestive cardiac failure (CCF). Reduced ventricular function leads to congestion of the venous system with increased volumes of blood; in essence the heart becomes a 'bottle neck' for the circulatory system.

This diagram illustrates the circulatory system as an integrated whole. From this it can be seen that reduced left ventricular function will cause congestion of the pulmonary veins while right ventricular failure will congest the systemic veins which drain blood from the body.

Treatment principles in cardiac failure

When patients are relatively well, endurance exercise should be encouraged, such as walking for 20-30 minutes, several times per week. However, during exacerbations, bed rest reduces cardiac workload and is useful. Any underlying contributory conditions should be treated, such as hypertension, diabetes mellitus or hypercholesterolaemia. Patients must not smoke and should not drink alcohol as this will depress myocardial function. If patients are overweight this should be addressed. Small meals also reduce the metabolic demand of the gastrointestinal tract and so the volumes of blood needed to perfuse the gut. Salt restriction is important as increases in plasma sodium concentration will lead to an increase in the volume of water in the plasma, increasing overall blood volume. If blood volume rises, the levels of venous congestion and cardiac preload will also increase.

Diuretic drugs increase the volumes of water excreted from the body and so reduce blood volume. This reduces venous return and cardiac preload which in turn reduces cardiac workload. Diuretics reduce peripheral oedema making the patients feel less bloated; they also reduce pulmonary oedema, which reduces dyspnoea. Some diuretics cause increased potassium excretion, explaining why potassium supplements may be required. The use of angiotensin-converting enzyme (ACE) inhibitors has greatly advanced the management of moderate and severe heart failure. ACE inhibitors work by preventing the conversion of angiotensin I into angiotensin II. This means there is less angiotensin II to cause release of aldosterone, as a consequence of this less sodium and water are reabsorbed by the kidney, so the volumes of sodium and water in the blood

Ace inhibitors prevent Angiotensin I turning to Angiotensin 2,

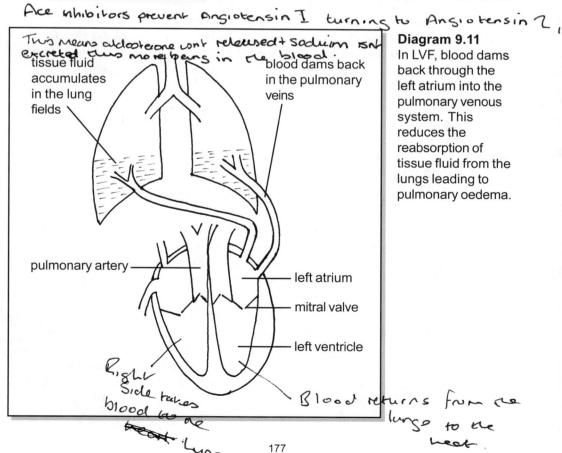

This means aldosterone won't released + Sodium isn't excreted thus more pens in the blood.

tissue fluid accumulates in the lung fields

blood dams back in the pulmonary veins

Diagram 9.11
In LVF, blood dams back through the left atrium into the pulmonary venous system. This reduces the reabsorption of tissue fluid from the lungs leading to pulmonary oedema.

pulmonary artery

left atrium

mitral valve

left ventricle

Right Side takes blood to the lungs.

Blood returns from the lungs to the heart.

will be reduced. This effect will reduce cardiac preload. Also less angiotensin II means there will be less constriction of the arterioles, an effect which will reduce afterload. Other useful drugs in cardiac failure include digoxin and some beta blockers.

Pulmonary heart disease

This is also termed cor pulmonale and describes right-sided heart disease which is caused by pulmonary arterial hypertension. Right ventricular failure therefore develops as a consequence of an underlying lung disease. The disorder may have an acute or chronic presentation.

Acute pulmonary heart disease (acute cor pulmonale)
Pathophysiology

Most acute cases are caused by pulmonary emboli (PE) which originate from a thrombus in a systemic vein. Less commonly, emboli may originate from the right side of the heart. An embolus lodges in a branch of the pulmonary artery and cuts off a section of the pulmonary blood supply. This means there is ventilation but no perfusion of the affected area of lung. After a few hours, non-infused areas of lung will collapse. As an embolus reduces the total cross sectional area of pulmonary arterial bed, the total resistance to blood flow is increased and this leads to pulmonary arterial hypertension. ↳Blockage causes BP to rise as pressure increases

As the lumen of the pulmonary artery is effectively reduced, the volume of blood the heart is able to pump out is also reduced. In other words there will be a reduction in right ventricular output. This is analogous to a car crash obstructing one or two lanes of a motorway; the number of cars which can filter past the obstruction is reduced. Reduced Cardiac output →Could Lead to cardiogenic Shock.

Clinical features

Sudden onset of dyspnoea with tachypnoea (rapid respirations) are the most common presentations of PE, tachycardia is also likely to be present. In some patients pleuritic chest pain and haemoptysis may also present. Clinical features of a deep venous thrombosis (DVT) are often not observed; this may be because emboli originated from the pelvic or abdominal veins. Fever may present; this can be explained by the release of pyrogens from damaged cells which comprise a component of the clot, or from the lung tissues which are deprived of their normal blood supply. DVT and PE are therefore non-infective causes of pyrexia.

A massive pulmonary embolism will cause immediate shock. This is because Cardiogenic Shock, lack of tissue perfusion blood is unable to pass through the lungs, so the venous return to the left atrium is massively reduced. This in turn will reduce left ventricular output leading to a fall in cardiac output and a consequent drop in systemic blood pressure. As there is an acute obstruction of the circulatory system, blood will not be able to return from the large systemic veins into the right atrium. This will be seen as an acute increase in jugular venous pressure (JVP), as the jugular veins become congested with blood, they will stand out on the side of the neck.

A massive PE is also likely to cause acute chest pain. This is explained by the fall in left ventricular output reducing perfusion pressure in the coronary arteries which supply blood to the myocardium. This leads to ischaemia, hypoxia and pain in the same way as myocardial hypoperfusion in angina.

A third possible presentation of acute cor pulmonale is progressive development of breathlessness over several weeks. This may be complicated by some chest pain from angina and syncope caused by exertion. This presentation can be explained via the mechanism of pulmonary hypertension caused by numerous small PEs.

Treatment principles

Oxygen should be given at high flow rates to saturate the blood which is still able to circulate. If possible oxygen saturations above 94% should be maintained. Low molecular weight heparin given subcutaneously in now known to be as effective as giving intravenous unfractionated heparin. Heparin is a fast acting anticoagulant which should prevent thrombi or emboli getting any bigger and should be given immediately. After the acute phase, this can be replaced with oral anticoagulants to prevent recurrence. Thrombolytic therapy may be given to break up any clots which are in the circulatory system. However, because of the possible dangers of dissolving blood clots this therapy should be reserved for more severe cases. Sometimes surgery may be used to remove thrombi or emboli. Various investigations may be ordered such as ultrasound, D-dimer, blood gas analysis, pulmonary angiography and a ventilation/perfusion (V/Q) scan.

Chronic pulmonary heart disease (chronic cor pulmonale)

Background physiology

Pulmonary arteries are able to dilate and constrict to regulate the volumes of blood which flow through particular areas of the lungs. This regulation of vasotone, and hence blood supply, is largely controlled by how much oxygen an area of lung receives. If part of the lung is well oxygenated, the blood supply to that area will increase to maximise the volumes of oxygen which can be absorbed. However, if oxygenation of an area of lung is poor, for example due to a localised infection, then there is no point perfusing that area with a lot of blood as there is no oxygen to pick up. In most circumstances this mechanism maximises the efficiency with which pulmonary blood flow is able to oxygenate the blood. However, if the entire lung is chronically poorly oxygenated, then there will be a global vasoconstriction of the branches of the pulmonary artery. This will lead to increased resistance and so increased pulmonary arterial pressure.

Pathophysiology

In chronic lung disease, such as that caused by COPD, fresh air is unable to efficiently enter and leave the alveoli resulting in reduced oxygen concentrations. In addition to reducing the levels of oxygen in the alveoli, there will be an increase in the concentration of CO_2 leading to areas of localised pulmonary acidosis. These factors cause localised reactionary vasoconstriction in branches of the pulmonary artery. This increases resistance to blood flow and so raises pulmonary arterial pressure. As the resistance offered by the pulmonary arterial system is increased, the right ventricle is obliged to pump harder in order to perfuse the lungs. In other words right ventricular work load is increased as a result of increased afterload. When the workload of a muscle is increased, over time it will enlarge. This is called hypertrophy. So in chronic lung disease right ventricular hypertrophy will develop. This will cause the heart to enlarge causing cardiomegaly. When muscle reaches a particular degree of hypertrophy, it is no longer able to contract efficiently and starts to fail. This causes right ventricular failure.

A reduction in right ventricular output means the ventricle is not able to pump out as much blood as it normally would. This means the right atrium is not able to pass as much blood through to the right ventricle as normal, leading to atrial congestion. As the right atria is congested, blood returning from the systemic veins is not able to flow into the heart as normal, which means the systemic veins become congested with blood, resulting in increased systemic venous pressure. This process dams back all the way to the systemic capillaries. When the pressure in the venous ends of systemic capillaries is increased tissue fluid reabsorption is inhibited and systemic oedema will develop, giving the patient a 'bloated' appearance. This process of congestion also affects the major organs, reducing their levels of efficiency.

Clinical features

Patients with chronic pulmonary heart disease (cor pulmonale) often feel tired; they become short of breath on exercise and may suffer chest pain. Many features develop as a result of the chronic systemic venous congestion, preventing the normal free flowing venous drainage of blood. As blood cannot flow freely from the jugular veins in the neck, back into the superior vena cava, the jugular venous pressure will be raised resulting in dilation. Inhibited return of blood from the lower limbs, into the inferior vena cava, will result in ankle and lower leg oedema which may be marked. Hepatomegaly (liver enlargement) develops as a result of chronic congestion of the liver with venous blood. Ascites (free fluid in the peritoneal cavity) is also possible as there is congestion of the mesenteric veins. Chest X-ray may show an enlarged heart as a result of the ventricular hypertrophy. Echocardiography will also demonstrate right ventricular dilation and hypertrophy.

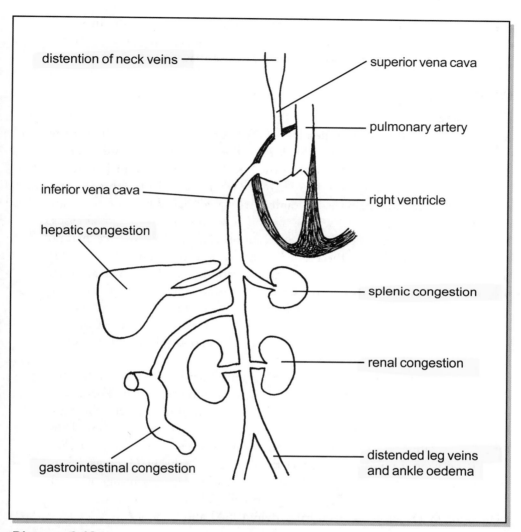

Diagram 9.12

Right ventricular failure will lead to congestion of the major organs with blood. Congestion in the inferior vena cava will dam back affecting the liver, spleen, gut, kidneys and lower limbs. Also increased jugular venous pressure will be seen on examination.

Management principles

Any primary pathology such as COPD should be corrected as far as possible. Diuretics may be given to reduce the volumes of water in the blood; this will reduce blood volume and so reduce the severity of the congestion. Long term oxygen therapy may help any underlying COPD and increase lung oxygenation. If lung oxygenation can be increased, the pulmonary arteries will dilate, reducing the degree of pulmonary hypertension and so reducing right ventricular workload. Warfarin may be used as an anticoagulant as it reduces the risk of venous thromboembolism and has been shown to improve the prognosis in severe cases. Unfortunately the overall prognosis in pulmonary hypertension is not good and sudden death may occur as a result of cardiac arrest.

Cardiac arrest

Diagnosis

In a cardiac arrest there is a sudden loss of cardiac output as a result of an acute cardiac event. The criteria recommended for the recognition of cardiac arrest are published by national bodies such as the UK Resuscitation Council. Current advice is that cardiac arrest should be diagnosed when the patient is unresponsive after a gentle shake and being asked loudly 'Are you all right?' It is also necessary to assess their breathing; this will be absent or feature so called agonal gasps. Loss of consciousness in a cardiac arrest is simply explained by the fact than no oxygen is being supplied to the brain as there is no cardiac output to provide cerebral circulation. Absent or abnormal respirations can also be explained by the lack of perfusion and oxygenation of the respiratory centres of the brain stem. In a cardiac arrest there will be no pulse as there is no cardiac output. Current guidelines for the diagnosis of cardiac arrest do not insist on this examination for signs of circulation; however it is a good skill for professionals to learn.

Before concluding the pulse is absent a central artery, such as the carotid, should be palpated for five to ten seconds with nothing being felt. This is why it is important to practice feeling central pulses in healthy subjects. We must be able to, quickly and reliably, put our fingers on the correct anatomical site for pulse palpation. If we are feeling in the wrong place we may wrongly declare there is no central pulse when in fact there is. Use of the ECG allows for an accurate assessment of the type of cardiac arrest which is presenting, of which there are four basic forms. These are ventricular fibrillation (VF), ventricular tachycardia (VT), pulseless electrical activity (PEA) and asystole.

Ventricular fibrillation (VF)

In this condition there is rapid, uncoordinated, ineffective contraction of the myocardium resulting in loss of cardiac output and absence of a pulse. The ECG shows chaotic and irregular ventricular activity. The deflections are often initially pronounced and the fibrillation is described as coarse, over time, if untreated it will become finer. Onset is sudden and the patient will lose consciousness, usually within a few seconds. VF has various possible causes; myocardial infarction, ischaemia or severe hypoxia are the most common. An infarcted or ischaemic area of myocardium can become electrically unstable and start generating rapid and abnormal electrical impulses. A lack of oxygen delivery to the heart muscle will lead to myocardial hypoxia. This again can lead to embarrassed areas of myocardium which generate abnormal electrical activity. This is why ventricular fibrillation may complicate conditions causing severe hypoxia. Other causes of VF include electrocution, poisoning, severe electrolyte imbalance and hypothermia.

Ventricular tachycardia (VT)

Ventricular tachycardia occurs when there is an ectopic electrical focus in the ventricular muscle. VT may be associated with a pulse and therefore some cardiac output. If this is the case the patient may remain conscious. On other occasions there may be no palpable pulse, resulting in a loss of consciousness. Typically the heart rate in VT is around 150 beats per minute, but the heart is working very inefficiently. If the patient remains conscious this is not technically a cardiac arrest, however VT will often progress to VF.

Pulseless electrical activity (PEA)

In this condition the electrical activity of the heart is relatively normal. The impulse is generated and propagated along the usual pathways from the sinoatrial node. Myocardial cells depolarise, but the depolarisation is not associated with contraction as normal. In this situation the electrocardiograph (ECG) trace may appear normal, but not be related to myocardial contraction. PEA is therefore usually diagnosed clinically; the ECG looks normal, but there is no central pulse. As there is little or no cardiac output the patient will soon become unconscious. There are numerous possible causes of PEA including: extensive myocardial infarction, acute hypovolaemia as might be caused by significant haemorrhage, cardiac tamponade, pulmonary embolism, hypothermia and tension pneumothorax. PEA used to be called electromechanical dissociation (EMD).

Asystole

Asystole is an absence of cardiac contractions. The heart is still, not generating any electrical activity or cardiac output at all. This may be caused by failure of the internal conducting system or massive ventricular damage after myocardial infarction. After a period of time all forms of untreated cardiac arrest will result in asystole. In fact all causes of death will ultimately lead to asystole.

Treatment of cardiac arrest

Many treatments have been employed to manage cardiac arrest over the years but the only interventions known to increase the probability of survival are cardiopulmonary resuscitation (CPR), oxygenation, defibrillation and for some indications adrenaline (epinephrine). The airway must be opened and basic life support (BLS) using CPR should be started as soon as the arrest is diagnosed. In CPR the heart is compressed between the sternum and thoracic vertebrae. This increases the pressure in the chambers of the heart and the valves ensure

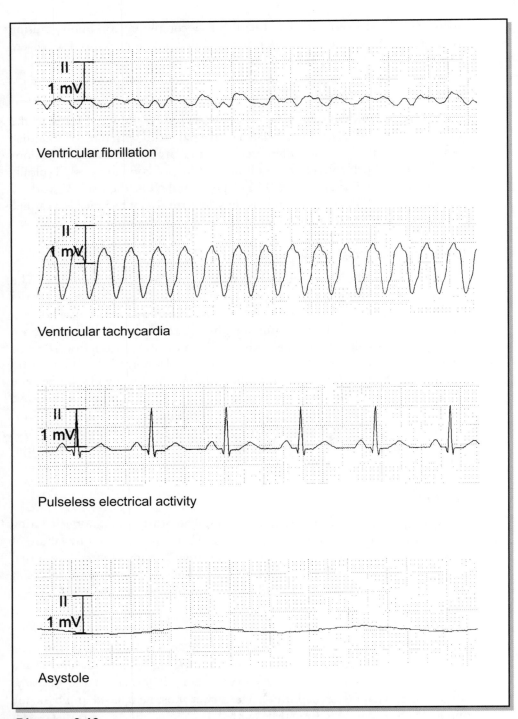

Diagram 9.13
Except in the case of PEA, the electrical activity of the heart reflects the movements of the myocardium.

the blood can only flow in a physiological direction. This will generate a cardiac output which can be felt as a central pulse. Air, or preferably oxygen, is blown into the lungs using positive pressure ventilation.

The arrest causing dysrhythmia should also be identified using the ECG. CPR does not restart the heart, but it does keep essential body organs perfused with blood and oxygen while advanced life support is arriving. Additional measures such as endotracheal intubation may be used to improve oxygenation. Good CPR using oxygen will also maintain the oxygenation of the myocardium itself, making subsequent defibrillation more likely to succeed. Defibrillation is indicated if the patient is pulseless, unconscious and when VF or VT is identified on the ECG. Defibrillation is the only effective treatment for ventricular fibrillation. In the UK resuscitation protocols are regularly updated and published by the Resuscitation Council.

CHAPTER 10

Hypertension

Introduction

Hypertension means an increase in blood pressure (BP); it affects up to 20% of the population in developed countries and is also common in developing countries. It is important to understand this topic as hypertension leads to a lot of pathology if unmanaged but when recognised it is usually eminently preventable or treatable.

Normal physiology

Blood pressure simply describes the pressure of blood on the vessel walls in which it is contained. The venous system is described as a low pressure system and the pressures generated by the right ventricle in the pulmonary arteries is usually about 25/8 mmHg. The term blood pressure as commonly used refers to systemic arterial pressure and this can be defined as cardiac output multiplied by systemic peripheral resistance. Cardiac output is the volume of blood pumped out by the left ventricle in a one minute period and is equal to heart rate multiplied by stroke volume (stroke volume is the volume of blood pumped out of the left ventricle per cardiac contraction). However, cardiac output and systemic peripheral resistance are both influenced by renal function and sodium homeostasis. Hypertension results from an imbalance between these factors.

Systolic blood pressure (SBP) is the highest pressure in the arterial system during cardiac contraction, i.e. during systole. Diastolic blood pressure (DBP) is the lowest pressure occurring in the systemic arteries during a cardiac cycle and occurs during diastole. Sixty percent of mean arterial pressure is determined by diastolic and 40% by systolic pressure. This is because arterial BP remains closer to the diastolic pressure than the systolic for more of the cardiac cycle.

Neuronal regulation of BP

Neuronal reflexes operate to regulate BP on a second by second basis. Pressure receptors, known as baroreceptors, are found in the arch of the aorta and in the carotid arteries. As BP in these arteries increases the baroreceptors are stimulated and generate nerve impulses which pass up sensory nerves to the medulla oblongata in the brain stem. In the brain stem these impulses inhibit the vasoconstrictor centre and stimulate the vagal parasympathetic centre. These effects lead to vasodilation of the arterial vessels (particularly the arterioles) and veins and reduction in heart rate and strength of cardiac contractions. Conversely, if the BP drops fewer impulses are generated by the baroreceptors resulting in vasoconstriction and increased cardiac output.

Renal regulation of BP

BP is partly determined by the volumes of water and salt the kidneys excrete or conserve. If salt and water are conserved blood volume will rise. This will result in increased volumes of venous return and so increase cardiac output. The kidneys also secrete renin which initiates the renin-angiotensin system. This is believed to be the dominant system regulating and determining systemic blood pressure.

When arterial pressure falls there is a consequent reduction in the perfusion pressure of the kidneys. This is detected within the afferent arterioles which then stimulate the adjacent granular juxtaglomerular (JG) cells, located close to the glomerulus, to release renin. Renin is an enzyme which acts on a plasma protein called angiotensinogen. Renin converts angiotensinogen into a small peptide sequence called angiotensin I. In the lungs there is a further enzyme called angiotensin converting enzyme (ACE) which converts the angiotensin I into a smaller peptide sequence called angiotensin II. This second form of angiotensin is a powerful vasoconstricting agent. As a result of this vasoconstriction there is increased peripheral resistance which increases blood pressure. Angiotensin II also stimulates the secretion of aldosterone which reduces the excretion of salt and water by the kidneys. This results in a progressive increase in blood volume and so blood pressure. Conversely, if systemic BP and hence renal perfusion pressures increase, less renin is secreted and so less angiotensinogen is converted into the active form. This will in turn allow peripheral vasodilation and increased excretion of salt and water by the kidneys.

Definition of hypertension

There is no clear agreement on what constitutes hypertension. The World Health Organisation has defined hypertension as a systolic BP over 160 mmHg and a diastolic BP above 90, or both. The International Society of Hypertension of the WHO goes on to define a systolic pressure of 130-139 mmHg and a diastolic of 85-89 mmHg as being 'high normal' BP. Others define hypertension as a consistent systolic of over 140 mmHg or a diastolic of over 90 mmHg. The British Hypertension Society considers an optimal BP to be a systolic of less than 120 and a diastolic of less than 80 mmHg. As the risk of hypertensive complications rises progressively with increasing systolic and diastolic pressures, perhaps the best definition of hypertension is 'that level of blood pressure above which investigation and treatment do more good than harm'.

Hypertension may be essential or secondary. In essential hypertension it is not possible to discover a cause of the problem, there is a primary elevation of BP. However, despite there being no clear cause, many factors are known to influence BP and some of these are open to modification. Conversely, acquired or secondary hypertension has an identifiable underlying disorder which causes the elevation in BP. Malignant or accelerated hypertension describes a rapid development of very high blood pressures associated with significant development of complications. Without treatment these patients have a short term high mortality from stroke, heart or renal failure.

Aetiology and prevention of essential hypertension

Genetic factors

A genetic factor is important in most cases of essential hypertension. No specific gene has been identified for essential hypertension and the genetic component is probably polygenic, i.e. caused by several different interacting genes. Children of hypertensive parents have an increased risk and hypertension tends to run in families. While this is likely to have a genetic explanation it is always worth considering that a family may have shared environmental risk factors.

Congenital factors

Low birth weight babies are more likely to become hypertensive as adults. This may be caused by fetal under nutrition affecting the development of the vascular system. This is sometimes referred to as the 'bad start' problem. Future cases of this problem can be reduced by good maternal nutrition and prenatal care.

Race

In Europe and the US hypertension is more common in people of African extraction compared to traditional European populations. It has been suggested that African populations, used to high temperatures and hence higher levels of sweating, have a 'salt thrifty gene' that allows them to conserve salt. This is supported by the observation that African people are generally more salt sensitive than European populations. In salt sensitive individuals blood pressure is increased when salt is eaten. This means it is particularly important for such high risk groups to eat less salt.

Obesity

Obese people generally have higher BPs than thin people and it is likely that obesity causes hypertension. Central obesity is a greater risk factor for hypertension than fat on the buttocks and legs. This may be because abdominal fat is more insulin resistant. This is why it is particularly important to advise people to have a relatively thin waist. If individuals who are obese lose weight, their blood pressure will be reduced.

Alcohol

Doses of alcohol over 21 units per week are associated with increased BP. All forms of alcoholic drinks may contribute to hypertension, with the systolic BP being affected more than the diastolic. BP readings are higher during a 'hangover' due to increased sympathetic activity. Reduction of alcohol intake should therefore be recommended. Some people may need to stop drinking altogether if they find it difficult to cut down. While small doses of alcohol may lower BP slightly we should not advise people to start drinking. In addition all alcohol consumption is calorific and so will contribute to obesity.

Sodium and potassium

Populations who have a high sodium intake have a tendency to have higher BP compared to low sodium consumers. While individual sensitivity to sodium varies, there are clear positive correlations between salt intake and systolic and diastolic BP. Many people in developed countries consume much more than the recommended maximum of 6g per day. Most dietary salt comes from processed and manufactured foods. It is unfortunate that food manufacturers add so much salt to many of their products. We should advise people to avoid manufactured foods with a high salt content. Also we should advise adding less salt to food in general. Once the palate becomes accustomed to low salt content foods they taste just as good. Conversely, high potassium intake will slightly lower BP. This seems partly to be due to a direct effect of the potassium but also because high potassium intake encourages sodium excretion. Fruit and tea are both sources of potassium.

Physical inactivity

Lack of physical exercise leads to increases in BP. People who are physically active have relatively lower BPs than their more sedentary counterparts. Exercise is also a factor in the prevention and correction of obesity. People should be advised to take regular aerobic exercise up to their individual advisable levels. Physical inactivity also contributes to the development of metabolic syndrome.

Metabolic (insulin resistance) syndrome

Metabolic syndrome (also called insulin resistance syndrome) is a collection of metabolic risk factors which promote the development of atherosclerosis with subsequent cardiovascular and cerebrovascular disease. Dyslipidaemia, hypertension, central (abdominal) obesity and hyperglycaemia caused by insulin resistance are the most widely recognised components of the syndrome. While it is unclear exactly how one component of metabolic syndrome inter-relates with the others, it is generally agreed that the underlying causative problems are central obesity and insulin resistance. One possible mechanism is that insulin resistance leads to hyperglycaemia which in turn stimulates hyperinsulinaemia. It is possible that high insulin levels stimulate the sympathetic nervous system in an attempt to use up excess glucose present in the blood. While this increased sympathetic activity will increase metabolic demand it also increases blood pressure, probably by stimulating vasoconstriction.

Smoking

Smokers typically have a slightly lower BP than average when they are not smoking, however when they are smoking BP is increased. This means in heavy smokers the BP may be increased for much of the day. Also hypertensive patients who smoke are more likely to develop accelerated or malignant hypertension in comparison to their non-smoking counterparts. Smoking is also a synergistic risk factor for ischaemic heart disease in the presence of hypertension, diabetes mellitus or hypercholesterolaemia. Clearly it is important for hypertensive patients not to smoke.

Psychological stress

It is certainly true that acute pain, anxiety or stress can significantly increase BP in the short term. However, there is very little evidence to suggest that psychological stress leads to the development of essential hypertension.

Other factors

It is normal for BP to fall during the night when a person sleeps. It may be that failure of the BP to fall overnight is a significant factor in the development of end organ complications. Oral contraceptive drugs may cause a mild increase in BP and in some predisposed women may cause a more significant increase. The prevalence of hypertension generally increases with age.

Acquired or secondary hypertension

There are several conditions which may cause hypertension as a secondary effect and it is important to identify these if present as they may be treatable. Most cases of secondary hypertension are caused by renal disease such as chronic glomerulonephritis, diabetic nephropathy or adult polycystic kidney disease. Initially the hypertension is typically caused by activation of the renin-angiotensin mechanism. Later, if renal function declines the kidney will no longer effectively excrete water and salt leading to their retention in the blood. This retention of sodium chloride and water will increase the blood volume leading to hypertension.

Renal arterial stenosis will reduce the blood supply to the kidneys; this will stimulate the release of renin resulting in hypertension. There are two forms of the stenosis. Firstly it may be caused by an accumulation of disorganised fibrous material in the walls of the renal arteries. This occurs in young patients, particularly tall white females. The second form of the problem occurs as a result of atheroma accumulation reducing the lumen of the renal arteries. This usually presents in middle aged smokers who often have evidence of generalised atherosclerosis. Renal arterial stenosis is an important cause of accelerated hypertension.

Other less common secondary causes of hypertension include increased levels of hormone secretion by the adrenal cortex. Primary elevation of aldosterone and Cushing syndrome both promote the retention of salt and water by the kidneys and therefore lead to increased blood volumes and hypertension. Pheochromocytoma describes a tumour affecting the adrenal medulla which secretes the catecholamines epinephrine and norepinephrine. Release of these may be paroxysmal leading to episodes of hypertension, headache, palpitations and sweating. Other patients with pheochromocytoma have sustained hypertension.

Coarctation of the aorta refers to a narrowing which results in a reduced blood flow to the kidneys and lower parts of the body. Hypertension may be caused partly by the increased resistance and partly by renal hypoperfusion leading to increased renin secretion. Other secondary causes of hypertension include hyperthyroidism and renin secreting tumours. Severe atherosclerosis may cause elevation of systolic BP as the sclerotic, hardened arteries cannot dilate to absorb the energy of the pulse wave.

Hypertension and pregnancy

Hypertension may develop in the second half of pregnancy. If this is associated with proteinuria and oedema it becomes pre-eclampsia. This should be closely monitored as it may lead on to eclampsia with severe hypertension, convulsions, cerebral and pulmonary oedema and coma. Once the baby is delivered the condition will resolve.

Clinical features of hypertension

It is important to know that essential hypertension does not generate clinical features, it is asymptomatic. Clinical features which do present are typically a result of the long term complications of hypertension. This means a diagnosis is made on the basis of recording blood pressure levels. As BP may vary significantly from time to time, a diagnosis should only be made if the BP is elevated on several occasions. Recordings should be made in a seated patient who has rested for five minutes and is feeling relaxed. The arm should be supported on a table at the same level as the heart. SBP should be recorded when the first sound is heard and DBP at the last sound that is audible.

The British Hypertension Society advises that everyone should have their BP measured at least every 5 years up to the age of 80. Individuals with readings which are high or in the 'high normal' ranges (i.e. SBP of 130-139 or a DBP of 85-89) should be reassessed annually. All hypertensive people should be monitored and treated for life.

'White coat' hypertension

Unfortunately the presence of nurses and doctors often leads to anxiety in our patients. This is counter-therapeutic. As part of our philosophy of doing no harm, our presence should relax and reassure patients, not frighten them. This means we need to examine how we interrelate with our patients and to empathise strongly with them. We should not put up barriers between 'us' and 'them', we are all people together and one is certainly not better or worse than the other.

In white coat hypertension the blood pressure increases via an alarm response. This makes hypertension very hard to diagnose because every time we take the patients BP it will be elevated. Sometimes the BP will drop when the patient becomes more relaxed after several recordings, over several visits. It may be found that readings are lower when taken by relatives or friends at home. Another approach is to use a 24 hour ambulatory monitoring device. This will record the BP automatically throughout the patient's normal day. This syndrome of course challenges us as health care workers, can we metaphorically 'take off our white coats'?

Pathological changes and long term complications of hypertension

It is well recognised that with ongoing, untreated hypertension there is increased overall morbidity and mortality from conditions including stroke, coronary heart disease, heart failure, peripheral vascular disease and renal failure.

Atherosclerosis

Hypertension is a major risk factor for the development of atherosclerosis in the larger arteries. This means all of the diseases associated with atheroma are more likely to develop; these include cerebrovascular, cardiovascular and peripheral vascular disease. The risk of these diseases developing also depends on interactions with other risk factors such as hypercholesterolaemia, smoking, poorly managed diabetes mellitus and obesity. Cerebrovascular and cardiovascular disease are the most common causes of death in which hypertension is a contributory factor. Aneurysm formation, affecting the aorta or cerebral vessels, may develop as a consequence of the high blood pressure weakening the arterial walls.

Lesions in smaller arterial vessels

Hypertension causes the slow accumulation of fibrous and elastic tissues in the intima (inner layer) of small arteries. This fibroelastic hyperplasia results in intimal thickening. This is in contrast to the accumulation of fatty, cholesterol based material which accumulates in atheroma of the larger arteries. Ongoing high pressure also causes hypertrophy of the media.

In addition to affecting the large and small arteries hypertension also damages the arterioles. Prolonged hypertension causes lipids and hyaline to be deposited in the arteriole walls. This results in thickening of the arteriole walls in the process of hyaline arteriolosclerosis. Hyaline literally means transparent, in this case it describes the accumulation of basement-membrane type material. As this material builds up the vascular walls are thickened and so take up more space, this will narrow the arteriole lumens reducing blood flow through the vessels. The thickened walls make it harder for the arterioles to expand and contract in order to regulate blood flow to various organs and tissues.

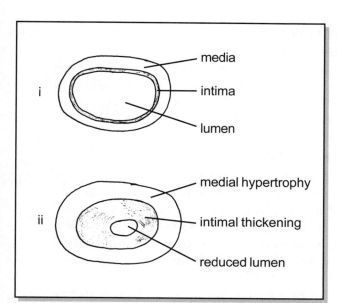

Diagram 10.1

i. Normal small arteries have a thin intima and a relatively thin media.

ii. Hypertension leads to intimal thickening as a result of fibroelastic hyperplasia. Ongoing high BP also causes medial hypertrophy. Both of these disease processes lead to hardening and narrowing of arterial lumens.
Hardening of arterial vessels is termed arteriosclerosis.

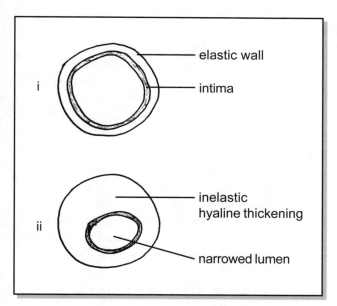

Diagram 10.2

i. A healthy arteriole has a relatively thin wall and is very elastic.

ii. The hyaline arteriole has a thickened wall resulting in a narrowed lumen and inelasticity.
Hardening of arterioles is termed arteriolosclerosis.

Cerebrovascular disease

Hypertension is a significant causative factor in stroke and transient ischaemic attack (TIA). Thromboembolic stroke is more likely as hypertension contributes to atheroma formation in the larger arteries. In addition hypertension increases the risk of a cerebral haemorrhage causing a haemorrhagic stroke. These may occur as a result of hypertension leading to aneurysm formation and rupture. Treating hypertension significantly reduces the risks of TIA and stroke.

Coronary and peripheral arterial disease

Coronary arterial disease may develop in hypertensive patients as atherosclerosis is more likely to be present. Angina may occur as a complication of coronary arterial disease exacerbated by the increased oxygen demand generated by myocardial hypertrophy. Peripheral vascular disease is also a possible complication of hypertension.

Left ventricular hypertrophy (LVH) and cardiac failure

When systemic blood pressure is raised the left ventricle must pump harder to overcome the increased outflow resistance generated by the arterial system. This increases the workload of the left ventricle. As with any muscle an increased workload leads to an increase in the size of muscle cells as a result of hypertrophy. This is one cause of cardiomegaly which describes an enlarged heart. In LVH there is an enlargement of the myocardial muscle cells (myocytes) as well as a change in the collagen matrix structure of the myocardium. Dysfunction of the left ventricle is caused by these collagen matrix changes which cause stiffening and reduced contractility of the myocardium. Eventually the condition is made worse by the loss of contractile fibres within the myocardial cells. As the disease progresses ongoing cardiac failure will develop. Left ventricular hypertrophy is a risk factor for cardiac dysrhythmias, such as atrial fibrillation, but there is also an increased danger of sudden cardiac death. If hypertension is controlled there may be regression of LVH. In untreated hypertension, atherosclerotic coronary heart disease is usually an additional contributing factor to heart failure.

Renal damage

Hypertension leads to vascular changes within the kidneys which in turn cause nephrosclerosis and reduced renal function. The vascular pathology within the kidneys occurs on three levels, affecting the small arteries, arterioles and capillaries. In the small arteries there is fibroelastic thickening of the intima with hypertrophy of the media. These changes result in ischaemia, reducing the blood supply to the afferent arterioles and glomeruli. Secondly, hyaline arteriolosclerosis develops and reduces the lumen of the arterioles. This further reduces the blood supply to the glomeruli. In addition the rigidity caused by the presence of the hyaline means the blood flow to the glomerulus can no longer be regulated by vasoconstriction and dilation.

Thirdly, there is thickening of the walls of the glomerular capillaries, which again reduces the flow of blood through the glomerulus and interferes with the process of ultrafiltration and glomerular filtrate formation. Disorder of the glomerular capillaries leads to protein escaping into the glomerular filtrate with consequent proteinuria. The changes in the renal vascular system all contribute to glomerular ischaemia, as a result glomerular cells are progressively lost and replaced by fibrous scar tissue. As blood volumes passing through the glomeruli are reduced, less blood passes into the efferent arterioles. This in turn reduces the blood supply to the renal tubules resulting in tubular atrophy. The kidneys become fibrous and small, ultimately resulting in end stage renal failure. Renal hypoperfusion may also cause increased secretion of renin, increasing the severity of the hypertension.

Retinal damage

Retinal arterioles and small arteries become thickened resulting in zones of retinal ischaemia. This causes hypoxia and reduces the ability of the light sensitive cells to function resulting in visual defects. Retinal haemorrhages often complicate retinal arteriosclerosis. Retinal haemorrhages also damage the light sensitive cells contributing to areas of visual loss.

At the point where thickened small retinal arterial vessels cross over small veins, the thickened small arteries can compress the small veins. As this will compress the veins it will lead to areas of venous obstruction. As a result the blood from the retinal capillaries will not be able to drain into the small veins as normal. This will increase the pressure within the capillaries resulting in oedema formation with possible haemorrhage. Again this will contribute to progressive retinal damage. The state of retinal vessels is a good indicator of the condition of the vessels in other organs such as the heart, kidney and brain.

Conclusion

Hypertension leads to pathology in many end organs and increases morbidity and mortality significantly. This means we need to identify people who have elevated BP. If a patient who is prone to hypertension is effectively managed to keep their blood pressure within acceptable limits these pathological changes can be prevented. Fortunately, highly effective treatments for hypertension are available, which are likely to be required for life.

Treatment principles

The first line of treatment for essential hypertension is lifestyle modification. Lifestyle changes such as those discussed above can lower SBP and DBP and significantly reduce the risk of morbidity and mortality. For many individuals these changes can bring BP down to acceptable levels. In the absence of other disease states, the aim of treatment is to achieve SBP below 140 and the DBP below 90. If lifestyle modification is not sufficiently effective, drugs may be used. It is important to realise drugs should be given in combination with a healthy lifestyle, i.e. drugs are 'as well as, not instead of'.

In chronic essential hypertension the principle factor increasing the blood pressure is increased peripheral resistance caused by vasoconstriction of the small muscular arteries and arterioles. This is why BP will drop rapidly in persons with hypertension when given vasodilators. Several drugs may be used to control hypertension and will need to be taken on an ongoing basis. Therapy should be titrated with BP remembering hypotension may be a possible side effect of BP lowering medications.

Thiazide-type diuretics, such as bendroflumethiazide, may be effective in relatively low doses. They promote a moderate diuresis which will have the initial effect of reducing total plasma volume; this will lower cardiac output and therefore lower blood pressure. However, when thiazide diuretics are given over time the blood volume will return to normal. Despite this the hypotensive effect persists indicating their principle mode of action is peripheral vasodilation lowering peripheral systemic resistance. At the time of writing the U.K. National Institute for Clinical Excellence (NICE) guidelines advise that in hypertensive patients aged 55 or over, or black patients of any age, the first choice for initial therapy should be either a calcium-channel blocker or a thiazide-type diuretic.

ACE inhibitors, such as enalapril, captopril and lisinopril, inhibit the conversion of angiotensin I to angiotensin II by blocking the action of angiotensin converting enzyme. As angiotensin II is a potent vasoconstricting agent this effect is reduced allowing more vasodilation. ACE inhibitors also suppress aldosterone secretion thereby reducing blood sodium levels. They also increase renal blood flow so promoting urine formation. NICE currently advises that in white hypertensive patients younger than 55, the first choice for initial therapy should be an ACE inhibitor. ACE inhibitors must not be used in pregnancy.

If the use of one drug does not bring the blood pressure down to desired levels a second hypotensive drug should be added in combination. Therefore NICE further recommend that if initial therapy was with a calcium-channel blocker or a thiazide-type diuretic and a second drug is required, add an ACE inhibitor. If initial therapy was with an ACE inhibitor, add a calcium-channel blocker or a thiazide-type diuretic.

Beta-blocking drugs such as propranolol, atenolol and nebivolol still have a place in some hypotensive treatments but are no longer recommended as a first line option. Other drugs used in hypertension may include angiotensin II receptor antagonists, alpha blockers and vasodilators such as hydralazine or minoxidil.

Orthostatic or postural hypotension

This occurs when there is an excessive drop in BP when a person stands up. Blood tends to pool in the lower parts of the body with resultant hypoperfusion of the brain. This causes dizziness with possible fainting (i.e. syncope). Postural hypotension is particularly noticeable when getting out of a hot bath. The heat leads to vasodilation and so further lowers BP. Pathological causes of postural hypotension include reduced blood volume and disorders of the endocrine or autonomic nervous system function. Hypotension may be a particular problem when patients start to take hypotensive medication to treat hypertension. However, this problem usually resolves once the correct doses are titrated and over time the baroreceptors adapt to the new lower blood pressure. Postural hypotension is also more common after prolonged bed rest and in the elderly.

CHAPTER 11

Respiratory Disorders

Bronchial asthma

This is a common condition primarily affecting the bronchioles. These are small airways which allow the passage of air from the larger bronchial tubes to the microscopic alveoli. Asthma is more common in developed, as compared to developing countries. The disorder is frequently seen, affecting more than 5 million people in the UK, over 1 million of who are children.

Aetiology

It is possible to classify asthma as extrinsic or intrinsic. In extrinsic asthma an attack has a definite external cause. In children, most sufferers have an underlying allergic disorder, and many are atopic. This means that patients have a tendency to produce allergic antibodies to everyday substances which act as antigens. Anything which the body recognises as foreign is called an antigen. Exposure to an antigen causes the immune system to produce specific antibodies to counter the foreign substance. If an antigen enters the airways of an individual who has antibodies to the substance, an immune mediated inflammatory reaction will be initiated. Antigens which may lead to an allergic reaction are often referred to as allergens i.e. substances which generate an allergic response. Common examples of allergens in asthma are house dust mite faeces, grass pollens, domestic pets, NSAIDs, occupational chemicals, tobacco smoke, air pollutants and viruses.

From this it can be seen that while extrinsic asthma has a definite external trigger, this trigger is acting on an allergic or atopic genetic predisposition. Another group who suffer from extrinsic asthma are people who present in adult life as a result of occupational exposure. These workers are exposed to a chemical or biological substance in the workplace to which they develop sensitivity. This is why nurses and doctors should avoid unnecessary contact with drugs, e.g. antibiotics, as repeated exposure can result in sensitisation.

As mentioned, atopy has a genetic component; however, the degree to which it is expressed may be modified by environmental factors. Factors which promote abnormal antibody production include early childhood exposure to potential antigens and tobacco smoke. A further factor seems to relate to the bacteria in the gut. Children who are brought up in a very clean environment are more prone to develop allergies. Probably those from 'dirty' environments, particularly with exposure to soil, have less allergic disorders.

Intrinsic asthma is sometimes referred to as cryptogenic. 'Cryptic' means hidden, so an external cause is not known. This condition usually starts in adult life. Despite the existence of intrinsic asthma, an external cause should always be searched for. If a trigger is identified this would mean the asthma would be reclassified as extrinsic but, more importantly, the trigger could be avoided.

Pathophysiology

When an allergen is inhaled into the airways it triggers the release of histamine and other inflammatory mediators from mast cells. These chemicals generate an inflammatory reaction which leads to swelling and increased production of viscous mucus from the epithelial lining. Histamine is also a bronchoconstricting agent and is part of the cause of the airway hyper-reactivity. This airway hyper-sensitivity leads to bronchoconstriction, swelling and increased production of secretions. All of these effects reduce the lumen of the airway and therefore restrict air entering and leaving the alveoli. As air exchange between the atmosphere and the alveoli is inhibited, fresh supplies of oxygen are no longer delivered. This means the concentration of oxygen in the alveoli will drop. As a result of this, blood passing through the pulmonary circulation is no longer fully oxygenated, giving rise to hypoxaemia. Oxygen saturations will therefore drop and all body tissues will become hypoxic.

Clinical features

The recurrent episodes of inflammation cause airway obstruction. Duration and frequency of attacks varies significantly between individuals. The common features are wheezing, difficulty in breathing (dyspnoea) with breathlessness, chest tightness and cough. Cough is often worse at night and in the early morning. Expiration is typically more difficult than inspiration. This is because inspiration is facilitated by active muscular contraction of the external intercostal muscles and diaphragm, whereas expiration is a passive recoil process. Wheeze is often more prominent during expiration, as air tries to pass through the narrowed bronchial passages. As air can enter the lungs more readily than it can leave, the alveoli and lungs become hyperinflated. In severe attacks the patients may become very distressed. Some have described an attack as 'like trying to breathe through a straw with your nose pinched'. Central cyanosis may be present, indicating potentially dangerous, low levels of oxygen in the blood and tissues.

Typically, bronchoconstriction and airflow limitation develops within a few minutes of exposure to a trigger. This rapid presentation of symptoms is called the early reaction. If the environmental trigger is withdrawn the attack usually resolves within an hour. However, sometimes a more prolonged attack will develop. This is termed the late phase reaction and may respond poorly to medications. Late phase reactions typically develop after 4-8 hours and may last for a day or more. Asthma is a potentially fatal condition. A severe asthma attack may progress to respiratory arrest. With treatment such a serious outcome is unlikely, but it does show that this condition must be taken seriously. Patients with intermittent asthma are usually asymptomatic between attacks.

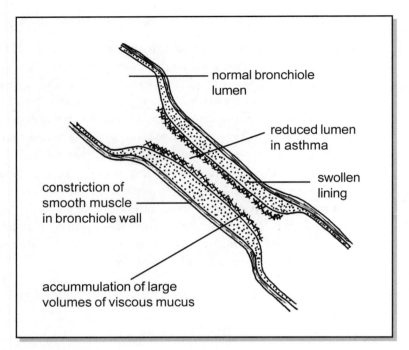

Diagram 11.1
The principle cause of asthma is inflammation which leads to
swelling of the lining (mostly from the submucosa), increased
volumes and viscosity of secretions and bronchoconstriction.
Swelling imposes into the lumen of the bronchiole reducing the
available lumen for air to pass through. Increased secretions
further obstruct the lumen, reducing air passage still further.
Bronchoconstriction also reduces the lumen of the airway. These
factors combine to generate an acute obstructive pathophysiology.

Treatment principles

Clearly trigger factors should be avoided whenever possible. Inhaled medications
are the basis of treatment. Basically there are two types of drug treatment.
Preventors (also called controllers) e.g. corticosteroids, are given to reduce the
inflammation which initiates the other pathophysiological features. Relievers,
e.g. salbutamol, are given to produce bronchodilation when symptoms occur.
In acute disease, high concentrations of oxygen may be given as required.

Acute severe asthma

This condition used to be described as status asthmaticus and refers to an
asthmatic attack which has not responded to the patient's self treatment. Such
patients have a respiratory rate of over 25 breaths per minute, a tachycardia of
110 beats per minute or more, and a peak expiratory flow rate of 33-50% of
their normal volume. The lungs become grossly hyperinflated as the patients

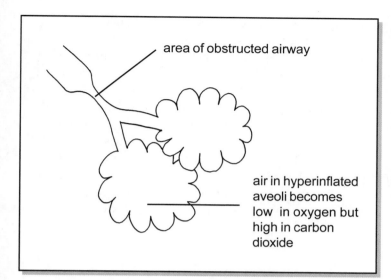

area of obstructed airway

air in hyperinflated aveoli becomes low in oxygen but high in carbon dioxide

Diagram 11.2
Obstruction in a bronchiole leads to a narrowed respiratory lumen; this inhibits the free passage of air to and from the alveoli. As a result the air trapped in the alveoli becomes stagnant.

can not breathe out effectively. Thick, tenacious mucus will accumulate in the airways and is likely to form plugs. Such patients should be admitted to hospital for treatment. Nebulised bronchodilators such as salbutamol will be given and in severe attacks adding ipratropium bromide provides further bronchodilation. Systemic corticosteroids will reduce the inflammatory response, common preparations include oral prednisolone or intravenous hydrocortisone. Attention should also be paid to fluid and electrolyte status. Arterial blood gases and pulse oximetry should be performed and high concentrations of humidified oxygen given. Patients who still fail to respond adequately may need mechanical ventilation.

Chronic asthma

In chronic asthma there are changes to the structure of the lungs as a result of long term inflammation. There will be thickening of the submucosa as a result of mucous gland enlargement, smooth muscle hyperplasia (an increase in the number of cells present) and an accumulation of inflammatory white cells with oedema. Patients suffer ongoing features which are essentially the same as those seen in chronic obstructive pulmonary disease (COPD).

Acute bronchitis

In acute bronchitis there is inflammation of the large and medium sized bronchi. Often the initial infection is viral but secondary bacterial infection may develop, especially in the presence of COPD or smoking. Initially there may be some chest discomfort, shortness of breath, some wheezing and an unproductive cough. A mild fever may develop with a degree of leucocytosis. Most patients recover completely within about a week.

Inflammation in the bronchial passages leads to increased production and viscosity of mucus. This is an important defense mechanism as viral particles and bacteria are caught in the mucus. Next, cilia propel the mucus containing the infective agents away from the small airways and alveoli, towards the trachea. Once in the trachea infected mucus can be coughed up, and so cleared from the respiratory system. This explains why a productive cough develops later on in an infection, as cilia waft the mucus into the trachea. An unproductive cough does not bring up mucus whereas a productive cough does. Antibiotics are not usually indicated in acute bronchitis. However, in debilitated or malnourished people infection may spread down to the small bronchioles causing bronchiolitis. This will normally be treated with antibiotics as there is a risk of developing life threatening bronchopneumonia. Repeated episodes of acute bronchitis can be a risk factor for chronic bronchitis.

Pneumonia

Aetiology

The cause of pneumonia is usually bacterial infection. While over 100 organisms have been identified as causes of community acquired pneumonia, Streptococcus pneumoniae (often simply called pneumococcus) is the most common. More cases occur in winter and smoking is probably an important risk factor. Patients who are immobile or generally ill are also at greater risk of developing pneumonia. This is a particular risk if patients are nursed lying down, which is why people should be managed sitting up whenever possible. Bacterial pneumonia is also more common in HIV infection compared to the general population.

Types of pneumonia

Pneumonia is sometimes referred to as community or hospital acquired. Community acquired simply means the condition was contracted in the community as opposed to in hospital. Traditionally pneumonia has been described anatomically as bronchopneumonia or lobar pneumonia. Bronchopneumonia is a diffuse infection, typically spreading over both lung fields, as well as the bronchi and bronchioles. Lobar pneumonia is an infection localised to one or more lobes. As the pleural membranes are in contact with the lung surface, infection in lobar pneumonia spreads to affect these membranes. Pain is caused by inflammation of the pleural membranes and occurs with respiratory movements. This has been described as a sharp pain, like being stabbed every time the patient breathes. Pleurisy simply describes inflammation of the pleural membranes.

Pneumonia is also sometimes classified by cause. In addition to Streptococcus pneumoniae (pneumococcus), it may be caused by other organisms such as Mycoplasma, Legionella or Mycobacterium tuberculosis (tuberculosis). Staphylococcus aureus can cause a very acute severe form of pneumonia. Pneumocystis carinii pneumonia (PCP) is caused by a protozoa and is found in immuno-compromised patients. For example, it is seen in developing countries in malnourished children, patients receiving immuno-suppressive treatments and in AIDS.

Aspiration of vomit is a danger if a patient inhales while vomiting. This is a particular risk in unconscious patients and explains why anaesthetists prefer to anaesthetise patients with an empty stomach. If inhaled, gastric contents such as hydrochloric acid, pepsin and food, will cause severe inflammation and secondary infection; this is often simply described as aspiration pneumonia. Also pneumonia which occurs as a complication of immobility and reduced mucocillary clearance is sometimes described as hypostatic pneumonia.

Pathophysiology

Pneumonia refers to inflammation of the lung tissue. Bronchopneumonia often develops after an acute bronchitis, as infection spreads down into the bronchioles and alveoli. Influenza or other viral infections also commonly precede pneumonia. Bronchogenic malignancy is another possible factor leading to pneumonia, as bronchial passages may be blocked by a tumour. This results in mucus stasis and the development of infection in the obstructed area.

The principle pathophysiological process in pneumonia is called consolidation. Literally this means to 'make solid'. In lobar pneumonia this affects a lobe and in bronchopneumonia the process is patchy over both lung fields. Inhaled bacteria such as pneumococci enter the lungs and generate a vigorous inflammatory response, with large volumes of inflammatory fluid being exuded from capillaries. In addition, the dilated capillaries allow fibrinogen and red cells to escape into the bronchioles and alveoli. Bacteria multiply in

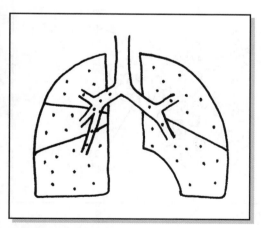

Diagram 11.3i
Bronchopneumonia involves both lungs and the airway passages.

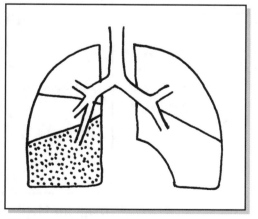

Diagram 11.3ii
In lobar pneumonia the infection is localised, in this case to the right lower lobe. Inflammation spreads to involve the pleural membranes, giving rise to pleurisy.

the inflammatory fluid, and white cells, mostly neutrophils, move into the area to combat the infection. The result of these processes is that alveoli fill up with fluid, fibrin strands, bacteria and blood cells. This means that instead of the alveoli being filled with air they are 'made solid' by being filled with this infective and inflammatory material. If the alveoli are filled with fluid normal gaseous exchange cannot occur, leading to possible respiratory failure.

Typically, after about 6-8 days, the immune system has made sufficient antibodies to the strain of pneumococcus causing the pneumonia that the condition starts to resolve. The bacteria are destroyed by antibodies and phagocytic cells, inflammatory exudate is reabsorbed and the lungs can usually repair themselves without any residual damage.

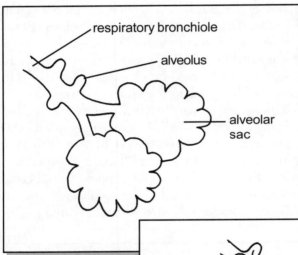

Diagram 11.4i
Healthy alveoli have a delicate structure and allow for gaseous exchange between alveoli and blood.

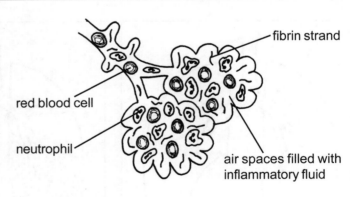

Diagram 11.4ii
In consolidated areas of the lung, alveoli fill with inflammatory fluid, bacteria, red cells, white cells and fibrin, prohibiting gaseous exchange. When the combination of red cells and other debris is coughed up this gives the sputum a rusty appearance.

Pneumonia and age

Lobar pneumonia is characteristically a disease of young adults. When antibiotics are not available, lobar pneumonia may rapidly result in the death of a previously fit, robust young person. Babies, children and old people are most at risk from bronchopneumonia. Chest infections remain one of the leading causes of death in children in developing countries. Bronchopneumonia is a significant cause of death in older people over the age of 70 years.

Some degree of bronchopneumonia is usually present at death, unless a patient has died suddenly. The illness and disability present in the hours and days before death predispose a patient to pneumonia. In some cases it may be the bronchopneumonia, rather than the actual terminal pathology, which is the ultimate cause of death.

Clinical features

Pneumonia has an acute presentation, usually with malaise, rigors, fever and a dry cough. There will be a tachypnoea with rapid and shallow respirations. Tachycardia usually presents as a consequence of the fever and hypoxia. Chest examination may reveal crackles and dullness on percussion. There may be a history of preceding viral infection. Severity of the disease varies considerably from a relatively mild infection to being life threatening within days of onset. It has been suggested that overall mortality for community acquired pneumonia is just under 14% so this is clearly a condition which must be taken seriously. With the common form of pneumococcal disease the patient quickly becomes very ill. If the pleural membranes are involved there will be pleuritic chest pain. Fever is often up to 39.5°C. After a few days the cough becomes productive and in pneumococcal disease the sputum is classically rust coloured. Blood tests will show an increase in white cell numbers and an increase in erythrocyte sedimentation rate. Chest X-ray shows white areas as a result of consolidation. Pneumonia can develop into life threatening severe sepsis and septic shock.

Treatment principles

Humidified oxygen should be given to all patients with hypoxaemia or tachypnoea with the aim of maintaining oxygen saturations at 92% or higher. Blood gases and pulse oximetry should be used to detect any respiratory failure and monitor the effectiveness of oxygen therapy. Sputum samples and possibly blood cultures should be collected for microbiology to determine the causative organism and recommend the most appropriate antibiotics which are the mainstay of treatment. In mild disease these may be given orally but intravenous administration will be needed in more serious cases. Antibiotics should be started at once, before the results of culture and sensitivity arrive.

Hydration should be maintained as this will help prevent excessive viscosity of bronchial secretions. Patients should be encouraged to cough as expectoration of sputum will help to clear the airways and alveoli of mucus and infection. If there is any pleural chest pain analgesics should be given as pain may inhibit coughing. Sitting up helps to dilate bronchial passages, encourages deeper breathing and aids expectoration.

Chronic obstructive pulmonary disease (COPD)

COPD is a collective term used to describe several conditions associated with damage to the lung tissue and airflow limitation. COPD includes two very common disorders which usually occur together in the same patient. These are chronic bronchitis and emphysema. Chronic asthma and bronchiectasis are also included in the COPD 'group' of disorders. Bronchiectasis refers to chronic dilation of the bronchi and is usually caused by chronic inflammation of these airways, tuberculosis is the most common global cause. In COPD the bronchial walls are inflamed and become thickened. Mucus is not effectively removed from the bronchioles making infections frequent. The alveoli become dilated and may fill with pus as a consequence of infection.

Aetiology

The main cause of COPD is smoking tobacco. Death rates are closely related to the number of cigarettes smoked. A person smoking 30 cigarettes per day is 20 times more likely to die from COPD than a non smoker. Cannabis smoke is also bad for the lungs. In developing countries many people are obliged to live in smoky conditions where solid fuels are often used for cooking and warmth. Again, such long term inhalation of smoke leads to COPD. Climate, dampness and living in areas of high air pollution probably play some role in disease development. Mortality from COPD increases during periods of intensified atmospheric pollution. Other risk factors include occupational exposure to air pollution and low birth weight. Impaired lung growth during childhood, as might be caused by passive smoking or repeated infections, results in reduced lung function in adult life.

Chronic bronchitis

Pathophysiology

Inhaled smoke, or other irritants, insult the lining of the bronchial passages leading to inflammation. In order to protect the lining from the irritating smoke, the body responds by increasing mucus production. Mucus works by lining the airways, and therefore protects the internal surface of the bronchial passages from the smoke. In the attempt to produce more mucus there is an increase in the number and size of mucus producing cells, i.e. there is a hyperplasia and hypertrophy of these secretory cells. However, this results in a persistent over production of mucus by mucous glands. As well as producing too much mucus,

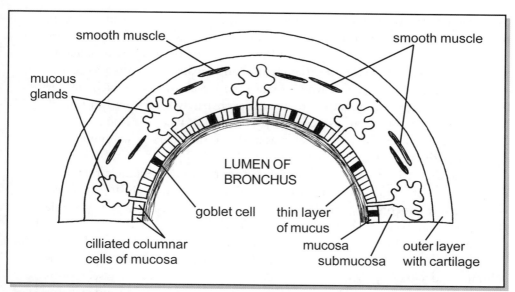

Diagram 11.5i
Cross section of a normal medium sized bronchus.

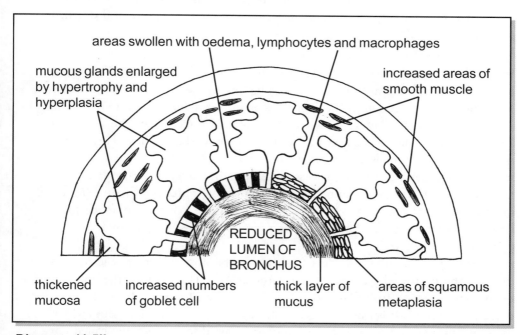

Diagram 11.5ii
Cross section showing a thickened submucosa. The submucosal layer is thickened by an increase in the size of the mucus producing glands it contains. As a result of the thickening of this layer the lumen of the bronchus is reduced which will restrict air flow. Reduction of lumen diameter is made worse by oedema and fibrosis, especially in the smaller airways.

the enlarged glands are bulky, resulting in a thickening of the bronchial wall; this in turn reduces the lumen of the airways causing a partial obstruction. This swelling of bronchial linings is made worse by the presence of oedema. In the smaller airways the cycles of inflammation and repair lead to the progressive accumulation of fibrous tissues which reduce the lumen through which air may pass. These factors act together to produce obstructive airflow limitation. Chronic inflammation may also cause a change in the type of tissue lining the airways. This is an example of a metaplasia; the normal ciliated columnar cells are replaced by non-ciliated squamous cells.

During the early stages of the disease, before the lungs become structurally damaged, the inflammatory changes are reversible, as long as the insulting smoke is removed. If patients stop smoking at this early stage full recovery is possible and even at later stages significant improvement can be expected.

In addition to increased volumes of viscid mucus there is loss of the cilia which normally line the bronchial passages. The combination of increased mucus volumes and viscosity, with reduced activity of cilia, means that secretions become relatively stagnant. This allows time for infection to develop and explains why episodes of acute bronchitis occur. These acute exacerbations are referred to as acute on chronic bronchitis. Superimposed bacterial acute on chronic bronchitis is potentially serious and may cause respiratory failure and death.

Clinical features

In order to remove excessive secretions the patient coughs a lot. This often begins in relatively young adult life with coughing in the mornings, often worse in winter. Smokers cough in the mornings as smoke reduces the activity of the cilia throughout the day. Only when there is no smoke, when the person is asleep, are they able to recover and waft mucus into the trachea. This means there are larger volumes of mucus in the trachea when the patient wakes up, stimulating coughing. As the disease develops, the cough persists all day. In fact, chronic bronchitis is defined as production of sputum and coughing on most days, for at least 3 months, over 2 consecutive years. In practice most patients go on coughing and producing large volumes of sputum for many years.

As the disorder progresses less fresh air containing oxygen is able to pass through the narrowed passages to reach the alveoli. This reduces the volumes of oxygen which diffuse from the alveoli into the blood resulting in lower oxygen saturations. It is this presence of deoxyhaemoglobin in the tissues which gives rise to cyanosis. Over time, pulmonary heart disease (formally called cor pulmonale) may develop. This right sided heart disease will lead to systemic oedema. The combination of cyanosis and oedema has led to the label 'blue and bloated' sometimes being used for these patients. Some patients become so short of breath on exertion that their mobility is severely limited; the term 'respiratory cripple' has been used to describe this severe condition.

Airflow limitation in the bronchial passages also means that less carbon dioxide is able to pass out from the alveoli to be exhaled. This results in increased levels of CO_2 in the alveoli, which in turn means this waste gas is unable to diffuse as effectively from the blood into alveolar air. As a result CO_2 is retained in the blood, a condition described as hypercarbia. In chronic bronchitis, the patient often does not appear to be short of breath. This is explained by the loss of the hypercarbic drive. As people with chronic bronchitis do not appear to be struggling to breathe they are sometimes described as 'non-fighters'.

Haemoptysis may be seen in acute exacerbations of COPD, but if it is seen other conditions such as tuberculosis or malignancy should be screened for.

Emphysema

Emphysema describes a loss of alveolar elasticity with a permanent enlargement of the air spaces due to destruction of the alveolar walls.

Pathophysiology

Smoke and other irritants reach the alveoli. Here they irritate the tissues and stimulate the migration of protective white cells into the area. This increases the numbers of neutrophils and macrophages in the alveoli, as part of a normal inflammatory reaction. Increase in the numbers of these white blood cells is to some degree protective, as they are able to phagocytose dangerous smoke particles. Smokers may have 6 times more macrophages in their alveoli than non-smokers. Unfortunately, as a result of the presence of smoke, these leucocytes do not work as efficiently as normal. In normal physiology all phagocytic cells contain digestive enzymes, required to digest foreign material, (such as bacteria or viruses) which have been ingested. However, in emphysema macrophages secrete a group of these enzymes called proteases, or protein digesting enzymes.

One of the proteases is an enzyme called elastase, which digests elastin. In normal physiology, it is the presence of elastic elastin which gives the alveoli their elastic properties. If this elastic tissue is lost the alveoli do not contract normally during expiration. In addition the other protease enzymes digest proteins in the wall of the alveoli, resulting in progressive destruction. As the walls of the alveoli are destroyed, the air spaces become larger. Larger air spaces mean that there is less surface area over which gaseous exchange can take place, reducing the efficiency of the lungs. These processes explain why there is a loss of elasticity with air space enlargement in emphysema.

Clinical features

Classically a patient with emphysema has been described as 'pink and puffing'. They have increased respiratory effort to compensate for reduced lung function. This is seen clinically as a marked dyspnoea. As a result of this they are able to maintain relatively normal levels of oxygen and carbon dioxide in the blood. As there is an increased respiratory effort in an attempt to compensate for reduced lung efficiency, emphysematous patients are described as 'fighters'.

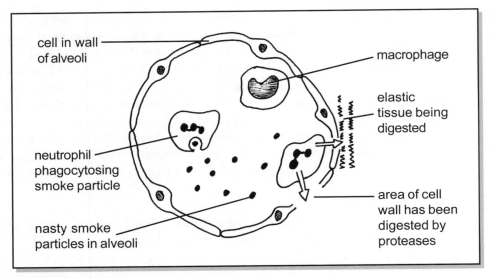

cell in wall of alveoli

macrophage

elastic tissue being digested

neutrophil phagocytosing smoke particle

nasty smoke particles in alveoli

area of cell wall has been digested by proteases

Diagram 11.6
The presence of smoke particles causes inflammation and attracts neutrophils and macrophages. To some degree these helpfully phagocytose smoke particles, but they also release harmful digesting enzymes. The arrows indicate the release of proteases, including elastase, by neutrophils which are destroying previously healthy tissues.

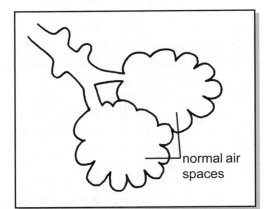

normal air spaces

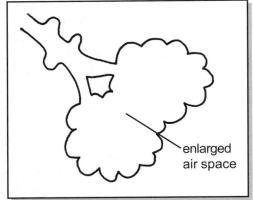

enlarged air space

Diagram 11.7i
Normal alveoli.

Diagram 11.7ii
Destruction of the walls of the alveoli, by proteases, increases the size of the air spaces and so reduces the internal surface area available for gaseous exchange. This process may be repeated several times resulting in the emergence of large air spaces. In addition, elastase will digest elastic tissue producing inelastic walls.

This difference, in comparison to chronic bronchitis, is explained by the preservation of the hypercarbic drive in emphysema. Emphysematous patients are able to maintain relatively low levels of carbon dioxide in the blood, and so preserve the sensitivity of the medulla oblongata to CO_2. This means that when CO_2 levels do increase there is massive stimulation of the respiratory centre, which in turn stimulates respiratory effort. People with emphysema do not usually develop pulmonary heart disease.

As the normal elastic recoil of the alveoli is lost, the pressure of exhaled air in the small bronchioles is not maintained by the outgoing flow of air. This results in collapse of the bronchioles at the start of expiration. As a result, air is not able to leave the alveoli which consequently become hyperinflated. Collapse of the small airways is exacerbated by pressure from other surrounding hyperinflated alveoli. Retained air in the alveoli in turn leads to whole lung hyperinflation. However, the trapped air in the lungs is not useful as it is low in oxygen and high in carbon dioxide. Via this mechanism of bronchiolar collapse, emphysema also causes airway obstruction, as was the case in chronic bronchitis. Another common observation is that people with emphysema often breathe out through pursed lips. This has the effect of increasing back pressure in the bronchial tree which helps to keep the bronchioles open, thus aiding expiration. Over time the hyperinflation of the lungs alters the shape of the chest making it deeper. This eventually results in a chest which is deeper than it is broad, a condition called a 'barrel' chest.

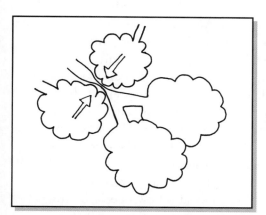

Diagram 11.8
As expiration begins, the lack of air pressure from the alveoli causes the bronchioles to collapse. This effect is increased by external pressure on bronchioles from surrounding hyperinflated alveoli. These processes make it difficult for the person to breathe out.

Chronic bronchitis and emphysema

These two conditions have been described separately and patients will present who suffer predominantly from chronic bronchitis or emphysema. However, many other patients present with characteristics of both clinical conditions. The reason why different individuals respond in these two patterns, to what appears to be the same underlying aetiology seems to be caused by genetic differences. These genetic factors are influential in how an individual responds to environmental insults and how disease processes develop and present.

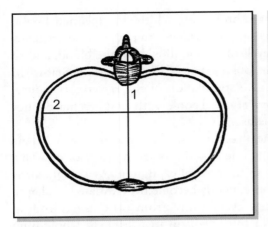

Diagram 11.9i
A normal chest is twice as broad as it is deep.

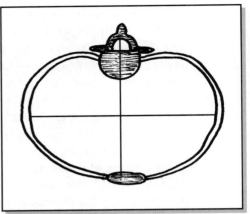

Diagram 11.9ii
In some cases of 'barrel chest' this normal ratio is reduced and may result in a chest which is deeper than it is broad.

Treatment of COPD

Bronchodilator therapy is central to the management of breathlessness. These may be given via inhalers or in nebulised form. Some bronchodilators work by stimulating the sympathetic nervous system while others work by inhibiting the action of the parasympathetic nervous system. Oral bronchodilators may also be used in patients who have difficulties with inhaler devices.

As previously discussed COPD patients are prone to respiratory infections. Acute infections should be treated quickly with appropriate antibiotics. Influenza vaccinations should be given to prevent this form of viral infection. Some patients with COPD respond well to a course of the steroid drug, prednisolone. This is probably explained by the anti-inflammatory steroid reversing the current inflammatory component of the condition. However, long term systemic steroids are associated with numerous side effects so patients who have benefited should go on to inhaled corticosteroids.

It is now well accepted that giving long term supplementary oxygen at home prolongs life. This is usually given via a nasal cannula at a flow rate of 2 litres per minute. Treatment aims to provide blood oxygen saturations at 90% or above. An oxygen concentrator should be installed in the home to provide the required oxygen. Ideally the patient should receive oxygen therapy for 19 hours or more per day. Oxygen given at higher concentrations via a mask seems to confer even greater benefits. In severe exacerbations ventilatory support may be required. This should preferably be by non invasive ventilation, (NIV). NIV uses a tight fitting mask or hood generating positive pressures to blow air into the patient's lungs. This often prevents the need for more invasive treatment using endotracheal intubation.

Health education has an important part to play in prevention of COPD. As symptoms worsen very slowly over many years, the patient is often at an advanced stage when they first seek help. However, if the condition could be identified at an earlier stage, the disorder is largely reversible and deterioration may be prevented. It is of course essential that the patient stops smoking. Smoking cessation at any stage has advantages, as there can be some recovery and prevention of further deterioration. In most patients, care at home should include a gradual exercise programme.

Risks of oxygen therapy in carbon dioxide retainers

Ventilations are controlled by the respiratory centre in the medulla oblongata of the brain stem. This is sensitive to increased levels of carbon dioxide present in the blood. In normal physiology, if the level of carbon dioxide rises, the respiratory centre sends impulses to the respiratory muscles to increase rate and volume of breathing. In health, it is the increase in CO_2 rather than the lack of O_2 which primarily stimulates breathing.

However, in some patients with chronic bronchitis, carbon dioxide is retained which results in a constantly high level in the blood. Chronic high blood levels of CO_2 overwhelm the respiratory centre, which therefore becomes unresponsive to these high levels. In other words, the medullary respiratory drive centre becomes CO_2 insensitive. These patients are therefore more dependent on the hypoxaemic drive generated by the peripheral chemoreceptors in the aortic arch and carotid bodies. In a minority of patients this hypoxaemic drive can be inhibited by giving high concentrations of therapeutic oxygen. This can result in hypoventilation meaning even more CO_2 is retained in the blood, leading to acidosis and drowsiness (known as carbon dioxide narcosis). Eventually these patients may stop breathing. While this potential complication only affects a minority of patients the British Thoracic Society recommend that for most patients with an acute illness oxygen should be prescribed to achieve a target saturation of 94-98%. However, for patients who chronically retain carbon dioxide, and are therefore at some risk of hypercarbic respiratory failure, the target saturations should be 88-92%.

There is also a danger in patients who have suffered from hypoxia for a period of time. Hypoxia causes sympathetic stimulation which over time causes the patient to become very tired. Upon admission to hospital, oxygen therapy will reduce the hypoxia and so reduce sympathetic activity. As the patient is usually tired at this time, and sympathetic stimulation is reduced, they are very likely to go to sleep. This combination of reduction in hypoxic drive, and sleep, increases the risk that a patient may hypoventilate. Therefore these patients must be closely monitored. If a patient hypoventilates or even stops breathing and we are aware of this straight away, artificial positive pressure ventilation may be given until their natural drive is restored. However if a patient stops breathing and we are not aware of it, they will die.

Tuberculosis (TB)

In the past, TB claimed so many victims that it was described as 'the captain of the men of death'. In developing countries it is still very common, and causes more deaths than any other single type of infection. Globally, the highest mortality rates are found in young adults.

Aetiology

Tuberculosis is a bacterial infection caused by Mycobacterium tuberculosis. These rod shaped aerobic bacteria have a waxy coat, which retains red dye when treated with acid. This is why they are referred to as acid-fast bacilli or AFBs. A bacillus is a rod shaped bacterium, as opposed to cocci which are spherical. TB is a droplet infection; people with active pulmonary tuberculosis secrete the bacteria into the air when they cough, sneeze or talk. Transmission is more likely in crowded, closed conditions. People who are immunosuppressed, such as those with HIV, are very much more likely to develop TB if exposed to M. tuberculosis. TB declined in incidence for many years in the West, primarily as a result of improved nutrition, living conditions and overall improvements in health. The development of BCG immunization and curative drug treatments also helped.

Primary infection

Primary tuberculosis occurs in people who have not been previously exposed to the bacilli. Inhaled droplets containing the bacilli pass down the bronchial tree to the small bronchioles or alveoli. Shortly after entering the lung, the tubercle bacilli are surrounded by macrophages and fibroblasts. These fibroblasts produce fibrous tissue around the collection of bacilli. This combination of bacilli, surrounded by macrophages, fibroblasts and fibrous tissue is called a tubercle. Despite this rapid activation of the bodies defence mechanisms there is spread to the regional lymph nodes.

Over the next 6-12 weeks, antigens from the bacilli stimulate the production of specific antibodies which act against the infection. This development of specific immunity can be demonstrated by a positive localized inflammatory reaction if some proteins from tubercle bacilli are injected intradermally. This is the basis of the tuberculin Mantoux skin test. The result of antibody production and the development of cellular immunity is that most (about 90%) primary infections resolve. During this process of developing immunity the patient usually remains well, and may only suffer mild symptoms such as a cough or wheeze. As the patient has now developed antibodies, they enjoy increased resistance to tuberculosis in the future.

Pathologically, the central area of a tubercle necroses generating a 'cheesy' material, a process referred to as caseation. Later, this area heals with fibrosis and may become calcified. In some cases the bacilli may be completely eradicated, but in others, a few survive within the scarred, calcified area. Here they lie dormant and cause no problems. However, they may revive, if the individual's level of immunity decreases in the future.

In a few cases of primary tuberculosis, (usually less than 10%) perhaps due to reduced levels of immunity, progressive primary tuberculosis may develop. The bacilli may spread out of the tubercle into the lumen of a bronchial tube. If the bacilli enter the sputum the patient may exhale the infection and so infect others. Infection may spread around the bronchial tree, causing life threatening acute bronchopneumonia. Another possible manifestation of progressive primary infection is miliary tuberculosis. This occurs when bacilli gain access to the bloodstream, and spread to other parts of the body. This is somewhat analogous to metastasis in malignant disease. In miliary disease, small tubercles form in all parts of the body and may be seen in the retina. Untreated, this complication is rapidly fatal. Miliary tuberculosis is so named because the numerous small tubercles resemble millet seeds.

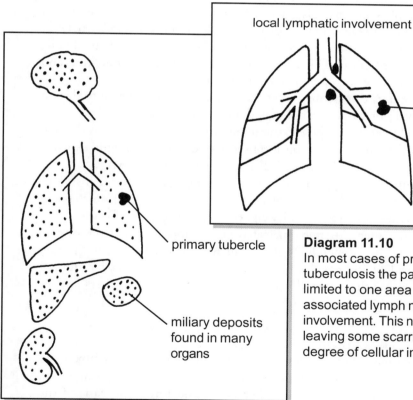

Diagram 11.10
In most cases of primary tuberculosis the pathology is limited to one area of the lung, with associated lymph node involvement. This normally resolves leaving some scarring and a good degree of cellular immunity.

Diagram 11.11
In a few cases of primary tuberculosis, the bacilli may gain access to the blood and form numerous miliary deposits all over the body, an acute life threatening complication.

Post-primary tuberculosis

Post primary tuberculosis is a term applied to any manifestation of tuberculosis which occurs after initial cellular immunity has developed. As previously mentioned, even after apparent complete resolution of primary tuberculosis, a few bacilli may survive within a fibrosed or calcified lesion. In this case, the disease is dormant. As bacilli are not secreted into respiratory mucus the patient is not infectious. If the level of immunity falls for any reason infection may be reactivated, the bacilli may multiply once more, and so the dormant tuberculosis becomes active. Post primary tuberculosis may also be caused by reinfection, but this is uncommon. Eighty percent of post primary tuberculosis affects the lungs, but 20% of cases result from infection of other sites in the body.

As in primary tuberculosis, a necrotic infected area of caseation forms. However, in post-primary infection, this leads to formation of a cavity within the lung, a process called cavitation. Several cavities may coalesce to form larger cavities of 10-15 cm in diameter. Other pulmonary complications such as pleural effusions and emphysema may also develop. Fibroblasts surround the area of infection with fibrous tissue. Often a situation develops where the body's defence cells and the process of fibrosis balance the ability of the bacilli to divide, leading to chronic infection. This is an example of chronic inflammation and as there is active disease the patient remains infectious.

Bacilli in secondary disease may enter the bloodstream and spread to distant sites such as the vertebrae or other bones, kidneys, joints, lymph nodes, meninges or gastrointestinal tract. Here, these extrapulmonary manifestations may develop and damage local tissues generating localised clinical features. This explains why tuberculosis is often a differential diagnosis with malignancy.

Clinical features in post primary tuberculosis typically have an insidious onset and commonly include fever, malaise, tiredness, anorexia, chronic cough, progressive shortness of breath and weight loss. In the past TB was called consumption; the patient became emaciated and it appeared that the disease process was 'consuming' the body. Night sweats may or may not occur. Sputum may be thick, purulent and possibly blood stained. AFBs can usually be cultured from sputum. During this active disease the patient may infect others as they expectorate the bacilli from their lungs.

Prevention

An essentially harmless, bovine (bovine means from cows) form of tubercular bacteria can be grown on potatoes. This can then be injected to promote the development of cellular immunity to tuberculosis and forms the basis of the BCG vaccination. The reason this injection leaves a scar is that the presence of the attenuated tubercular bacteria produce a small tubercle in the skin where they are injected. A tubercle will also develop in the lymph nodes of the axilla (armpit). The end result of this is that the vaccinated person will have about a 70% increased resistance to tuberculosis infection in the future.

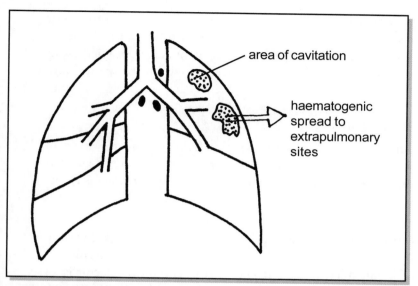

area of cavitation

haematogenic spread to extrapulmonary sites

Diagram 11.12
Post primary tuberculosis. Latent infection persists in the lungs, possibly for many years. When reactivated the infection most commonly involves the lungs, but there may be spread, via the blood, to almost any other area of the body. Extrapulmonary sites include the lymph nodes, meninges, urinary system, gastrointestinal tract, joints or bones, particularly the vertebrae. Extrapulmonary spread is more likely in HIV infection.

Perhaps the main way to reduce the incidence of TB is to improve living conditions and fight poverty. Good nutrition helps to maintain high levels of natural immunity. If patients do have active disease they should be treated to prevent spread to others and to cure the individual. HIV infection is currently leading to many people with immunosuppression, many of whom live in areas where TB is endemic. This is leading to many more cases of TB and is one more reason why we need to reduce the transmission of HIV.

Treatment

In the past bed rest was considered essential, but in fact this does not help. Today, most cases of tuberculosis may be treated with drug protocols. Courses of drugs need to be taken daily, for 6 months to a year depending on the disease presentation. The World Health Organisation publishes guidelines and protocols for the treatment of tuberculosis using rifampicin, isoniazid, pyrazinamide, ethambutol and streptomycin. The key to effective treatment is compliance. Poor compliance probably accounts for most cases of unsuccessful treatment. For this reason some patients may need directly observed therapy (DOT) to make sure they follow the protocol and take the full course. In some parts of the world patients who cannot be relied on are more or less imprisoned until treatment is completed. Failure to complete a full course is one factor leading to the development of drug resistant strains of tuberculosis. Multiple drug resistant tuberculosis (MDRTB) clearly has the potential to pose a significant public health threat. Nosocomial MDRTB is a recognised threat to nurses and doctors.

Bronchial carcinoma

Bronchial carcinoma is the second most common form of primary cancer in the West and is also widespread in many developing countries. In the UK it is still more common in men, but unfortunately the incidence in women is rising.

Aetiology

Tumours arising from the bronchial passages are by far the most common respiratory tract malignancy. Some carcinomas do arise from the alveoli and trachea but these are much less common. The most important risk factor is, of course smoking. Passive smoking also increases risk, particularly if there is regular exposure, such as from a spouse who smokes, or working in a smoky environment. Risk increases with number of cigarettes smoked and the tar content of the tobacco. If a smoker stops, the risk declines, but only slowly over many years. This demonstrates the importance of stopping as soon as possible. People who live in cities are somewhat more prone to bronchial carcinoma than country dwellers. Some occupational exposure also increases risk. Asbestos exposure can cause lung cancer, pulmonary fibrosis or a mesothelioma which is cancer of the pleural membranes. Exposure to asbestos and tobacco smoke act synergistically to greatly increase the risk of lung cancer. In some geographical areas radioactive radon gas may collect in cellars and basements. As this is radioactive it can cause malignancy. Eating plenty of vegetables probably has some protective effect.

Pathophysiology

As the name suggests bronchogenic carcinoma begins in the bronchial passages. Bronchial carcinoma may be classified as small-cell or non-small-cell. Small-cell (formally called oat cell) carcinoma accounts for about 20% or more cases of bronchial carcinomas. This form of carcinoma is highly associated with cigarette smoking. The cells which turn malignant in small-cell disease are endocrine neurosecretory and called Kulchitsky cells. They are found in the bronchial lining. In addition to local effects of the tumour, patients with small-cell carcinoma suffer from a range of paraneoplatic effects; at least some of these may be caused by abnormal hormone secretion from the increased number of small (Kulchitsky) cells. Small-cell carcinoma is very malignant; cell division, tumour growth and metastasis are all rapid processes. However, small-cell carcinoma does respond to chemotherapy.

Non-small-cell carcinomas include tumours which arise from, and are composed of, several other types of cell, the main ones being squamous, adenocarcinoma and large cell. Injuries to the bronchial lining, such as those caused by cigarette smoke, cause the normal columnar epithelium to change to squamous cells. This change in the normal type of tissue found in a location is an example of metaplasia. It is these metaplastic cells which give rise to squamous cell carcinoma and account for up to 35% of all cases of bronchial carcinoma.

Bronchogenic adenocarcinoma usually arises from glandular tissue in the smaller airways and causes about 30% of all cases. Alveolar cells may also become malignant but these only cause about 1-2% of cases. Large-cell carcinoma causes about 15% of all bronchogenic carcinomas. Histologists use this large cell classification when the malignant cells are not squamous or glandular and have been shown not to be small-cell.

Secondary tumours of the lung are also common. In a third of all cancer deaths, multiple metastatic tumour deposits are found in the lungs.

Clinical features

Persistent cough, with or without some chest pain, is the most common presentation. As a tumour mass may cause obstruction in a bronchial passage, normal sputum clearance may be inhibited or blocked and this will cause an area of stasis behind the obstruction. This may lead to a presentation of chest infection. As tumours may cause haemorrhage into the lumen of the respiratory tract, blood may be coughed up, a sign referred to as haemoptysis. Some patients feel generally unwell and present with general malaise. Weight loss may also be present. This develops partly because malignant cells and tumours are metabolically active and use up the bodies energy reserves. Pain is not an early feature. Typically, clinical features only present when the condition is already well established conferring a poor prognosis. Around 80% of patients die within a year of diagnosis.

Later features may occur due to direct spread of the tumour, as it invades local structures. Some tumours may invade the brachial plexus. As this bundle of nerve fibres supplies the arm and shoulder, severe pain may be felt in these areas. If the phrenic nerves are damaged there may be partial paralysis of the diaphragm. The pleural membranes and ribs may be infiltrated with tumour. This causes pain as the parietal pleura and periosteum are very sensitive. Involvement of the pleura may also lead to large pleural effusions; in this complication there is an accumulation of excess fluid in the pleural cavity. Fluid exudate accumulates in the potential pleural space, leading to partial lung collapse and breathing difficulties. Such effusions often need to be drained to improve breathing. If a tumour erodes into a large blood vessel, severe haemorrhage and massive haemoptysis will occur. Many other clinical features of bronchial tumours can be explained as a result of pressure effects as tumours press on other structures in the chest.

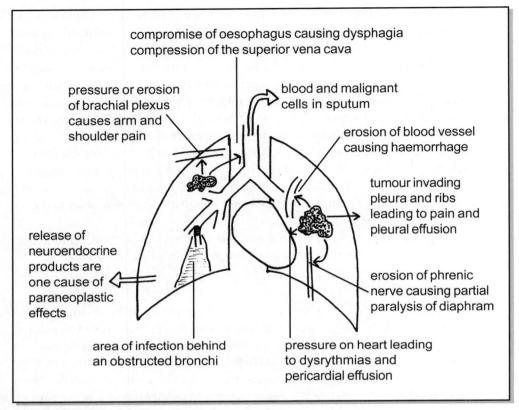

compromise of oesophagus causing dysphagia
compression of the superior vena cava

pressure or erosion
of brachial plexus
causes arm and
shoulder pain

blood and malignant
cells in sputum

erosion of blood vessel
causing haemorrhage

tumour invading
pleura and ribs
leading to pain and
pleural effusion

release of
neuroendocrine
products are
one cause of
paraneoplastic
effects

erosion of phrenic
nerve causing partial
paralysis of diaphram

area of infection behind
an obstructed bronchi

pressure on heart leading
to dysrythmias and
pericardial effusion

Diagram 11.13
Some possible effects of bronchial tumours.

Pressure on the oesophagus, as it passes through the chest, can cause progressive dysphagia as swallowing becomes more and more difficult. Involvement of the pericardium may lead to pericardial effusion and compression of the heart. Abnormal cardiac rhythms may also occur as a result of pressure and local invasion. Tumours which press on the superior vena cava obstruct the normal return of blood from the upper body back to the heart. This leads to congestion of the head and arms resulting in headache and swelling with congested jugular veins.

Metastatic, secondary spread via the blood or lymphatics to distant sites in the body will also occur. This may involve the bones, giving rise to severe pain and possible pathological fractures. Spread to other sites, such as the brain or liver, is also possible.

Management principles

When bronchial carcinoma is suspected a chest X-ray will be ordered. This is usually able to detect tumours of 1 cm or more in diameter. Other investigations include CT scanning and direct viewing using bronchoscopy. Sputum samples should be sent for cytology and AFBs. Cytology may give a definitive diagnosis and if AFBs are found tuberculosis is present. In some cases tuberculosis may be a differential diagnosis for bronchial carcinoma.

As bronchial tumours generate clinical features comparatively late in the disease process, the outcome is often poor. Only a few cases are suitable for surgical resection. In some patients radiotherapy may be part of a curative treatment but more often is used as a palliative intervention. Small-cell malignancies treated with chemotherapy may well go into remission. Various chemotherapy combinations are used for non-small-cell cases but these have a very limited effect. Overall five year survival is less than about 6% in the UK, which means that palliative care is very important in bronchial carcinoma. Given the current unsatisfactory nature of treatment, prevention becomes even more important.

Cystic fibrosis (CF)

Aetiology

CF is entirely genetic. It is autosomal recessive, caused by a defective gene on chromosome 7. The disease presents when a child is homozygous, i.e. has 2 copies of the CF gene. Defective genes cannot produce normal proteins; therefore the protein which the CF gene codes for becomes abnormal, and so does not function as it should. The abnormal protein in CF is called cystic fibrosis transmembrane regulator (CFTR) protein. CF is a disease of white people; it is very rare in black populations and almost unheard of in Asians. In white populations about 1 in 25 people carry one copy of the defective gene, i.e. are heterozygous. These carriers do not suffer from the disease.

Pathophysiology

CFTR protein is located in the membranes of epithelial cells. In the airways, this protein normally exports chloride from inside the cells into the respiratory lumen; therefore in CF this process is inhibited. Reduced secretions of chloride also result in reduced levels of sodium in bronchial secretions. As water osmotically follows sodium, the result is that bronchial secretions become dehydrated. Lack of water in secretions means that they are too thick and therefore too viscous. This is why CF is sometimes described as mucoviscidosis. In addition to affecting bronchial secretions, the lining of the gut and exocrine glands also produce abnormally thick secretions.

Clinical features

Although these children are born with normal lungs, the viscous secretions are not effectively transported by cilia. This is described as reduced mucociliary clearance. Sputum is viscid and difficult to cough up, leading to stasis and repeated chest infections. Over time the lungs deteriorate and bronchiectasis develops leading to further infections. Eventually pulmonary heart disease and respiratory failure develop. Overall, respiratory complications account for most of the morbidity and mortality associated with CF.

Pancreatic secretions are also too viscid. This prevents normal drainage of digestive enzymes from the pancreas into the duodenum. Viscid mucus plugs in the pancreatic ducts cause progressive atrophy, destruction and secondary fibrosis of the digestive enzyme producing exocrine tissue. Subsequent lack of pancreatic digestive enzymes results in poor digestion of food with reduced absorption of digestive products. This in turn leads to nutritional deficiencies which result in retarded growth and delayed puberty. As poorly digested fat is not absorbed, steatorrhoea will present. Steatorrhoea describes bulky, greasy,

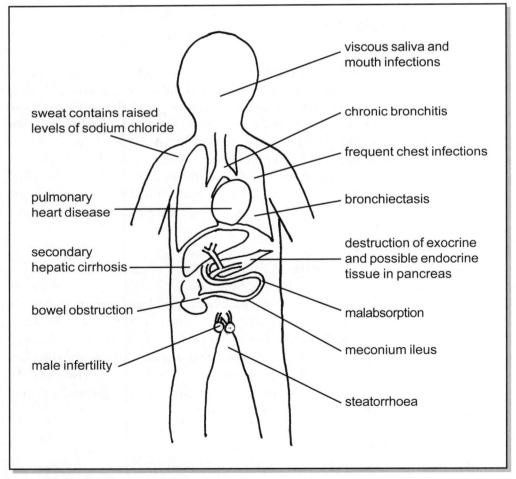

Diagram 11.14
Overview of possible clinical features in cystic fibrosis.

offensive stools which contain undigested fat. Pancreatic fibrosis may involve endocrine tissue and so lead to diabetes mellitus in some older patients.

Bile ducts may also become plugged by viscous secretions. This leads to an increased incidence of gall stones, and in a minority of older patients, hepatic cirrhosis, which may be complicated by portal hypertension. Saliva is more viscous than normal, leading to a dry mouth and a predisposition to oral infections. About 97% of males are infertile, due to viscous secretions causing atrophy and fibrosis of the seminal ducts.

Sweat glands excrete more sodium chloride (common salt) than usual. It is often noted that people suffering from CF taste salty when kissed. It seems strange that other exocrine glands do not secrete enough chloride and sodium while sweat glands secrete too much. This is because sweat glands normally reabsorb some chloride, and therefore sodium, from sweat before the fluid leaves the gland. However, in CF this process is inhibited. The most reliable diagnostic test for CF uses this knowledge to assess the concentration of salt in sweat, which may be 2-5 times higher than normal. CF may be formally diagnosed when sweat sodium or chloride exceeds 70 mmol per litre.

In newborn babies a meconium ileus may present. This is a form of intestinal obstruction caused by a viscous meconium plug in the small bowel. This may be explained by a reduced secretion of the enzyme trypsin from the pancreas, which normally digests and softens the meconium. A further form of potential bowel obstruction occurs in children of all ages when gumlike masses in the caecum obstruct the bowel causing nausea, vomiting and pain.

Treatment principles

Respiratory infections should receive prompt and aggressive antibiotic treatment. Inhaled antibiotics and corticosteroids may also be indicated. Physiotherapy, postural drainage and percussion should be used to increase expectoration. Aerosols of mucolytics can help to hydrate mucus and some new treatments acting on the DNA of inflammatory cells have been helpful. Humidified oxygen may be needed during acute respiratory episodes. Lung or heart lung transplantation has been effective for some individuals.

In order to compensate for the lack of pancreatic secretions, enzymes in capsule or powder form may be given orally with food. A well balanced high protein, high calorie diet of 150% of recommended daily amounts is often needed for normal growth and vitamin supplements may also be helpful. Adequate salt must be eaten to compensate for the losses in sweat. This is especially important during hot weather when more is lost.

The severity and progression of CF in individuals is very variable. Some may die as neonates from meconium ileus while others may occasionally live into their late 40s. Typical life expectancy in CF has risen over the past 30 years, from childhood or teens to mid thirties, or beyond. However, there is still no curative treatment.

Common acute respiratory infections

The common cold

The common cold is correctly termed acute coryza. It is caused by infection of the lining of the nasal cavity with one of many possible rhinoviruses. Viruses may spread from person to person by direct contact or droplet infection. This occurs as viruses are found in small water droplets, given off in large numbers during coughing and sneezing. Typical clinical features are nasal irritation and watery discharge, sneezing, malaise, sore throat and a slight pyrexia. Over a few days the discharge becomes thicker, but the condition usually resolves within a week. Severity of clinical features probably depends on the degree of immunity a person has to the causative virus. After infection with one virus an individual should be immune to the particular strain involved. The problem is there are many possible rhinoviruses and they also change their genetic makeup. These problems result in most people in the UK suffering from 2 or 3 colds per year. Antibiotics are not usually indicated as secondary bacterial infection is not very common.

Sinusitis

This is inflammation of the sinuses around the nose, usually caused by bacterial infection. A sinus is a hollow cavity in a cranial bone. Secretions produced by the lining of the sinuses normally drain via a channel into the nasal cavity. This drainage channel also provides a communication through which bacteria can ascend to cause the infection. If the inflammation blocks the normal drainage channel, pressure builds up within the sinus giving rise to pain. Antibiotic treatment may become necessary.

Influenza

Most people call this flu. Many strains are highly transmissible, in the 1918-1919 pandemic it is estimated that 70 million people died. Such a pandemic, as illustrated by 'Swine Flu', may well occur again and will probably spread around the world rapidly due to frequent international travel. Aetiology is the influenza virus which can infect the upper and lower respiratory tract and occurs in two main forms. Influenza B causes a milder form of the disease and occurs in local outbreaks. Influenza A causes more severe disease and may spread globally, causing a pandemic. Clinical features start with fever, aching joints and limbs, there can be headache and cough and malaise can be severe. Incubation period is normally 2-5 days and the person is ill for around 3 to 5 days. The initial viral infection may be complicated by secondary bacterial infection which may cause pneumonia.

Treatment is mostly supportive. The person must rest completely. Traditionally, plenty of fluids have been advised which sounds reasonable. Antibiotics are not usually necessary unless the patient has an underlying COPD or other chronic disease. Some antiviral drugs help to limit the duration and severity of symptoms and should be given as early as possible after the onset of symptoms. Giving antipyretic drugs to reduce fever is very effective in lowering body temperature and making the patient feel much better. However, pyrexia is a normal defence mechanism which inhibits replication of the virus and also improves the function of the immune system. Prophylaxis by influenza vaccine is reasonably effective but needs to be repeated every year as it must be specific to the prevalent forms of virus.

CHAPTER 12

Hypoxia

Introduction

Hypoxia means a deficiency of oxygen in the body tissues. This is in contrast to the term hypoxaemia, which describes low levels of oxygen in systemic arterial blood. Another term people sometimes use is anoxia. Technically this means a complete absence of oxygen.

Oxygen physiology

In any clinical situation it is always essential to ensure that a patient is oxygenated. Oxygen is required on a continuous basis by every cell in the body. This is why airway, breathing and circulation are always the first priority in any emergency situation. The airway must be patent; the person must be breathing and the blood circulating.

Oxygen is present in the air at a concentration of 20.84% and is required by the mitochondria. These mitochondria are organelles present in all cells, and are sometimes referred to as the 'power house' of the cell. Their function is to combine fuels, such as glucose or fatty acids, with oxygen. When this happens, oxygen breaks down fuel molecules, releasing the energy they contained. The more metabolically active a tissue is, the more oxygen and fuel it will need. Metabolically active cells, such as those in muscles, brain, kidneys or the liver, contain more mitochondria than less metabolically active cells such as those in the skin. Without the energy released by the oxidation of food fuels, there can be no activity in the cell; this is because all of the processes of life require energy to facilitate them. The mitochondria work by converting ADP (adenosine diphosphate) into the energy rich molecule ATP (adenosine triphosphate). It is this ATP which is then used to provide the energy for all physiological processes. The process of oxygen use by the mitochondria is often referred to as internal respiration and is outlined using the equation of respiration below;

$$C_6H_{12}O_6 \quad + \quad 6O_2 \quad \rightarrow \quad energy \quad + \quad 6CO_2 \quad + \quad 6H_2O$$

$$glucose \quad + \quad oxygen \quad \rightarrow \quad energy \quad + \quad carbon\ dioxide \quad + \quad water$$

Significant volumes of oxygen cannot be stored in body tissues. This means that people need a constant supply. Without oxygen there will be no energy, resulting in no physiological processes, resulting in death. In fact a useful definition of death could be the absence of physiology.

Oxygen is essential

As oxygen is needed to produce energy, and all physiological processes need energy, hypoxia will stop a tissue performing normal physiological functions. In addition, if the hypoxia continues, tissues will start to die. In the words of the medical researcher J.S. Haldane (1860-1936) 'Oxygen lack not only stops the machine but wrecks the machinery'.

Hypoxic injury

When a cell is deprived of oxygen it is no longer able it produce energy using oxygen. When energy is produced using oxygen the process is termed aerobic metabolism. As a hypoxic cell will not be able to use this normal form of metabolism it will start to produce energy in the absence of oxygen, a process called anaerobic metabolism. This will produce lactic acid as a waste product which will reduce the pH of the cell, leading to increased acidity. This acid environment has a damaging effect on the chromosomes, cellular organelles and membranes.

As a cell loses its energy supply it is no longer able to pump sodium out of the cell. This means sodium accumulates inside the cell. As sodium is osmotic, water also accumulates within the cells causing them to swell. Despite these changes, cells at this stage have the ability to recover as long as the oxygen supply is restored. However, if the hypoxia persists the damage caused by the acid and swelling will become irreversible. Eventually the membranes around the lysosomes will rupture and the cells will be killed.

Oxygen transport from air to mitochondria

If mitochondria are to be supplied with oxygen, there must first be enough oxygen in the air around us. Next we must be able to breathe this air into our lungs. After this oxygen must be able to diffuse from the alveoli, across the respiratory membranes, through the walls of pulmonary capillaries and into red blood cells. After this, red blood cells must circulate from lungs to tissues. Oxygen must then pass from the red cells, through the capillary membrane and into tissue fluids. Next, oxygen must be able to diffuse through the tissue fluids, into individual cells. Finally, the mitochondria in the cells must be able to use supplied oxygen to oxidise fuel molecules.

This chain of events must occur before the cells of the body can produce energy. If any one part of the chain is absent, or not working properly, the transport of oxygen will stop or be reduced at that point. This will mean the tissues do not receive enough oxygen and will become hypoxic. From this brief review of oxygen physiology it is clear that for hypoxia to be prevented, the oxygen chain must be maintained. If any part of this oxygen pathway is interrupted, this must be rapidly recognised and corrected. Maintaining patient oxygenation is absolutely fundamental.

Classification of hypoxia

A useful way to describe hypoxia is according to the cause. A cause may affect any part of the oxygen chain outlined above. The classifications of hypoxia below are based on this sequence of oxygen delivery; from air to mitochondria. Classifications used will be extrinsic, pulmonary, anaemic, stagnate and histotic hypoxias.

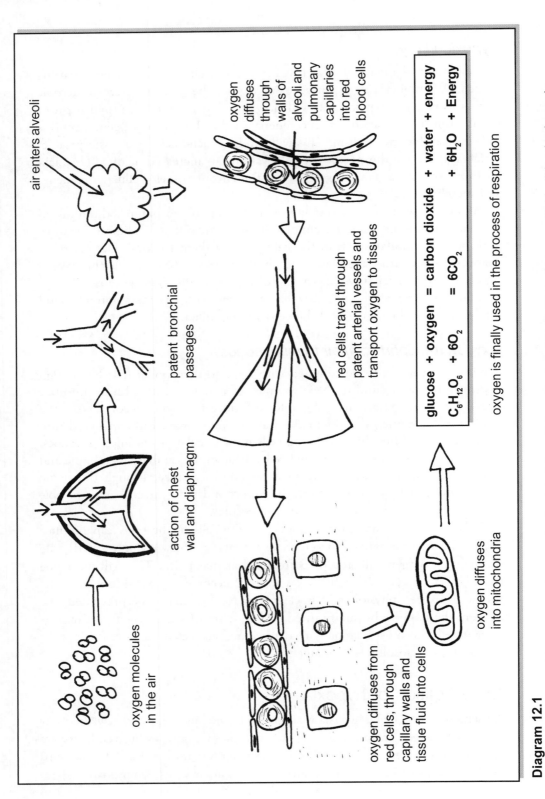

Diagram 12.1
The oxygen pathway from external atmospheric air to intracellular mitochondria. Failure of any one 'link' will lead to hypoxia.

Extrinsic hypoxia

Extrinsic hypoxia describes inadequate oxygenation of the lungs for extrinsic reasons; that is outside of the lungs. This means that the tissues of the body become hypoxic because there is not enough oxygen entering the lungs.

Altitude

Levels of oxygen in the air decrease with increasing altitude. As air pressure is lower at altitude, the part of the total air pressure generated by oxygen is correspondingly reduced. At heights above 2500 metres people can experience problems caused by the altitude. 'Extreme altitude' is described as heights above 5800 metres. If climbers and treckers do not take enough time to acclimatize, the lack of air pressure and oxygen causes a condition called altitude illness or acute mountain sickness (AMS). The sufferer feels ill; the malaise suffered from has been described as having similarities to a severe 'hang over'. Clinically the two common presentations are pulmonary oedema and cerebral oedema. These conditions are described as HAPE (high altitude pulmonary edema) and HACE (high altitude cerebral edema). Both of these disorders can lead to death. People suffering from altitude related illness must rapidly descend until recovered. Altitude related problems may also occur in aviation.

A degree of adaptation to altitude will develop in the process of acclimatization. More erythropoietin will be secreted by the kidney which will stimulate erythrocyte production in the red bone marrow; this will increase the numbers of red blood cells in circulation and so the oxygen carrying capacity of the blood. The number of mitochondria in cells will increase as will the amounts of myoglobin in muscle cells. In many hypoxic tissues more capillaries will grow to increase blood supply and so oxygen delivery. There are also a range of poorly understood intracellular biochemical adaptations which allow people to function on very low partial pressures of oxygen in the blood.

Lack of oxygen in the air

Even at sea level there may be a lack of oxygen in the air. This may be an occupational risk, for example in the alcohol brewing industry a large amount of carbon dioxide is produced. If this displaces enough normal air, workers may be overcome in poorly ventilated areas. There is a similar risk for farmers working in silage pits. The danger from carbon dioxide arises because the gas is much heavier than air, and so settles out in low confined spaces. Drowning is also a situation where there is not any external gaseous oxygen.

Problems causing hypoventilation

Extrinsic hypoxia may also occur as a result of conditions which prevent normal chest and diaphragm movements, so oxygenated air is not drawn into the lungs to take part in gaseous exchange across the alveolar membrane. This hypoventilation may occur in neurological conditions causing paralysis, such as myasthenia gravis and Guillain-Barre syndrome. In addition it may occur after elapid snake bites. Elapids are such snakes as cobras, mambas and krates. The venom from these snakes interferes with neuromuscular transmission, so the respiratory muscles will lack motor innovation. As a result, the victim dies because they are unable to breathe.

An inability to breathe for neuromuscular reasons will also occur with muscle relaxing drugs used by anaesthetists. These drugs cause neuromuscular blockade, preventing transmission of an action potential from the axon of the motor neurone to muscles. Patients receiving muscle relaxing drugs will need to be maintained by artificial positive pressure ventilation. Residual effects of muscle relaxants may cause hypoventilation and consequent hypoxia in the post operative period.

It is important to be aware that respiratory depression may occur as a result of opioid overdose. Opioid drugs were originally based on sap from opium poppies. Currently used examples include, morphine, diamorphine, alfentanil and pethidine. Some people may suffer respiratory problems, even with normal doses of opiates, especially if they have pre-existing chronic hypoxia. This is why patients on opiate analgesics should be monitored for their respiratory and oxygen status.

If a patient does stop breathing, or hypoventilates as a result of opioids, they may be artificially ventilated while an antidote is prepared. Naloxone is the antidote for overdose, or respiratory depression induced by opioids. The dose of naloxone should be titrated for each patient in order to achieve sufficient respiratory response; an initial dose may be 100-200 micrograms, intravenously. Unfortunately naloxone also reverses the analgesic effects of opioids as well as respiratory depressant effects.

Respiratory paralysis can occur as a result of pressure on the chest and abdomen which restricts normal ventilatory movements. This may occur when a person is trapped under fallen masonry or in a car after an accident. Inability to breathe as a result of external pressure has occurred in crowds and in cases where a person has been sat upon by someone else. This is also how constricting snakes such as pythons and anacondas kill their prey. When the prey breathes out, the snake tightens up around the chest to prevent them from breathing in again.

Chest injuries can be severe enough to generate sufficient mechanical deficiency to prohibit normal lung ventilation. This can happen when several ribs are fractured at the same time, especially if some ribs have two or more fractures each. This can lead to an area of chest wall which is not mechanically secured to the rest of the chest wall, described as a flail segment. These patients often need some form of positive pressure ventilatory support while the fractures heal, possibly using a CPAP (continuous positive airway pressure) system. Positive pressure ventilation is when a ventilator blows air into the lungs in order to inflate them, rather than depending on the negative pressures normally generated by the chest wall and diaphragm.

Breathing may also be inhibited by pain; this may be the case in pleurisy, where inflammation of the pleural membranes can cause severe pain with respiratory movement. Pain can inhibit lung ventilation postoperatively or after chest trauma. Pain can also inhibit coughing; this results in the accumulation of bronchial secretions, predisposing to infection. When pain presents as a problem it should be covered with adequate levels of analgesia.

Airway obstruction

If the airway is blocked, air will not be able to enter the lungs and the patient may asphyxiate. Airway obstruction should be suspected in any patient who has noisy breathing or stridor. Stridor describes the abnormal sound generated as air passes a partially occlusive obstruction in the airway. It is also important to remember that if there is a complete obstruction of the airway there will be no breathing sounds at all and the individual will not be able to speak.

Airway blockage may occur for a number of reasons. For example, if a patient is unconscious, the airway may become narrowed or blocked due to lack of tongue and pharyngeal innervation. This allows the tongue to fall back, leading to obstruction. Airway obstruction in these patients can be corrected by extending the airway to 'open' it. Two fingers should be placed under the chin and lifted upwards, to extend the neck. This must be done very carefully in unconsciousness, as the patient is unable to protect their neck as normal. If there is any possibility at all of cervical vertebral damage, the airway should be opened using the jaw thrust manoeuvre. This is done by placing the forefingers of both hands behind the angle of the mandible (lower jaw) and pulling the mandible forward. This movement will also move the tongue forward, away from the airway.

Once the airway is open, an unconscious patient should normally be managed in the recovery position, on their side. This will prevent the tongue falling backwards again; it will further allow saliva to run out of the mouth, instead of into the trachea.

Other causes of obstruction include vomiting during unconsciousness. If a patient is lying on their back when they vomit, gastric contents can be inhaled. As well as the risk of acute airway obstruction, the patient will develop a condition called aspiration pneumonia. Inhalation of vomit is a common problem in cases of drug and alcohol overdose and is frequently fatal. Risk of aspiration is reduced if the patient is positioned head down, or on their side. If vomiting does occur, suction should be used to clear the mouth as soon as possible. If vomiting is considered a particular risk in an unconscious patient, they may be intubated to protect the airway. As a general principle patients with a GCS of less than eight should be intubated 'less than eight, intubate'. Nasogastric aspiration can sometimes be used to remove material from the stomach as a prophylactic measure.

Food may also block the airway causing choking. Again this is a life threatening condition and requires emergency treatment. Some obstructions may simply be removed using suction. In a first aid situation the patient should be placed in a head down position and given up to five sharp blows between their shoulder blades using the heel of the hand. Often the vibrations caused by this can loosen an obstruction. If this is not effective in removing the airway obstruction the patient should be given up to five abdominal thrust manoeuvres. If these measures are ineffective and the patient is unconscious, cardiopulmonary resuscitation may become necessary. If the obstruction is above the level of the larynx appropriately trained people may consider a cricothyroidotomy. This involves making an opening through the centre of the cricothyroid ligament, below the thyroid cartilage, above the cricoid cartilage.

Inflammation of the airway may cause swelling so is another possible cause of obstruction. This may occur in burns patients, as a result of inhalation of hot gases. This is why very careful observation of these patients is vital. Sometimes steroid drugs are given to reduce inflammatory swelling to keep the airway open. Oedema and swelling of the airway may also occur in some forms of severe allergic reaction. Intramuscular adrenaline may need to be given to reduce this swelling. Airway obstruction is also a risk after some forms of surgery, particularly if the face or neck is involved.

In children airway obstruction may develop as a complication of acute epiglottitis. This is a bacterial infection which causes the epiglottis to swell; as a result it may block the glottis which is the opening to the airway. Children are at risk of this because the volume of the pharynx is still physically small. Acute epiglottitis may develop over a few hours. The child feels ill, develops a high fever, has a very sore throat and stridor. Some children lean forward in an attempt to keep their airway open. These children may need to be intubated in order to maintain their airway. Steroid medication may be given to reduce swelling and antibiotics such as cephalosporin used to combat the infection.

For the first six months of life babies can only breathe through their noses. They are described as obligate nose breathers. This means that if the nasal passages are blocked the baby will be unable to breath. After the age of six months a baby is able to breath through their mouth as well as their nose.

Pulmonary hypoxia

Lung disorders are perhaps the most obvious causes of hypoxia; if the lungs are not working properly the process of breathing can be adversely affected. Pulmonary hypoxia may occur as a result of increased airway resistance, disorders affecting alveoli, or reduced membrane transport of oxygen. Virtually any lung disease may lead to hypoxia, such as bronchial asthma, pneumonia, bronchiolitis, lung cancers, chronic obstructive pulmonary disease and cystic fibrosis. Pulmonary oedema will also prevent normal gaseous exchange, as parts of the lungs fill up with fluid. Lung contusion may occur as a result of chest trauma;

this is associated with blood and inflammatory fluid in the tissue spaces which will reduce oxygen absorption. Lung collapse, secondary to pneumothorax, haemothorax or hydrothorax will also cause hypoxia.

Lung collapse

This may occur whenever the potential pleural space is converted into an actual space. There are two pleural membranes, the outer or parietal pleura is adherent to the inside of the thoracic cavity and superior surface of the diaphragm. The inner or visceral pleura is adherent to the surface of each lung. In the potential space between the two membranes there is a slight negative pressure and some lubricating serous fluid. The negative pressure sucks the two pleural membranes together and so ensures lung expansion when there is chest or diaphragmatic expansion. When the ribs move up and out, and the diaphragm moves down during inspiration, the lungs expand to occupy all available space. This lowers the pressure in the lungs causing atmospheric air to be drawn in.

Any injury or pathology which interferes with the integrity of the pleural membranes can lead to lung collapse. Air in the pleural space is referred to as a pneumothorax. Penetrating chest trauma will cause a traumatic pneumothorax and a pathological lesion in the pleural membranes will cause a spontaneous pneumothorax. Damage to the pleural membranes can allow air to enter the potential space from the outside atmospheric air or from within the lungs. This means the visceral pleural membrane is no longer being sucked onto the parietal pleura so the lung will collapse. Chest injuries may lead to bleeding into the pleural space causing a haemothorax. Often after penetrating chest trauma there will be a haemopneumothorax with both blood and air present.

An open wound in the chest wall will allow air to be sucked into the pleural space. This is why such injuries are described as sucking wounds. As the patient exhales some or all of the air passes back out of the wound. In traumatic and spontaneous cases, patients may also complain of pleuritic chest pain and breathlessness. As the lung is collapsed, or partly collapsed, it will no longer be possible to hear breath sound on the effected side. This is because the normal breath sounds are generated by air passing through the bronchial passages. As the space which was formally occupied by lung tissue is now occupied by air, the effected side of the chest will sound more hollow than usual with percussion; this is termed hyper-resonance.

A collapsed lung can be restored to normal function if the foreign material is removed from the pleural space. This is normally achieved using a chest drain. A plastic drainage tube is inserted between the pleural membranes, into the pleural space, and the blood and/or air is allowed to drain out. In order to prevent air being sucked back into the pleural space a valve is attached to the drainage tube. The traditional way to do this is to form a valve by placing the end of the tube under water forming an underwater sealed drain. Such drains can usually be removed after a few days as the original injury heals over.

Diagram 12.2i
In health the visceral pleural membrane is sucked onto the parietal. This means the lung will fill all of the available space in the thoracic cavity. (Pleural membranes are actually much thinner than illustrated.)

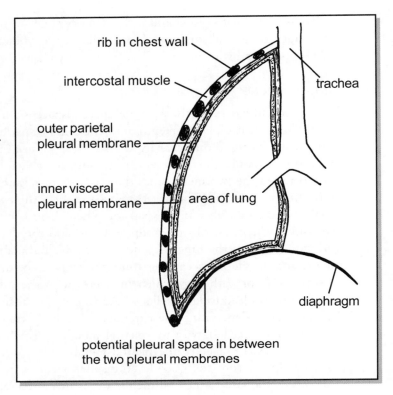

rib in chest wall

intercostal muscle

trachea

outer parietal pleural membrane

inner visceral pleural membrane

area of lung

diaphragm

potential pleural space in between the two pleural membranes

Diagram 12.2ii A pneumothorax with a partially collapsed right lung. Note the parietal membrane remains attached to the chest wall and the visceral is still attached to the lung surface. The potential pleural space has become an actual space.

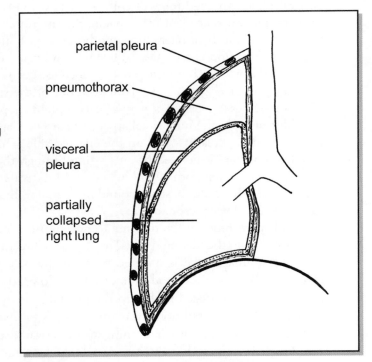

parietal pleura

pneumothorax

visceral pleura

partially collapsed right lung

Some cases of pneumothorax may be complicated by tension effects. In a tension pneumothorax the air in the pleural space is under tension (i.e. pressure). This develops if the injury to the pleura does not seal itself but acts as a valve, allowing air in but not out. Each time the patient breathes in a little more air is sucked in and sealed within the pleural space. This will completely collapse the lung on the affected side. The pressure also pushes the heart and large blood vessels over to the uninjured side, a condition referred to as mediastinal shift. Pressure on the heart and large vessels can close off the vena cava which will prevent venous return to the heart and so reduce cardiac output. Without treatment a tension pneumothorax can be fatal within minutes.

Progressive lung collapse may also complicate some malignant conditions where malignant inflammatory exudate accumulates in the pleural space. Although the inflammatory fluid is not in fact water, this complication is termed a hydrothorax. Aspiration of the fluid using a syringe and two way tap can significantly relieve the symptoms.

Anaemic hypoxia

Even if the atmospheric air is clean and fresh, the lungs are working perfectly and oxygen is diffusing efficiently through the walls of the alveoli and pulmonary capillaries, the tissues can still be hypoxic. This can occur as a result of impaired oxygen delivery by the blood. Erythrocytes (red blood cells) are needed to transport oxygen from lungs to tissues. If there are not enough red cells, or they are defective in some way, oxygen transportation will be impeded. Any cause of anaemia, as discussed in chapter 17, or blood loss can therefore lead to anaemic hypoxia.

Stagnant hypoxia

Sluggish circulation, often referred to as stagnant hypoxia, may occur in congestive cardiac failure or shock, both of which are discussed in separate chapters. If blood is not able to circulate around the lungs and body freely, clearly the transport of oxygen will be impeded.

Venous-to-arterial shunts

A shunt in this context describes a communication between the arterial and venous circulation. If there is mixing of deoxygenated venous blood with oxygenated systemic arterial blood, then some deoxygenated blood will be pumped to the tissues, without first circulating through the lungs to be oxygenated. This may occur in two congenital conditions. Firstly, in septal defects there is a communication between the two sides of the heart. This commonly affects the atria and is called an atrial septal defect (ASD). The communication through the atrial septum will allow deoxygenated blood from the right atrium to enter the left atrium. From the left atrium it will enter the left ventricle and be pumped into the systemic circulation. Surgical correction may be necessary.

Secondly, in patent ductus arteriosus, there is a communication between the pulmonary artery and aorta. During fetal life the lungs are collapsed. This means it is not desirable to have large volumes of blood flowing through the pulmonary circulation until the baby starts to breathe. The ductus arteriosus is a special fetal artery which connects the pulmonary artery with the aorta. Blood ejected from the fetal right ventricle enters the pulmonary artery, but instead of going to the lungs, it passes through the ductus arteriosus into the aorta to join the systemic circulation. Normally blood flow through the ductus arteriosus stops at or shortly after birth. In about 1 in 5500 babies the ductus arteriosus does not close. Surgical closure is indicated in these patients during which the duct is tied off at each end.

Localised causes of stagnant hypoxia

Localised circulatory deficiency may reduce arterial perfusion to regional areas of tissue. This problem may occur secondary to arterial disease or trauma. As a reduced blood supply is referred to as ischaemia, this effect may be referred to as ischaemic hypoxia. This abnormality may lead to clinical features such as intermittent claudication, acute limb ischaemia, angina and cerebral transient ischaemic attacks. Thrombosis will completely occlude an area of its blood supply so will also cause an extreme localized hypoxia, often leading to necrosis, depending on the level of collateral circulation. Local pressure effects, possibly caused by a constrictive bandage, may also cause an acute regional hypoperfusion and hypoxia.

Tissue oedema is another mechanism leading to localized tissue hypoxia. Oedematous fluid in the tissue spaces has the effect of increasing the diffusional distance between oxygenated blood in the capillaries and tissue cells. As oedema increases the distance oxygen must diffuse across to reach tissue cells, the amount of oxygen they receive is reduced. This is one reason why pressure sores are more likely to develop in oedematous areas, as poor oxygenation of tissue cells reduces viability.

Histotic hypoxia

Finally, even if lots of oxygen arrives at the tissue cells, in some conditions the cells may be unable to use the oxygen in the process of tissue respiration. This occurs in some poisonings of cellular enzymes, which is how cyanide works. All of the stages in the generation of energy from oxidation of food molecules require enzymes to facilitate biochemical reactions. Cyanide blocks the enzyme which catalyses the last reaction of this process, so prevents all energy generation, this is why it causes rapid death if enough is taken. In sepsis or SIRS (systemic inflammatory response syndrome) shock the mitochondria are unable to take up or effectively use oxygen. This results in damage to many tissues and contributes to multiple organ failure. Reduced cellular metabolic activity may also complicate vitamin deficiencies such as beri-beri, caused by lack of B vitamins. Some of the vitamin B group act as so called co-enzymes which combine with other enzymes to facilitate biochemical transformations needed in the energy production process. Alcohol and carbon monoxide may also reduce the efficiency of energy production in the mitochondria.

Response of the body to hypoxia

Oxygen flux

The flow of oxygen from lungs to tissues is described as oxygen flux; this is defined as follows;

Oxygen flux = cardiac output x arterial oxygen saturation x haemoglobin concentration x 1.39 (1.39 is the volume of oxygen in mls carried by 1g of haemoglobin).

From this equation we can see that oxygen flux may be increased by increasing cardiac output, oxygen saturation or the amount of haemoglobin in the blood. This explains why we see rapid cardiovascular and respiratory responses to hypoxia and in the longer term a haemoglobin response.

Cardiovascular compensatory response

In hypoxia the heart rate and stroke volume will increase, both of these will increase cardiac output. If cardiac output is increased, oxygen flux will also be increased because oxygen flux is partly determined by cardiac output.

There are chemoreceptors scattered along the underside of the arch of the aorta, these are called the aortic bodies. In addition, there are two carotid bodies, one located at the bifurcation of each of the common carotid arteries. These aortic and carotid bodies are called peripheral chemoreceptors, as opposed to those in the medulla which are classified as central. Peripheral chemoreceptors are sensitive to oxygen lack. The anatomical position of the oxygen lack chemoreceptors under the arch of the aorta and near the carotid arteries allows blood circulating towards the brain to be sampled.

When oxygen lack in the blood is detected, the chemoreceptors are stimulated. These in turn send nervous messages to the cardiac and vasomotor centres in the medulla oblongata of the brain stem. These medullary centres initiate sympathetic activity which increases cardiac output and causes peripheral vascular vasoconstriction. Both of these measures increase blood pressure. These effects mean the red cells are circulating more rapidly between the lungs and body tissues, and so may deliver more oxygen to the tissues in a given amount of time. Even if each red cell is carrying less oxygen than usual, the higher throughput of red cells can make up the difference. The increased sympathetic activity can also cause sweating.

Cerebral hypoxia also directly produces dilation of the blood vessels supplying the brain; in other words hypoxia causes cerebral vasodilation. Again this vasodilation will increase cerebral blood flow and therefore oxygenation, this is another compensatory mechanism.

However, if the degree of hypoxaemia increases, (i.e. the levels of oxygen in the blood continue to drop), energy production in the myocardium will eventually be reduced. This will lead to a reduced cardiac output resulting in a consequent reduction in blood pressure. This will lead to failure of the compensatory increase in blood flow around the body. In addition, as the blood pressure falls there will be a reduced perfusion of the myocardium itself. Hypoxia, and the accumulation of respiratory waste products in the myocardium cause electrical instability. Initially there may be dysrrythmias and this will lead on to cardiac arrest, usually ventricular fibrillation. This is why hypoxic patients should have their ECG rhythm continuously monitored.

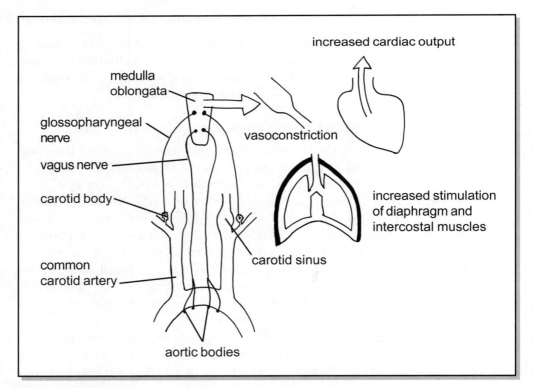

Diagram 12.3
Peripheral chemoreceptors detect hypoxaemia and send impulses to the medulla oblongata. This generates increased sympathetic outflow which stimulates vasoconstriction, increased cardiac output and respiratory effort.

Respiratory compensatory response

In hypoxia there will be tachypnoea (increased rate of respirations) with increased respiratory volumes. This makes perfect sense; if the body is short of oxygen it attempts to compensate by increasing respiratory effort. When O_2 levels decrease, the peripheral chemoreceptors in the aortic arch and carotid bodies are strongly stimulated. These chemoreceptors then send messages, via sensory nerves, directly to the respiratory centre in the medulla oblongata to stimulate respiratory activity and drive.

In normal physiology, the principle stimulus of breathing is an increase in the amount of carbon dioxide (CO_2) in the blood. Increase in blood CO_2 is detected in the medulla oblongata of the brain stem. This central chemoreceptive area then stimulates respiratory drive to increase pulmonary ventilation. In hypoxia blood CO_2 levels may be raised or may be normal, depending on the underlying cause. Clearly, if CO_2 is retained in an otherwise healthy person there will be a massive urge to breathe as respiratory drive is stimulated.

Even if CO_2 levels remain constant the pulmonary ventilation rate will be increased to 15 litres per minute at an oxygen saturation (SaO_2) of 90%. If SaO_2 falls to 80% the pulmonary ventilation rate rises to 25 litres per minute. At lower SaO_2 levels, that is in more extreme hypoxaemia, ventilation rates may be stimulated to even higher volumes. These figures compare to a normal ventilation rate of about 6 litres per minute at rest. In terms of the oxygen flux equation, increased respiratory effort will increase oxygen saturation (SaO_2) of the blood. Increase in SaO_2 will increase oxygen flux meaning more oxygen will be delivered to the tissues of the body.

Increase in red cell numbers response

From the oxygen flux equation we notice that flux is partly dependent on haemoglobin concentration. If haemoglobin concentration is increased, hypoxia will be reduced. Ongoing hypoxia will stimulate the production of more red blood cells which contain haemoglobin. This mechanism works by chronic oxygen lack being detected in the kidneys. They respond by increasing the secretion of erythropoietin. This hormone stimulates erythrocyte production in the red bone marrow. If the number of red cells is increased, so will the oxygen carrying capacity of the blood. This is a very useful mechanism to improve oxygenation at altitude or to improve fitness and aerobic capacity with exercise. Clearly, it will take time to increase red cell production, unlike the cardiovascular and respiratory compensations which work within seconds.

Any disease condition which causes prolonged hypoxia will also have this effect. This means red cell production will be stimulated, in anaemia, cardiac failure and chronic respiratory diseases. Smoking will reduce the oxygen carrying capacity of the blood as a result of the accumulation of carboxyhaemoglobin leading to hypoxia. This will also stimulate red cell production. If there is an

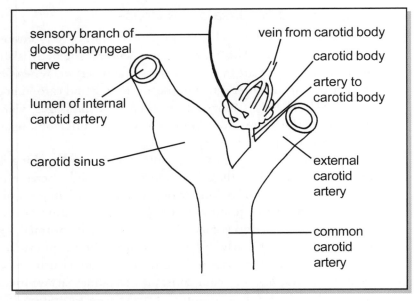

Diagram 13.4
The carotid bodies are located between the internal and external carotid arteries. Despite being very small, they have a high blood flow from the external carotid artery. This allows the sensitive cells in the carotid bodies to detect any reduction in blood oxygenation. If blood oxygen levels fall this information is sent to the medulla oblongata via sensory fibres of the glossopharyngeal nerve.

abnormal increase in the number of red cells in the blood the condition is described as an erythrocytosis or polycythaemia. As there are more red blood cells the blood becomes more viscous and organ perfusion can be reduced. There may be an increase in blood pressure and symptoms caused by reduced perfusion of the brain such as headaches, dizziness or blackouts. Thromboembolic disorders also become more likely.

Other clinical features of hypoxia

Cyanosis

Cyanosis describes the bluish tint seen in skin and mucous membranes which occurs as a result of the accumulation of dark red deoxygenated haemoglobin in the blood. When seen through the skin or mucous membranes this appears as a dark blue to the eye. Cyanosis is often described as central or peripheral. Central cyanosis is caused by hypoxaemia and is seen in the centre of the body in areas such as the lips, tongue, face, neck and chest. Peripheral cyanosis is seen in areas such as the ear lobes and fingers and is often caused by reduced or sluggish circulation. If the blood is going through the peripheries at a slow rate there is more time for it to become deoxygenated.

Central cyanosis is perhaps the best known clinical feature of hypoxaemia. However, it is not a sensitive clinical indicator; even experienced staff often fail to detect any cyanosis in hypoxic patients. When cyanosis is clinically apparent, the oxygen saturation has probably already dropped to 85%. It has been estimated that clinical cyanosis is not present until there is 5g of deoxyhaemoglobin per 100mls of capillary blood. With good monitoring of patient oxygen status using oximetry, cyanosis is a feature we would hope to prevent, rather than treat.

Central nervous system effects

Effects on the CNS vary depending on the severity of hypoxia. Mild hypoxia, with saturations of below 85% may cause fatigue, lethargy, headache, nausea, vomiting, dizziness and confusion, as the thinking parts of the brain no longer work properly. Moderate hypoxia with saturations below 75% will make these features worse causing severe mental impairment; there will also reduce pain sensitivity. Severe hypoxia, with saturations below 65% will lead to coma, convulsions and eventually to death of the brain.

Central nervous system cells may recover after a short period of oxygen deprivation, but neurones are very prone to hypoxic damage. Nerve cells require a constant supply of oxygen to metabolise glucose, on which their energy requirements almost exclusively depend. As the central nervous system contains very few stem cells (i.e. cells capable of mitosis to produce new cells) damaged neurological tissue does not effectively regenerate.

In addition to hypoxaemia, cerebral hypoxia may occur as a result of a reduced blood supply (ischaemia) to the brain. During a feint (i.e. a syncope) the brain becomes unconscious as a result of a transient cerebral hypoperfusion. If blood circulation stops completely, as would be the case in cardiac arrest, brain damage begins after one minute and may be irreversible after three. A complete loss of the supply of oxygen to the brain results in loss of consciousness in about 10 seconds.

Hypoxia and cerebral oedema

In order to improve oxygen delivery in cerebral hypoxia, blood vessels to the brain dilate, increasing blood flow. However, if this hypoxia is severe or prolonged, dilation of cerebral capillaries will lead to increased capillary permeability. In other words they become leaky, increasing the volume of tissue fluid. This vasogenic process will eventually lead to the development of cerebral oedema and raised intracranial pressure. Cerebral hypoxia also leads to disruption of axonal cell membranes. This can result in a loss of intracellular proteins into the extracellular environment. As proteins are very osmotic molecules, they suck water from neurones and capillaries into the tissue spaces. This process dehydrates neurones and further exacerbates cerebral oedema occurring secondary to hypoxia. Hypoxia will also inhibit he normal function of the sodium-potassium membrane pumps. This will cause an increase in the concentration of sodium ions within the cells. This sodium osmoticaly attracts water into the cells leading to cytogenic cerebral oedema.

Hypoxic damage to other organs

All tissues and organs will be damaged by oxygen lack however, the amount of time taken to cause damage varies. CNS tissues can be damaged after one minute. Myocardial tissue is damaged after about 5 minutes when deprived of an oxygen supply. Kidney and liver tissues are adversely affected after about 10 minutes. Skeletal muscles may survive for about 2 hours in the presence of hypoxia.

Treatment of hypoxia

Ideally, hypoxia should be treated by removing or treating the underlying cause. However, this is not always possible. Normally oxygen therapy is indicated. In acute hypoxia it should be ensured that the airway is open and the patient is able to breathe, they can be given oxygen. The saying is 'A and B and oxygen first'.

Aspects of oxygen therapy

Aim of oxygen therapy

The aim of oxygen therapy is to supply enough oxygen to the tissues to allow them to continue functioning normally and to prevent any hypoxic damage. In acute hypoxia we can give 100% oxygen without fear for a period of time, certainly until help arrives. In fact an hour or two on pure oxygen will be safe for most people. What is certain is that if oxygen is not given, hypoxia can be rapidly fatal. For longer term oxygen support, concentrations usually vary from 24-40%, depending on the clinical picture, oximetry and arterial blood gas results. Oxygen should therefore be given at a level which maintains satisfactory oxygen saturations. When patients are ill the target oxygen saturations should be 94-98% (88-92% for patients who chronically retain carbon dioxide). There should be continuous assessment of the patient's oxygenation status with titration as indicated.

It is best to manage patients receiving oxygen therapy sitting upright if possible. This will maximise the efficiency of the respiratory muscles, promoting effective pulmonary ventilation. Sitting up will also help to drain excess tissue fluids from the lung fields. Upright posture promotes dilation of the bronchial passages, also increasing ventilatory volumes.

Oxygen flow rates

The key to good oxygen therapy is a tight fitting mask and adequate total flow rates. A normal inspiration takes one second and inhales 500 mls of air. This means an impractical flow rate of 30 litres per second would be needed if all of the air inhaled was to contain the appropriate percentage of oxygen. Various manufacturers produce masks where this problem is accounted for by mixing oxygen with air before it is supplied to the mask. An alternative method is to pipe oxygen into a reservoir bag with a valve, which allows oxygen rich air from the bag to be inspired.

Warming and humidification

If oxygen therapy is prolonged it should be warmed if possible as this prevents the airways being cooled. Longer term therapy should also use humidified oxygen. This is usually achieved by bubbling the oxygen supply through warmed sterile water. Humidification prevents the respiratory surfaces from drying out. Dry secretions become more viscous or even hardened which reduces normal clearance by the action of cilia and coughing. Retained secretions are at increased risk of becoming infected. This is another example of the general principle that stasis leads to infection.

It is important to remember that ill patients are more prone to opportunistic infection, so we need to make sure the delivery system is not infected. Water particles in humidified oxygenated air may transport bacteria into the lungs, so we need to observe for any early clinical indicators of infection. Expectoration should always be encouraged to remove any potentially infected mucus. Chest physiotherapy is usually indicated. People on oxygen therapy will also appreciate regular mouth care, normally using toothbrush and paste.

Mechanical ventilation

If physiological mechanical ventilation is not able to provide adequate minute volumes, it may become necessary to use some form of positive pressure ventilation. This can be done by use of a positive pressure ventilation sealed face mask or hood, without the need for intubation. However, on other occasions patients need to be sedated and intubated to allow full intermittent positive pressure ventilation for a period of time.

Oxygen toxicity

In clinical practice this is not usually a problem but it is worth knowing about as a potential issue. If high levels of oxygen are given for prolonged periods it can become toxic. After 6 hours on high concentrations over 50%, there can be respiratory features such as cough, reduced clearance of sputum and decreased vital capacity. Over longer periods of time, accumulation of free radicals causes pulmonary endothelial and macrophage damage. Progressive inflammation will lead to pulmonary oedema and ultimately death. Oxygen toxicity is a particular risk in premature babies and neonates where it may cause retinopathy.

Safety aspects of oxygen therapy

Oxygen is odourless and colourless, it is not flammable and it does not burn. However oxygen aids combustion of anything which is burning, so is especially dangerous when mixed with a flammable gas. Ward oxygen cylinders should be stored upright and secured to the wall as they cause a lot of pain if one falls on your foot.

Pulse oximetry

Pulse oximetry is an excellent method for monitoring the oxygen saturations of the patient's blood; it is often referred to as the 'fifth vital sign'. It gives a readout of the pulse rate and oxygen saturation of arterial blood at the level of the tissues. Pulse oximetry is easy to use and completely non-invasive.

Oxygen saturation

Oxygen saturations (SaO_2) are measured as a percentage of blood which is completely (100%) saturated with oxygen. Saturations as recorded using oximetry are often referred to as SpO_2. S stands for saturation and p indicates it is measured in the periphery of the body. O_2 describes the two atoms which comprise an oxygen molecule, so SpO_2 is the saturation of oxygen in the peripheral arterial blood circulation.

Background physiology

The normal range for oxygen saturation in arterial blood is 95-100%. A normal figure of 97% is often quoted. If the oxygen saturation is below 94% the patient is defined as being hypoxaemic. Approximately 98% of the oxygen carried in arterial blood is transported by haemoglobin molecules in red blood cells. As blood passes through the tissues some of this oxygen is given up. Venous blood has a typical oxygen saturation of 75%

How oximetry works

Oximetry probes have two sides which are positioned over the site to be monitored, e.g. a finger. One side contains light emitting diodes which shine a red and an infrared light. These two lights then pass through the finger and are picked up by detectors in the other half of the probe. These detectors measure the intensity of the light that has passed through the finger, and from this a microprocessor is able to calculate how much of each form of light has been absorbed. These two lights are differently absorbed by oxyhaemoglobin and deoxyhaemoglobin. From this the machine is able to calculate the relative proportions of oxygenated and deoxygenated haemoglobin. Pulse oximetry is able to differentiate between the pulsatile blood in arteries and arterioles from the smoothly flowing blood in capillaries, venules and veins. This is why the oxygen saturations recorded reflect arterial oxygen saturation levels.

Recording sites

To give a valid reading an oximetry probe must be positioned so the lights pass through the blood in a vascular bed. The probe is usually placed over the end of a finger or a toe. Sometimes an ear lobe or the nose may also be used. However, some probes are designed for use specifically with digits, so should only be used on fingers or toes. Fingers give the most accurate readings, so should be used as the site of choice. In addition to using oximetry to determine systemic oxygen saturation status it may be used regionally. For example, if there was suspected, or actual, reduced perfusion of a limb this can be assessed by placing the detector on a digit. In babies and children the continuous light generated by the diodes may burn the skin. This may be avoided by removing the probe in-between readings. In adults the position of the probe should be changed every few hours.

Anaemic and histotic hypoxia

Pulse oximetry differentiates between the levels of oxygenated and deoxygenated haemoglobin in the blood. However, in anaemia there may be a simple lack of haemoglobin. This may mean that high saturation levels are displayed, as the blood contains little deoxyhaemoglobin, but the overall oxygen supply to the tissues may be reduced. In other words in anaemia there may be hypoxia in the absence of apparent hypoxaemia. In histotic hypoxia the tissues are unable to use supplied oxygen. This means the oxygen saturations may be high, but the tissues hypoxic.

Carboxyhaemoglobin

As the current generation of machines only use two diodes they are unable to compensate for the presence of carboxyhaemoglobin. This means the saturation readouts may be inaccurate in cases of carbon monoxide poisoning. Even relatively small amounts of carboxyhaemoglobin in the blood can cause an oximeter to overestimate oxygen saturation. In fact carbon monoxide in the blood can give rise to erroneous readings of 100% oxygen saturations. This is a dangerous situation as it gives a false sense of security. This information must be remembered when caring for patients who have been in smoky environments. This is clearly the case with many burns victims. Smokers and people who work in traffic fumes may also give falsely high SpO_2 readings.

Pigments on the nails or skin

Finger nail polish or other pigments on the nails or skin may distort the results of pulse oximetry. These should be removed if present. This is why patients who require surgery should never wear finger nail colouring. Distortions may also occur if there is dried blood or other material on the inner surfaces of the probe. These should therefore be cleaned whenever required.

Alarm settings

Pulse oximeter devices should be used with default alarm settings. This means an alarm will sound if readings fall below, or rise above, the default parameters. Default setting will mean there will be an alarm if the pulse rate falls below 60 or rises above 100. If saturations drop below 95% the alarm should also be triggered. In particular cases we may choose to alter the default settings which should return to normal when the machine is switched off.

CHAPTER 13

Nervous System Disorders

Motor neurone disease

Pathophysiology

In motor neurone disease (MND) there is progressive degeneration of the upper and lower motor neurones. Upper motor neurones are nerve pathways which initiate and control movement; these are located in the brain and spinal cord. Lower motor neurones carry impulses from the spinal cord via peripheral nerves to the muscles. In MND there is no involvement of the sensory neurones which continue to function normally. In some parts of the world MND is referred to as amyotrophic lateral sclerosis (ALS).

Aetiology

The cause of MND is unknown. Slightly more men than women are affected and the onset is usually in middle age. Occurrence of MND is sporadic; cases just seem to occur for no particular reason. There may be an underlying genetic predisposition which results in abnormal biochemistry in the motor neurones, leading to a relentless degeneration. Suggested environmental factors include viral infection, trauma and exposure to toxins.

Clinical features

Progressive muscular wasting (i.e. atrophy) occurs. This process of atrophy often begins in the hands and then spreads up the arms. Muscle atrophy develops when muscles lose their nerve supply and are no longer able to exercise. In addition to atrophy, loss of motor supply to muscles causes a progressive weakness and paralysis. Paralysis eventually affects all four limbs resulting in tetraplegia (tetra means four; all four limbs are involved and plegia means paralysis). Sometimes patients complain of muscle cramps but the disorder is not painful.

Many patients suffer from bulbar palsy which describes a progressive paralysis of the muscles of the mouth, pharynx and larynx caused by cranial nerve involvement. Defective swallowing allows saliva, food and drink to be aspirated into the trachea. This may lead to aspiration pneumonia which is a life threatening condition. Interestingly eye movements remain unaffected in MND. The disorder is always progressive, there are never any remissions. Survival for more than three years is unusual and death typically occurs from bronchopneumonia.

Treatment

There is no curative treatment but good nursing care can prevent the complications of immobility. Feeding via gastrostomy and ventilatory support may extend life.

Multiple sclerosis (MS)

This is a relatively common disorder and is the leading cause of neurological disability in young adults. In Europe and North America the prevalence is 1 in 800 and in the UK 50,000 people are disabled as a result of MS. Onset of symptoms is typically between 20-40 years of age.

Aetiology

The exact cause of MS is not known but the presence of activated T lymphocytes in areas of CNS inflammation suggests an autoimmune mechanism. There is some genetic tendency with an increased prevalence in first degree relatives of sufferers. The condition seems curiously related to the latitude where people live. MS is rare at the equator but becomes more common in people who live nearer to the poles. Children immigrating from near the equator into Northern Europe acquire the same prevalence of disease as people born in the area indicating a possible environmental factor.

Pathophysiology

In MS there is loss of the myelin sheath which normally protects, insulates, and nourishes nerve fibres. Myelin is also necessary for the normal transmission of nerve impulses. Peripheral nerves are never affected in MS; the pathology is limited to the central nervous system (CNS) and optic nerve. In the peripheral nervous system myelin is formed by specialised cells called Schwann cells.

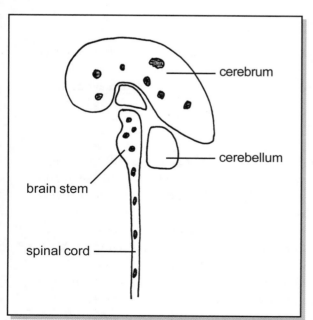

cerebrum

cerebellum

brain stem

spinal cord

Diagram 13.1
Areas of plaque formation occur in various places within the CNS. Lesions are restricted to areas of white matter; areas of grey matter such as the cerebral cortex are not affected.

However, in the CNS it is formed by oligodendrocytes. MS can therefore be seen as a disease of these oligodendrocytes and the myelin they produce.

Lesions in MS are patchy areas of demyelination, mostly forming in the white matter of the CNS. White matter is composed primarily of nerve fibres, as opposed to the grey matter which is largely neuronal cell bodies. Multiple lesions which may form throughout the CNS are visible to the naked eye at post mortem or on MRI scans.

The presence of activated T lymphocytes in an area of white matter triggers an inflammatory cascade with the release of cytokines. This acute inflammation causes loss of neuronal function resulting in a clinical relapse. The particular clinical features suffered during a relapse, and the location of symptoms in the body, will be determined by the anatomical location of the inflammatory lesion within the CNS. Remission occurs when the inflammation subsides. Further remission can occur as oligodendrocytes which survive a period of inflammation recover and resume myelin production, effectively repairing some of the damage.

However, immune mediated inflammation also leads to activation of macrophages which damage and eventually kill the oligodendrocytes and myelin. The end result of this destructive inflammatory process are areas of hardened, demyelinated lesions called plaques. The old name for MS was disseminated sclerosis because the areas of hardened plaques are found in various parts of the CNS. When damage to the myelin reaches a certain point, areas of axons will be permanently damaged. This pathophysiology explains why the disease often has a relapsing and remitting course with an overall downward direction with developing persistent disability.

Diagnosis

This is largely by clinical presentation and is classically described as lesions separated by both space and time. This means that a patient suffers symptoms in different parts of the body at different times. If available, MRI imaging can confirm the diagnosis.

Clinical presentations

Multiple sclerosis takes three main forms; these are relapsing and remitting, primary progressive and secondary progressive. Most patients present with relapsing and remitting disease (about 85-90% of MS cases); the patient suffers symptoms for a period of time which then resolve. However, over a ten year period after initial diagnosis, 50% of these patients go on to develop secondary progressive disease. In this form, after a period of relapsing and remitting MS, there is a steady worsening course with or without flare-ups from time to time.

Primary-progressive MS is less common affecting about 10% of patients. In this form there is an almost continuous worsening of the condition from the onset, with no distinct relapses or remissions.

Clinical features

Lesions of the optic nerve lead to blurred vision in one eye which develops over a few hours or days. This is referred to as optic nerve neuropathy. Vision usually recovers within two months. Often the optic discs of the eyes appear normal as the inflammation is behind the retina; this is referred to as retrobulbar neuritis which is an inflammation of the nerve behind the eyeball.

Motor symptoms include skeletal muscular weakness and spasticity. Spasticity means a state of increased muscle tone which may give rise to painful cramps. There is also sensory involvement when patients may experience areas of numbness or altered sensation.

Bladder dysfunction is common in MS as there is delayed or blocked transmission of nerve signals in parts of the CNS that control urinary function. There may be frequency during the day or night (night time frequency is termed nocturia), hesitancy in starting urination and urinary incontinence. Failure of the bladder wall muscle to contract normally can lead to urinary retention and infection.

Inflammatory episodes affecting the brain stem give rise to clinical features such as double vision (diplopia), facial sensory loss, facial weakness and vertigo. Vertigo describes feeling dizzy with a whirling sensation. Brain stem involvement may also affect lower parts of the body as the motor and sensory nerve tracts pass through this structure on their way to and from the brain.

Swallowing and speech may be affected as a result of lesions in areas of the brain controlling these functions. As swallowing is difficult, choking is a risk. Patients may have emotional lability meaning their emotions can change rapidly. In the later stages of the disease frontal lobe involvement can lead to impairment of memory and reduced intellectual function.

Treatment

There is no cure and there are no treatments which have been proved to alter the long term outcome. Short courses of steroids such as methylprednisolone may sometimes reduce the severity of a relapse. Immunosuppressants are sometimes used but are not of clear benefit. A very expensive drug called beta-interferon has been shown to reduce the relapse rate by one third. It may also delay plaque development. However, long term outcomes do not seem to be improved.

Most treatment consists of good nursing to manage the clinical features of the disease and prevent complications. Prompt recognition of urinary and chest infections is important. Cannabis has been claimed to help nausea and muscle spasms caused by MS. Muscle relaxants such as baclofen are a more established treatment for spasticity. Physiotherapy, occupational therapy and taking time to listen are all very helpful.

Despite all of the problems associated with MS, life expectancy is not greatly reduced and the disease may have a course of 30 years or more. Death may ultimately occur from complications of infection such as renal failure or bronchopneumonia.

Epilepsy

A fit or seizure (both words describe the same thing) occurs as a result of abnormal electrical activity in cerebral neurones. Epilepsy describes a tendency for fits to occur.

Aetiology

In most people who suffer repeated epileptic fits the condition is described as idiopathic which means the cause is not known although genetic factors are often important. Idiopathic epilepsy usually presents in childhood. In the remaining cases some cause can be identified. This may be anything which causes an anatomical or physiological abnormality in the brain such as scarring after injury, congenital or genetic abnormalities, tumours, infection, or cerebral ischaemia. When an underlying cause can be identified the epilepsy is termed secondary or symptomatic. In other words the fits are occurring as a symptom of the underlying disorder. When epilepsy presents in adult life it is highly likely to indicate the presence of focal cerebral pathology.

Pathophysiology

In a normal brain small groups of neurones depolarise together to generate some aspect of brain activity, e.g. motor neurones will depolarise to generate movement in part of the body. The summation of physiological neuronal electrical activity generates the normal electroencephalograph (EEG) trace. In health, spread of electrical activity is inhibited by the action of inhibitory synapses. These reduce the transmission of electrical activity between adjacent neurones. Inhibitory synapses therefore reduce the overall levels of electrical activity in the brain.

In epilepsy the inhibitory synapses do not work properly allowing electrical activity to spread. This results in large groups of neurones depolarising together. When large groups of nerve cells are switching on and off together in this way it is referred to as hypersynchronisity; many neurones are synchronized as opposed to just a few. This abnormal pattern of neuronal electrical activity gives rise to the characteristic 'spike and wave' pattern on the EEG. Epilepsy has been described as 'an electrical brain storm'.

Seizure threshold

All people are capable of having a seizure. If the brain is electrocuted, or certain drugs are given, everyone will fit. In addition non-epileptics may start having fits as a result of an anatomical lesion in the brain such as a tumour,

Diagram 13.2
The origin and spread of abnormal electrical activity in primary generalised epilepsy. Most of these seizures probably originate in the area of the diencephalon. This area contains fibres which communicate upwards to both cerebral hemispheres, explaining why the seizure begins synchronously throughout the cerebral cortex. From the

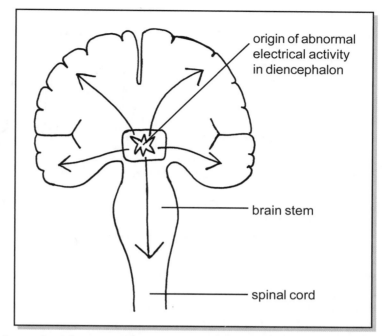

origin of abnormal electrical activity in diencephalon

brain stem

spinal cord

diencephalon, fibres also project downwards to the brain stem and spinal cord. These nerve fibres convey excessive, abnormal electrical activity down to the spinal cord and on to the skeletal muscles. Arrows indicate spread of electrical activity.

Diagram 13.3
Partial (also called focal) epilepsy originates in a localised area of the brain, in this case the temporal lobe. If the abnormal electrical activity is confined to one brain area the seizure remains partial. However, the abnormal electrical activity may spread to the diencephalon, from where it can spread upwards to the cortex, and down to the brain stem and spinal cord. If this spread occurs there will be a generalised secondary seizure.

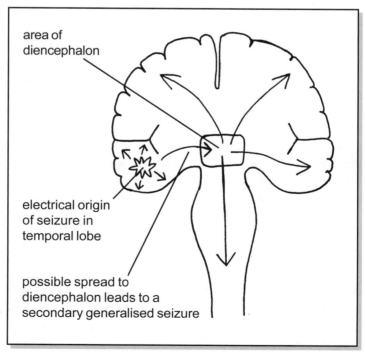

area of diencephalon

electrical origin of seizure in temporal lobe

possible spread to diencephalon leads to a secondary generalised seizure

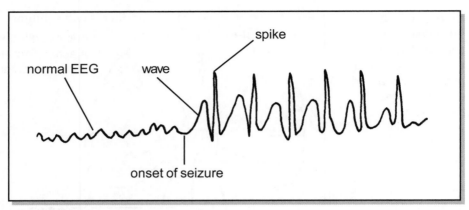

Diagram 13.4
A normal EEG suddenly becomes a spike and wave pattern as a seizure begins.

cerebrovascular disease or after trauma. The difference between an epileptic and a non-epileptic is seizure threshold. People who are epileptic have a low threshold compared to the normal situation. For example, in some patients a flashing light of a particular frequency may be enough to bring on a seizure.

Classification of epilepsy

Seizures can be classified as partial or generalised. In a partial seizure the abnormal electrical activity is restricted to a localized (focal) area of the brain. For example, if the abnormal electrical activity is confined to part of the left cerebral hemisphere the clinical features would be limited to part of the right side of the body.

However, a local event may spread to affect all of the brain, in which case the seizure progresses to becomes generalised. This effect is called a secondary generalization of a partial seizure. A generalised seizure affects both hemispheres of the brain and so the clinical features are seen to affect all of the body. The greater the area of cerebral cortex affected by abnormal electrical activity, the less capable the brain will be of generating normal consciousness. So in a partial seizure there should be no, or limited loss of awareness, whereas in generalised seizures consciousness is lost.

Partial seizures

Partial seizures may be subdivided into simple or complex. In simple partial there is no loss of consciousness. In complex partial there is some disturbance of awareness. Before the attack begins there may be an event called an aura. This is usually a sensation the person experiences which warns that a seizure is about to begin. An aura is usually a sensory experience such as a characteristic smell, taste in the mouth or tingling.

In Jacksonian (also called partial motor) seizures there are involuntary jerking movements, often beginning in the thumb and fingers. These movements then spread to affect the limbs on one side of the body. The seizures are simple in that consciousness is preserved. For a few hours after such a seizure, the affected limbs may be very weak. This is called Todd's paralysis.

Other areas of the brain may be affected by partial seizures giving rise to the experience normally generated by the area of brain involved. For example, visual abnormalities may occur if the occipital lobes are affected. Temporal lobe epilepsy may give rise to mystical experiences and feelings of unreality. There may be déjà vu, the feeling that something is familiar or has happened before. Some people even find temporal lobe seizures pleasurable.

Generalised absence seizures

There are two common forms of generalised seizure; these are absence seizures (also called absence attacks) and tonic clonic seizures. Absence seizures used to be referred to as petit mal fits. In this form of epilepsy the person seems to be 'absent' for a short time, often just a few seconds. Individuals affected by absence seizures almost always present in childhood.

During an absence seizure the child stops their activity and appears to be staring into space. As the abnormal electrical activity causing the absence seizure does not spread out of the cerebral hemispheres the posture is maintained and there is no muscle spasm or shaking. After a few seconds normal activity is usually resumed as if nothing has happened. Sometimes the seizures present in such a mild way they may be missed or dismissed as 'day dreaming'. If an EEG is recorded during an attack, global spike and wave activity will be seen. It is important for people who work with children to be aware of the possibility of this form of generalised epilepsy.

Absence seizures are never caused by lesions of the CNS such as tumours or scarring, they occur as a result of abnormal development of neuronal synaptic inhibition. Children who suffer absence attacks unfortunately often go on to develop tonic-clonic fits in adulthood.

Generalised tonic-clonic seizures

In this form of seizure (previously termed grand mal) there are clearly defined stages. Often there is an aura where the patient has some unusual feeling or sensory experience. It is useful if patients can recognise an aura as they can lie down so they do not fall and hurt themselves.

Shortly after an aura, the tonic phase begins. If an EEG is in place there will be generalised spike and wave activity in both hemispheres. The whole body becomes rigid as all of the antagonistic pairs of muscles contract together. This happens because the generalised abnormal electrical activity generated in the brain passes down the spinal cord and out to the muscles via the motor neurones. Patients may cry out due to involuntary contraction of the diaphragm, expelling air through the vocal cords.

At the start of the tonic phase consciousness is lost and the patient falls over. Nasty injuries are often sustained as a result of these falls as the muscles are rigid. Clearly the life of a patient is at risk if they are driving, up a height, beside a fire or in water at the time of tonic onset. Sometimes the patient also bites their tongue. There may be incontinence of faeces or urine, depending on what is in the rectum or bladder at the time. The tonic phase may last from a few seconds up to a minute.

The tonic phase then passes directly into the clonic. In the clonic phase there is rhythmic jerking of skeletal muscles giving rise to a 'shaking fit'. Increased stimulation of salivary glands combined with involuntary muscular activity gives rise to frothing at the mouth. This stage may last for a few minutes. Once the clonic stage is over the patient remains in a coma for a variable amount of time and this is usually followed by a few hours of confusion and drowsiness.

Status epilepticus

In this condition repeated epileptic fits occur one after another without recovery of consciousness between seizures. This is a medical emergency and carries a risk of death from cardiac or respiratory failure. Status epilepticus is usually treated with intravenous benzodiazapines and anticonvulsants.

Treatment principles in epilepsy

During a seizure the aim is to stop the patient harming themselves. If possible their fall can be controlled in some way to prevent injury. Physical restraint is not necessary and it is appropriate just to hold their hand and wait for the fit to finish. It is clearly essential to maintain the airway during and after the fit as the patient is unconscious. They should be nursed in a semi-prone recovery position and the airway continuously monitored. When recurrent seizures occur they need to be prevented by using anticonvulsant drugs. In the UK people are not allowed to drive unless they have been clear of seizures for one year.

Guillain-Barré syndrome

Aetiology

Guillain-Barré develops 1-4 weeks after a viral infection which is often trivial. Gastrointestinal infection with campylobacter is also known to be a cause in some people.

Pathophysiology

This condition is caused by an acute inflammatory demyelinating polyneuropathy. This means that many peripheral nerves become inflamed and do not work properly. Motor and sensory nerves are involved.

Initially, the immune system produces antibodies to combat an incidental infection. The immune system is able to identify invading organisms as foreign antigens by recognising non-self material. Invading microorganisms have particular shaped molecules on their surfaces. These foreign molecules are referred to as epitopes and have a particular molecular shape. In order to counter the infection the immune system produces specific antibodies which are immune proteins. These are individually engineered to be able to bind onto specific foreign epitopes. Once bound to the epitope, antibodies are able to destroy the invading antigenic organism.

The problem is that some of the molecules on the surface of nerves, and their myelin sheaths, have a similar shape to the foreign epitopes. This means the body's own antibodies may bind to and damage it's own nerves and myelin sheaths (so called molecular mimicry). In other words there is a failure of the body to be self-tolerant and not immunologically attack its own tissues. This leads to the release of inflammatory cytokines which block nerve conduction leading to the acute neurological deficit. In severe cases there may also be complement mediated destruction of the myelin sheath and the associated length of nerve fibre.

Clinical features

Symptoms usually begin in the feet or hands and work towards the centre of the body. In other words initial features are usually distal with proximal progression. There is muscular weakness and abnormal tactile sensations with limb pain. The condition progresses over several days to three weeks. About 20% of patients rapidly develop respiratory failure caused by paralysis of the respiratory muscles. Without respiratory support these patients may die from not being able to breathe. Eighty percent of patients make a complete recovery over 3 to 6 months, but a minority suffer from varying degrees of ongoing neurological disability.

Treatment principles

Treatment basically consists of keeping the patient alive until they spontaneously recover. Respiratory function should be closely monitored with a minority of patients requiring mechanical ventilation for a period of time. Good nursing can prevent the complications of immobility. Subcutaneous heparin should be given to guard against the development of deep venous thrombosis. Corticosteroids do not help.

Meningitis

Aetiology

There are a variety of causes of inflamed meningeal layers; these include infection with bacteria, viruses, fungi and protozoa. Malignant cells in some cases of cancer are another possible cause. Inflammation may also be caused by drugs or contrast media given into the CSF (intrathecally) and by blood after a subarachnoid haemorrhage.

Bacterial meningitis is an acute life threatening disease. The 3 most common bacterial forms are meningococcal, streptococcal and haemophilus meningitis. A variety of viruses may lead to the viral form of the disease. Viral meningitis may initially present a similar picture to the bacterial form but is usually less serious and is self limiting. Possible aetiological viruses include enteroviruses (e.g. echo, coxsackie and polio), mumps, herpes simplex and HIV.

Transmission

Spread occurs via airborne droplet transmission from the nasopharynx of people suffering the disease or from carriers. A carrier is an individual who carries the pathogen which causes the disease but does not suffer from the condition themselves. Kissing is another possible mode of transfer. In the case of enteroviruses spread is via the faecal-oral route. Although meningitis may occur at any age it is most common in young people and children under the age of 14 years. The increase in incidence in late teenage and early twenties is probably due to close contact between young people in schools, colleges, residences and clubs.

Pathophysiology

Inflammation of the meninges is referred to as meningitis. Inflammation in the meninges will lead to increased blood flow in the meningeal vessels. There will also be an increase in capillary permeability leading to the formation of inflammatory exudate. In bacterial meningitis large numbers of neutrophils accumulate in the CSF, arachnoid and pia mater, often leading to the development of a layer of pus. These factors lead to cerebral oedema and raised intracranial pressure.

Clinical features

Meningism is a frequently used term which describes the group of symptoms which accompany inflammation of the meninges from any cause. The principle clinical features are headache, neck and back stiffness, nausea, vomiting and photophobia. Malaise in meningitis is often intense. The headache is global and usually severe. Fever with rigors occurs as a consequence of infection.

Neck and back stiffness and a positive Kernig's sign (inability to fully extend a leg with the hip joint flexed without extreme pain) develop within a few hours of feeling unwell. When the neck is flexed in an attempt to touch the chest with the chin, the neck muscles will tighten. The patient will not be able to curl up enough to touch their nose on the knees. These physical signs are generated by stretching of the inflamed meninges and the muscle guarding this produces.

Other possible features of meningitis include confusion, drowsiness, joint pain and fitting. There may also be disorientation and acute confusion. Importantly meningitis should be considered in all patients who have headache and fever.

Meningism may occur in the absence of meningitis but should always receive a rapid clinical assessment. In babies the presentation is different; there is rarely evidence of neck and back stiffness, they usually appear flaccid and there may be a bulging fontanel.

Clinical features in bacterial meningitis

This is usually of sudden onset with a high fever. A petechial haemorrhagic rash often develops but the rash may well be sparse and not develop for some time. Rash is a very serious sign as it means there is a septicaemia. Petechial describes small red or purple spots caused by leakage of blood into the skin. The rash does not fade or blanch when pressed on with a glass because the red blood cells are in the tissue spaces. This is in contrast to a rash caused by inflammatory vasodilation which will blanch under pressure. If the septicaemia is not treated the rash gets bigger and looks like bruising.

Clinical features in other forms of meningitis

Viral meningitis is typically less severe than the bacterial form of the disease and is usually self limiting in 4-10 days. Tuberculosis meningitis causes chronic meningitis with vague headache, lassitude and anorexia. Malignant meningitis causes a chronic meningitic process which may cause other neurological features such as cranial nerve palsies.

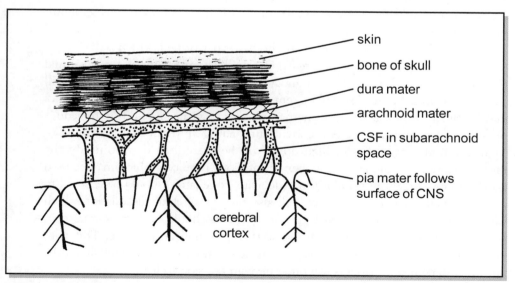

Diagram 13.5
The meninges are composed of the three layers which surround the CNS; they are the dura mater, arachnoid mater and pia mater. As the meninges form a continuous surface around the brain and spinal cord infection is able to spread around these areas. In pyogenic meningitis the CSF contains purulent exudate.

Complications of bacterial meningitis

The probability of serious complications or death increases rapidly with time. This is why very prompt treatment is so vital. The bacteria causing the meningitis or its toxins may damage the brain and major nerves.

There is a risk of rapidly developing septicaemia with acute septic shock. Septicaemia means bacteria are proliferating in the blood. This condition is correctly referred to as fulminating meningococcaemia if caused by meningococcus. There is overwhelming shock, often complicated by renal infarction. It is important that the disease is detected well before septicaemia develops as death occurs within 6-18 hours.

Hydrocephalus may develop as a result of purulent material obstructing the flow of CSF. Further complications include cerebral infarction, cerebral abscess and subdural empyema. Patients may be left with neurological problems such as deafness, blindness, learning difficulties, paralysis or intractable epilepsy. Septicaemia caused by meningococcal infection may present in the absence of meningitis and therefore without the usual meningitic clinical features. Meningococcal septicaemia can also be complicated by gangrene of the hands and feet which in severe cases can necessitate amputations.

Management principles

Meningitis has a high mortality and therefore must be treated as an emergency. Minutes count, literally minutes. Clinically diagnosed bacterial meningitis or septicaemia should be immediately treated with intravenous benzylpenicillin prior to transfer into hospital.

Once in hospital a lumbar puncture should be performed, which is diagnostic for meningitis. In bacterial meningitis this will reveal a cloudy cerebrospinal fluid with increased numbers of monocytes and neutrophils. Protein levels will also be increased. Some CSF will be sent for microscopy and culture. Analgesics may be given for headache. Dexamethasone may be given in children to reduce neurological complications. Anticonvulsants may be prescribed for fitting.

Intravenous antibiotics in high doses will be prescribed depending on the microbiology. There are also a number of antibiotic protocols which may be used if the causative organism is unknown. Adequate oxygenation should be ensured to prevent hypoxia. Good oxygenation will also prevent cerebral vasodilation which will exacerbate raised intracranial pressure. Patients should be barrier nursed in isolation for 24-48 hours until antibiotic therapy has been effective. This is to prevent the spread of the disease to other patients and staff. The room should be quiet and darkened as patients will often have an aversion to light.

Prevention

Haemophilus (Hib) vaccine is now available. Parents should be informed that Hib vaccine will not mean that children are immune to all forms of meningitis. Currently the meningococcal vaccine is effective against serogroups A and C. Public education is important to alert people to the risks of delaying treatment. The danger signs need to be understood so early medical help may be sought. People who have come into close contact with people suffering meningococcal infections should be given a short course of prophylactic rifampicin or ciprofloxacin.

Prion disease

Prion diseases have been known for a long time but were wrongly believed to have been caused by a 'slow virus'. They have recently come to prominence with 'mad cow disease' correctly termed bovine spongiform encephalopathy; 'bovine' means to do with cattle.

Pathophysiology

Prion diseases lead to spongiform encephalopathies. 'En' means in, 'ceph' relates to the brain and 'pathy' is disease of, spongiform describes a brain which has many small holes – like a sponge. Prion is short for proteinaceous infectious particle. These particles of protein may transmit prion disease with no bacteria, viruses or other infectious agents involved. The discovery that proteins alone can transmit disease was a surprise.

Once a prion protein gets into the nervous system it converts normal proteins into more prions. So in an infected person the volumes of normal protein decline while the amount of prion type protein increases. The abnormal prions formed in a sufferer are in themselves infectious, and may trigger the prion formation process if they are able to enter a second person. Creutzfeld Jacob disease (CJD), new variant CJD and Kuru are all prion diseases.

Clinical features

The diseases are characterised by loss of motor control, dementia, paralysis, wasting and eventually death.

Transmission

Infection may be acquired by eating foods infected with prions or following procedures such as certain forms of surgery with infected instruments, growth hormone injections, corneal transplants and possibly blood transfusions. Normal methods for the sterilisation of surgical instruments may not remove potentially infective prions.

Alzheimer's disease (AD)

Alzheimer's disease is the most common form of dementia. In dementia there is a progressive irreversible loss of intellectual function. Dementia is irreversible as neurones cannot divide to replace areas of lost brain. Alzheimer's disease may progress rapidly or slowly but the overall direction is to decline. Death occurs after about 10 years if the patient is well nursed and does not die of something else first. If a dementia begins before the age of 65 years it is described as presenile, but the pathology and clinical pictures are the same as in senile dementia, which begins after the age of 65.

Aetiology of Alzheimer's disease

AD is primary, that is it does not seem to occur as the result of an underlying disease process. The cause is unknown and the majority of cases are sporadic, but there is a genetic component in about 10% of cases. Alzheimer's is more likely to occur with a history of head injury or Down's syndrome. Smoking, hypertension and hypercholesterolaemia seem to somewhat increase risk.

Clinical features

Onset is insidious with progressive loss of intellect and memory. There are also personality changes. Often the first feature which is noted is memory loss and an inability to learn new things. Memories for recent events are lost first, while distant memories from childhood and youth may be preserved for longer. Language function declines, often beginning with difficulty remembering names. In early disease there may be distress and agitation as the person realises what is happening to them but later in the condition insight is often lost. Wandering and aggression are also possible.

Disorientation begins with time, and then progresses to place and person. This means they will not know when, in time, they are, which might begin with the hour, day or month but can progress on to the year and decade.

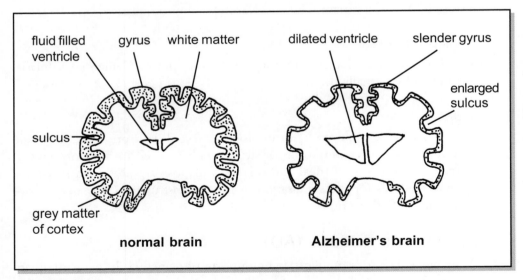

Diagram 13.6
A section of normal brain in comparison to one with features of AD. Note the loss of cortex and dilation of the ventricles in the diseased brain. The gyri become slender and the sulci wide and prominent.

Disorientation for place means patients do not know where they are. Patients in hospital often think they are living at home. In disorientation for person, patients are confused about who someone is; patients may believe a nurse to be their daughter, wife or mother.

Pathophysiology

In AD there is a general loss of neurones resulting in a cortical atrophy, most notable in the parietal and temporal lobes. Loss of brain tissue also leads to enlargement of the ventricles; this means brain tissue is replaced by cerebrospinal fluid. Microscopically there are extracellular deposits of abnormal amyloid found in the brain; this is a protein which accumulates in the tissues. Amyloid is found in numerous senile neurotic plaques which are surrounded by damaged neurones. Amyloid deposition may also damage the walls of blood vessels in the brain.

Within the cytoplasm of abnormal neurones are pathological structures called neurofibrillary tangles. In a normal cell there is an internal framework composed of microtubules. These are composed of a protein called tau. In AD these microtubular proteins get all tangled up causing affected cells to die off. Severity of the disease is largely related to the number and distribution of these plaques and tangles. Reduction in production of acetylcholine may partly account for memory disturbance.

Other causes of dementia

The second most common cause of dementia has a vascular aetiology and is usually called multi-infarct dementia. This usually develops after a series of cerebrovascular events as a result of arterial occlusions. Unlike Alzheimer's which is primary, multi-infarct dementia is clearly secondary to cerebrovascular disease. Third most common is Lewy bodies dementia. Lewy bodies are collections of abnormal protein found inside neurones. Other forms of dementia are Pick's disease, Creutzfeldt-Jacob and Huntington's diseases. In Parkinson's disease mental function is initially well preserved but dementia often presents in the later stages.

Parkinson's disease

This disease was first described by James Parkinson in 1817. The disease is more common in the elderly but may present in middle or even young adult life.

Aetiology

Parkinson's disease is idiopathic meaning the cause is not known. It occurs all over the world. Early onset Parkinson's disease may have a slight genetic tendency. Interestingly, a few epidemiological studies have shown a reduced prevalence in smokers.

Pathophysiology

In the substantia nigra and basal ganglia there is progressive death of cells which produce the neurotransmitter dopamine. The substantia nigra is a strip of dark pigmented cells located in the midbrain and the basal ganglia are collections of nerve cell bodies located near the base of the cerebrum.

Motor impulses which initiate movement of the body all originate from the motor cortex. However, these often need to be modified by the basal ganglia and substantia nigra. These structures are involved in planning, initiating, maintaining and terminating many aspects of motor activity and therefore movement. The substantia nigra and basal ganglia therefore monitor and modify motor activity initiated by the motor cortex. They are also involved in maintenance of muscle tone, posture and making fine adjustments to movements. Collectively these structures comprise the extrapyramidal motor system.

All of the motor nerve pathways in the brain can be classified as pyramidal or extrapyramidal. The pyramidal motor system consists of the nerve pathways which arise in the motor cortex and pass directly through the midbrain, pons and medulla in the bundles of motor fibres called the medullary pyramids. These bundles were named because they form elevations, which are vaguely pyramid shaped in cross section, passing down the front of the medulla oblongata.

Conversely, the extrapyramidal system involves the passage of motor impulses through the basal ganglia and substantia nigra where they are modified as described above. These extrapyramidal tracts do not pass through the pyramids of the medulla.

The extrapyramidal system needs the neurotransmitter dopamine to function normally. For an unknown reason these dopamine secreting cells die in Parkinson's disease. This means that nervous impulses cannot be transmitted through the structures of the extrapyramidal system normally. It is this abnormality which gives rise to the clinical features of Parkinson's disease. This anatomy and physiology also explains why Parkinson's signs and symptoms are sometimes described as extrapyramidal features.

Clinical features

The principle features are generalised slowness of movement, stiffness and tremor at rest. Activities such as dressing can become very slow processes; it is a bit like watching a film in slow motion. The correct term for slowed movements is bradykinesia, 'brady' means slow and 'kinos' refers to movement. Slowness comes about because the dopamine producing neurones in the substantia nigra have an indirect effect on the function of the motor cortex. Lack of activity in the substantia nigra results in inhibition of the rate at which the motor cortex functions, leading to slow movements.

As a result of muscular stiffness the joints feel stiff when moved by an examiner. Stiffness of movement is present equally in opposing muscle groups. Opening or closing an arm has been compared to straightening a length of lead pipe; this is why such stiffness is sometimes called 'lead pipe rigidity'. Stiffness of muscles may be explained as a consequence of the reduced ability of the extrapyramidal system to control muscle tone.

Akinesia refers to absence of movement and this may develop in more severe cases. Inability to move facial muscles generates a typical 'mask like' appearance as facial expressions can no longer be generated. Blinking rates are also reduced giving the impression that the patient is staring.

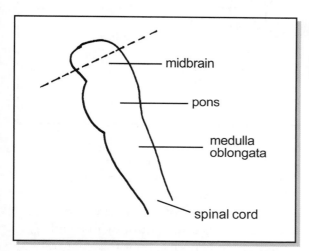

Diagram 13.7
The brain stem is in three sections, the midbrain, pons and medulla oblongata.

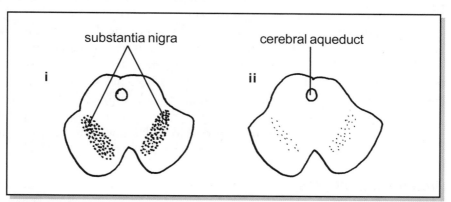

Diagram 13.8
i. This shows a section through a normal midbrain at the level shown in the previous diagram. Note the dark staining of the healthy substantia nigra. These cells release dopamine.
ii. A section through the midbrain in an advanced case of Parkinson's disease, note the lack of the dark stained dopamine producing cells of the substantia nigra. The cerebral aqueduct contains cerebrospinal fluid.

Diagram 13.9
This diagram illustrates an extrapyramidal pathway from the cerebral cortex through the basal ganglia and substantia nigra. In Parkinson's disease these structures do not produce enough dopamine so the transmission is absent, reduced or abnormal.

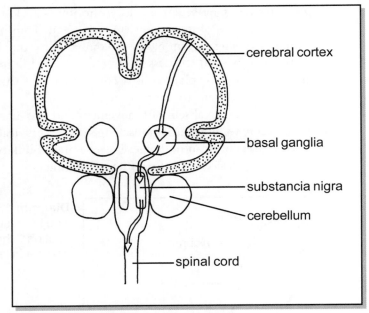

- cerebral cortex
- basal ganglia
- substancia nigra
- cerebellum
- spinal cord

In addition to stiffness it becomes difficult to initiate movements such as walking or getting up from a chair. This feature is consistent with the role of the basal ganglia in the planning and initiation of movements. The characteristic Parkinsonian tremor is present at rest; it has a frequency of 4-7 Hertz or cycles per second. As the extrapyramidal system is involved in control of fine and precise movements the tremor may be seen as an abnormality of this control mechanism, again caused by lack of dopamine.

Features develop slowly over months and years as the dopamine producing cells gradually reduce in number. Over time there is also a change in posture, which is not surprising as part of normal extrapyramidal function is to control posture. The patients develop a stoop. Walking becomes shuffling with small steps. Balance is also impaired causing frequent falls and accidents.

Speech is usually monotonous and later becomes slurred. Difficulty in swallowing, often with dribbling also develops. Handwriting becomes small (technically referred to as micrographia) and spidery.

Treatment principles

Good nursing and physiotherapy can delay adverse effects of immobility. No drug treatments slow down the evolution of the disease. Drugs which enhance dopamine activity in the brain have a dramatic short term effect in reducing the clinical features. Especially in early drug treatment, flowing movements can be regained. Levodopa is often used as it is a precursor to dopamine; the problem is that after some time it can produce excessive movements and hallucinations. Anticholinergic agents also have a place in early management.

Parkinsonian syndromes

Various other conditions may give rise to Parkinson type features. These include some viral infections, damage caused by certain toxins and as a side effect of some major antipsychotic tranquillisers.

Cerebrovascular accident (Stroke)

Stroke is defined as a focal neurological deficit due to a vascular lesion which lasts for more than 24 hours. Stroke is the third most common cause of death in most developed countries, after heart disease and cancer. It is also the major cause of disability in adults.

Thromboembolic pathophysiology

There are two main types of stroke; thromboembolic and haemorrhagic. As the name implies thromboembolic stroke is caused by an occlusion of the normal blood supply by thrombosis or embolism. This cause of stroke is most common accounting for about 85% of cases. Thromboembolic stroke occurs mostly as a compilation of atherosclerosis with atheroma leading to thrombus formation. As in other forms of arterial disease a thrombus will develop on a ruptured plaque of atheroma. The presence of a thrombus will occlude an arterial lumen and so fully or partly cut off the blood supply to an area of the brain. Parts of a thrombus may break away from the main clot generating emboli. When an embolus reaches a vessel it is too large to pass through, the embolus becomes jammed, occluding blood flow. Thromboembolic pathology may arise from the heart and large extracranial arterial vessels supplying blood to the brain or from smaller intracerebral vessels.

Extracranial emboli

Emboli may arise from thrombus formation in the heart. Emboli from the left side of the heart can pass into the cerebral circulation via the aorta and account for about 20% of thromboembolic strokes. Emboli may be generated in the heart as a complication of atrial fibrillation, endocarditis or from a mural thrombus which may complicate myocardial infarction.

The most common cause of stroke is emboli which arise from thrombus development in the extracranial arteries such as the aorta, carotid or vertebral arteries. These vessels transport blood from the left ventricle to the cerebral arteries in the brain. The most common cerebral artery which becomes occluded as a result of embolism is the middle cerebral artery. This artery carries high volumes of blood from the circle of Willis to large areas of the brain. As a result any thromboembolic occlusion of this vessel will potentially deprive a significant area of brain of its normal blood supply resulting in a large cerebral infarction.

Diagram 13.10 Sources of emboli which may enter the cerebral circulation and so lead to stroke. In atrial fibrillation there are stagnant areas of blood which may clot, mural thrombosis may complicate myocardial infarction and the arch of the aorta and carotid arteries are both common sites of atheroma formation. Emboli from extracranial vessels are the most common cause of cerebrovascular accidents. Arrows indicate the direction of emboli travel towards the brain.

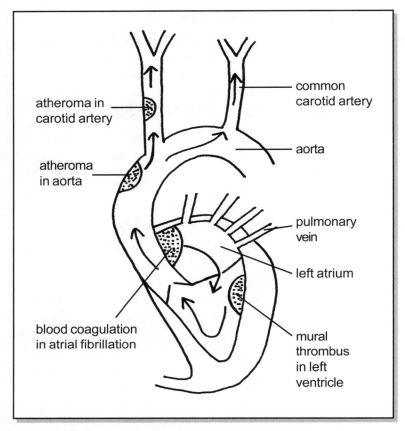

atheroma in carotid artery

atheroma in aorta

blood coagulation in atrial fibrillation

common carotid artery

aorta

pulmonary vein

left atrium

mural thrombus in left ventricle

Disease in intracerebral arteries

A further 20% of infarctions are due to disease within the smaller intracerebral arterial vessels within the brain. These small penetrating arterial branches carry blood from the larger vessels, such as the middle, posterior or anterior cerebral arteries into the brain tissue. Disease in these smaller vessels is most likely to develop in patients with diabetes and hypertension. When one of these arteries becomes occluded it will infarct a small area of the brain giving rise to a highly localised stroke. For example, the patient may present with only loss of motor or sensory function, as opposed to most strokes when both are lost in the same area of the body. The relatively small lesions generated by disease of these penetrating vessels are termed lacunar infarcts. Because they do not involve a large area of the brain they are unlikely to cause impairment of cognition, memory, speech, or level of consciousness. Despite only affecting relatively small areas of the brain the effects of a small infarct can be significant, especially as they may affect the nerve fibres within the internal capsule.

There is an internal capsule in both hemispheres of the brain. These capsules carry nerve fibres between the cerebral cortex and brain stem. All of the motor fibres from the motor cortex pass through this capsule. All of the sensory fibres travelling to the sensory cortex also pass through the internal capsule.

These nerve pathways carry on through the brain stem and down the spinal cord to the body. This means that if part of the blood supply to the internal capsule is occluded, many nerve fibres can be infarcted which will no longer be able to carry nerve impulses. As a result sensory information will not be able to pass from the body to the sensory cortex and motor impulses will be unable to pass from the cortex to the body.

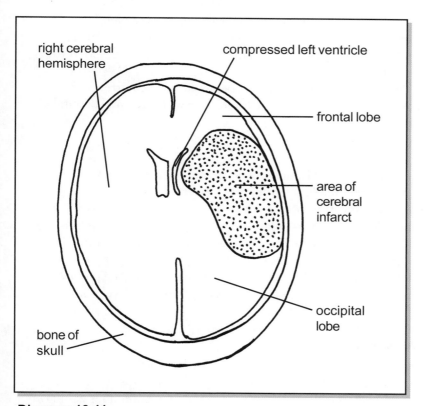

Diagram 13.11
Thromboembolic stroke caused by occlusion in a large arterial vessel. This diagram shows a large area of infarct in the left cerebral hemisphere affecting the parietal and frontal lobes. The cause is a thromboembolic occlusion of the middle cerebral artery. Motor loss will occur on the right side of the body as a result of involvement of the left motor cortex in the frontal lobe. Sensory loss on the right side can be explained by involvement of the sensory cortex in the left parietal lobe. It is also likely that this patient will be aphasic as the speech centre is usually in the left hemisphere.

Haemorrhagic pathophysiology

Haemorrhage is the other main cause of stroke. Haemorrhagic stroke caused by intracerebral (within the cerebrum) bleeds account for about 10% of cases. Bleeds may occur as a result of a ruptured aneurysm, which is a weakness in the wall of a blood vessel. The explosive entry of blood into the tissues of the brain immediately prevents the normal function of the neurones in the affected area. The haematoma caused by the haemorrhage may be reabsorbed over time and there may be varying degrees of patient recovery. Large bleeds may lead to raised intracranial pressure, shifting of intracranial contents and death from coning.

In addition to cerebral haemorrhage causing stroke it is also possible for a thromboembolic stroke to be complicated by haemorrhage. Ischaemia or infarction caused by an arterial occlusion may damage the walls of blood vessels as well as neurological tissue. Bleeding may then occur through this damaged vascular wall leading to haemorrhage into the infarcted area. This is referred to as haemorrhagic transformation.

The remaining strokes which are not thromboembolic or haemorrhagic may be caused by cerebral hypoperfusion, subarachnoid haemorrhage and subdural or extradural haematoma.

Aetiology and Prevention

As stroke is most commonly caused by underlying arterial disease, the risk factors are the same as those for the development of atherosclerosis. People should be given all of the health education advice and treatments necessary for the prevention of atherosclerosis. In particular, hypertension is a significant risk factor for stroke. This is important to know as high blood pressure can usually be effectively managed, therefore reducing the risk. If heart disease is present this should be treated as far as possible. If atrial fibrillation is an ongoing problem then anticoagulants are important to reduce the risk of thrombi developing in the atria.

Clinical features of stroke

There will be a sudden onset (over a few minutes) of focal neurological deficit. Features may continue to develop over the next few hours; this is called a stroke in evolution. Usually the clinical features reach a maximum after about 6 hours when the stroke is said to be completed.

As most nerve fibres cross over at the level of the medulla oblongata, a stroke affecting the left side of the brain will cause neurological deficit on the right side of the body. Likewise a stroke in the right side of the brain will affect the left side of the body. Therefore limbs on the opposite side to the cerebral lesion become weak and may be completely paralysed. In severe cases there may be a complete hemiplegia (paralysis of one side of the body). Other cases may show a hemiparesis (muscular weakness on one side of the body). Often the facial muscles on one side will be paralysed giving rise to a droop.

Sensation is also usually lost; the patient is unable to feel affected areas of the body. Indeed the situation is often more extreme than this, patients neglect, or even fail to acknowledge the existence of one side of the body. Some patients may try to push their hand out of bed because they do not believe it belongs to them.

Centres which generate speech are usually located in the dominant cerebral hemisphere. In right handed people the dominant hemisphere is the left. This means that if the left hemisphere is involved the speech centres may no longer function normally. An impaired ability to generate speech is termed a dysphasia and a complete loss of speech as aphasia. Other patients know what they want to say but find it difficult to articulate words as a result of loss of motor function. This feature is described as dysarthria. There may also be involvement of the parts of the brain that facilitate the understanding of language, described as receptive dysphasia. Dysphagia (difficulty in swallowing) is also common after stroke. If the occipital lobes or tracts are involved there may be a sudden deterioration of vision in one or both eyes.

Most patients remain conscious during a stroke making it a very frightening experience. Confusion is possible but loss of consciousness usually indicates a large lesion or the involvement of the brain stem. While severe headache and

Diagram 13.12
From the cerebral cortex (including the motor and sensory areas) numerous fibres pass down into the white matter of the brain. Collectively these fibres are called the projection tracts (they are also called the corona radiata). These fibres are all collected together in an internal capsule to be carried through the brain to the brain

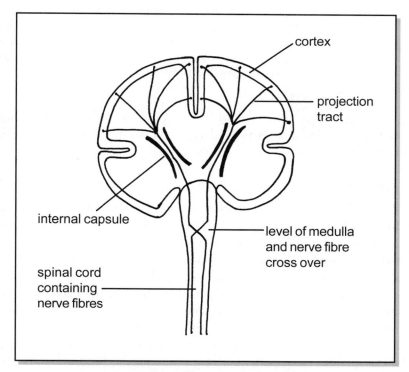

stem. Most nerve fibres cross over at the level of the medulla oblongata, before communicating with the body via the spinal cord.

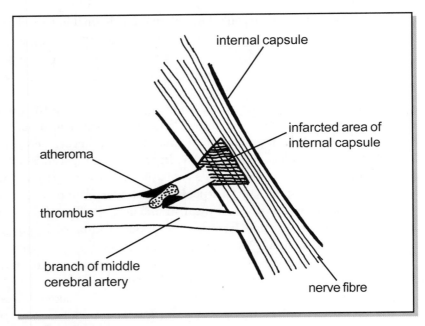

Diagram 13.13
Branches of the middle cerebral artery supply blood to the internal capsule. Disease in these small arteries can therefore infarct some of the nerve fibres in the internal capsule. Infarcted fibres will die and so be unable to carry nerve impulses. A large infarct may affect many fibres leading to an extensive stroke. (Only four fibres are illustrated, in reality there would be tens of thousands).

vomiting at the onset of a stroke are possible indicators of a haemorrhagic cause, brain imaging is needed to diagnose thromboembolic as opposed to haemorrhagic strokes.

Prognosis

Patients have very varied recovery after a stroke. Initial recovery may be rapid for a few days. This initial recovery can be explained by the existence of a zone of ischaemia and inflammation around the cerebral infarction. This area of ischaemia and inflammation, caused by the stroke, can be severe enough to prevent normal electrical activity in the cells involved, but not severe enough to cause them to necrose. Short term adaptations in the circulation can allow the ischaemic area to regain an adequate level of blood perfusion and so result in a restoration of function. If an area of brain recovers, the motor and sensory function will be restored to the represented parts of the body. Following this initial period, most patients show a gradual improvement and some recovery may continue for 2-3 years. Overall about a third of patients make a good recovery, a third are likely to die and the final third are left permanently disabled.

Management principles

Initial management must pay careful attention to maintenance of a clear airway. Swallowing must also be assessed to prevent aspiration of saliva, food or drink into the airway. Specialist stroke units now give thrombolysis to suitable patients as soon as a diagnosis of thromboembolic stroke is confirmed, usually by CT or MRI. Clearly, if a stroke has a haemorrhagic component thrombolysis would be contraindicated. CT and MRI scanning can readily distinguish between a haemorrhagic or thromboembolic stroke. In thromboembolic stroke aspirin started within 48 hours has been demonstrated to improve long term outcome. This reduces platelet aggregation and so reduces the likelihood of thrombus or emboli formation in future. Lowering blood pressure reduces the risk of recurrent stroke. Statins should be given to lower high plasma cholesterol and are associated with improved outcomes. Rehabilitation is often a long process in stroke management but can be very rewarding. Speech therapists, physiotherapists and occupational therapists all have an important role in addition to good nursing.

Transient ischaemic attack (TIA)

This refers to the clinical features generated by an episode of cerebral ischaemia. Once blood flow and oxygen delivery fall below a minimum threshold neurones will be unable to generate normal electrical activity. At this reduced level of blood flow the neurones remain viable so infarction will not develop. Function will recover as blood flow increases after the ischaemic episode. Traditionally a TIA has been defined as neurological deficits which resolve within 24 hours. The neurological deficit is caused by reduced blood flow through a partly occluded vessel or a small thromboembolic event. While recovery is complete, the patient should be regarded as being at risk of a future stroke.

Subarachnoid haemorrhage

In this condition there is spontaneous bleeding into the subarachnoid space which means blood enters the cerebrospinal fluid. Most bleeds occur from small 'berry' aneurysms which develop on the circle of Willis, the arrangement of arteries located at the base of the brain. Other bleeds may come from congenital abnormalities of blood vessels within the brain, referred to as arteriovenous malformations (AVMs).

Onset is sudden with extreme headache, most commonly at the back of the head. There is usually vomiting and some patients lose consciousness. Neurosurgeons can clip off the bleeding aneurysm, or insert stents into the weakened segment of artery involved with good results.

CHAPTER 14

Head Injuries

Brain Injuries

Injuries to the head which may affect the brain can be caused by any form of trauma such as falls, road traffic accidents or assaults. In practice the terms head injury and brain injury are used synonymously.

Primary brain injury

Primary brain injury describes the damage inflicted on the brain at the time of trauma. This means that when a patient arrives at the point of care the injury already exists. As adult neurones do not have significant mitotic abilities these primary injuries are probably not amenable to treatment.

Focal brain injuries

Penetrating injuries clearly may cause localised, i.e. focal damage to the brain directly. Focal injuries may be complicated by a depressed skull fracture with consequent risk of infection.

Diffuse brain injuries

Minor trauma to the head typically does not lead to brain injury. This is because the brain floats within the layer of cerebrospinal fluid, between the arachnoid and pia maters, which surround the CNS. This fluid acts as an excellent shock absorber which cushions the brain. However, with more severe blunt trauma diffuse brain injuries will result as a consequence of contusion and shearing forces.

Trauma to the head will cause the brain to impact on the inner surfaces of the skull. This will damage small blood vessels leading to cerebral contusion (i.e. bruising). External forces cause the skull to accelerate rapidly and impact on the area of brain below the point of contact. This causes injury to the underlying area of the brain and is referred to as a coup injury. When the inside of the skull hits the brain, this force also causes the brain to accelerate rapidly causing it to hit the inside of the skull on the opposite side of the head. This causes the brain to decelerate rapidly leading to a further primary injury referred to as a contrecoup injury. Inflammatory changes associated with cerebral contusion will also lead to the release of inflammatory fluids causing cerebral oedema.

The other principle mechanism of diffuse brain injury is stretching and tearing of nerve fibres. These are inflicted by shearing forces set up as the brain moves within the cranial cavity. This damage to the white matter of the brain leads to the microscopic development of features termed retraction balls.

Diffuse brain injury and concussion

Concussion describes a usually reversible loss of cerebral function with or without a period of unconsciousness. Mild concussion is caused by some diffuse stretching of the white matter caused by sheering forces, which leads to a reversible disruption in the function of some axons. In mild concussion there is no loss of consciousness but there is a deficiency in attention and memory functions for a period of time. Classic cerebral concussion is caused by diffuse axonal injury (DAI) which results in some disconnections between the brain stem reticular activating system (RAS) and the cerebrum. As consciousness is generated by the RAS, the patient will be unconscious for a period of time, often more than 24 hours. This more severe form of concussion causes memory loss (amnesia) for the events around the time of the accident.

In cases of severe diffuse axonal injury the condition may not be fully reversible and consciousness may be impaired for a prolonged period. Patients with more severe DAI may be left with long term cognitive impairment and physical deficits such as spastic paralysis, swallowing difficulties, sight and hearing problems and dysarthria (difficulty in articulating words).

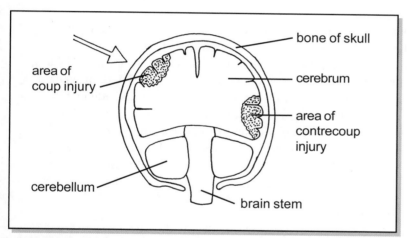

Diagram 14.1
In this case there is an area of cerebral contusion in the region of brain under the point of impact. The same force has caused a further area of contusion on the opposite side of the cerebral cortex which is a contrecoup injury. Arrow indicates direction of force.

Secondary brain injury

Secondary brain injury describes any further damage to the brain which occurs after the initial trauma. This is vital for us to understand as secondary brain injury typically develops while a patient is under our care. This means we are in a position to prevent secondary brain injuries. If secondary brain injuries are allowed to develop this can lead to permanent cognitive, motor and sensory loss, as the dead neurones do not significantly regenerate. It is useful to divide secondary causes into extracranial and intracranial.

Extracranial secondary brain injury

This describes factors which relate to the patient's systemic condition. These are external to the cranial cavity and may lead to brain injury development after the initial trauma.

Hypoxia

Neurones need a constant supply of oxygen to metabolise glucose in order to generate the energy necessary for living processes. If there is a reduced delivery of oxygen to the cerebrum, function will acutely decline and permanent neuronal damage will rapidly ensue. In addition to compromising neurones directly, a fall in the concentrations of oxygen in the arterial blood supplying the brain will lead to a reactionary cerebrovascular vasodilation. Physiologically, this will lead to an increase in cerebral blood flow and so is a useful mechanism to protect the brain against hypoxia. However, in patients who have a head injury it can contribute to further increases in cerebral oedema and therefore intracranial pressure (ICP).

Cerebral hypoxia must be prevented by ensuring the patient has a patent airway. This is particularly likely to be compromised if the patient is unconscious when intubation may be needed to guarantee the airway is fully secured. As a general principle intubate if the Glasgow coma scale (GCS) is less than eight. Once the airway is patent it must be ensured the patient is breathing adequately. This may be compromised by chest injuries or a pneumothorax. Additional oxygen may be given to maintain high blood saturation levels. In an unconscious patient with a head injury the possibility of a cervical spinal injury must always be accounted for. Unconscious patients should be treated as if they have an unstable cervical spine until proved otherwise.

Increased carbon dioxide

If there is an increase in the concentration of carbon dioxide in the blood perfusing the brain this will also lead to a significant cerebrovascular vasodilation with consequent increase in cerebral blood flow. Physiologically, this can be seen as a process to protect the brain against high levels of CO_2 as this will be carried away in the increased blood flow. This vasodilation will also protect the brain against acidosis as carbon dioxide combines with water to form carbonic acid. However, in patients with head injury the increased cerebral blood flow may contribute to cerebral oedema and raised ICP. In order to maintain relatively low levels of CO_2 in the blood the airway must be clear and the patient must be breathing with adequate ventilatory volumes.

Cerebral hypoperfusion

In a traumatised patient the systemic blood pressure may be low as a result of haemorrhage. If a patient is systemically hypotensive there will be a corresponding cerebral hypoperfusion. If the volumes of blood perfusing the brain are reduced there will be a corresponding cerebral hypoxia.

The pressure of blood flowing through the brain is termed the cerebral perfusion pressure (CPP). This is determined by the mean arterial blood pressure (MABP) and the resistance encountered as a result of intracranial pressure (ICP). As the pressure within the cranial cavity tends to resist the entry of arterial blood, this relationship can be summarised as CPP = MABP minus ICP. This means that a fall in MABP or a rise in ICP will reduce the CPP. In traumatised head injury patients there may be a reduction in MABP as a result of blood loss. There may also be an increase in ICP as a result of a brain injury. Cerebral ischaemia is therefore a particular danger if there is a combination of a reduced MABP with an increased ICP.

This is why it is important to correct any causes of hypotension, such as haemorrhage, and to replace blood volume as required. Correction of hypotension will probably involve the administration of intravenous fluids or blood. As discussed ICP can be lowered by ensuring the patient is fully oxygenated and does not become hypercarbic. Other extracranial factors which may contribute to secondary brain injury include acidosis, pyrexia and hyperglycaemia.

Intracranial secondary brain injury

This describes any cause of secondary brain injury, within the cranial cavity of the skull, which develops after the initial trauma.

Extradural (epidural) haematoma

An extradural haematoma is a collection of blood external to the dura mater. The blood therefore collects between the dura and the skull. Usually this is caused by rupture or tearing of the middle meningeal artery as a complication of overlying skull fracture. Sharp, jagged fracture ends may cut into the underlying arterial walls leading to significant haemorrhage. A minority of extradural haematomas may be caused by injuries to meningeal veins. The most common sites for an extradural haematoma are the temporal or temporoparietal regions. All intracerebral haematomas can be clearly seen using CT or MRI scanning. Treatment involves surgical ligation of the bleeding vessel and evacuation of the haematoma.

Subdural haematoma

This is a blood clot which develops under the dura mater, just above the arachnoid mater. Bleeding is from veins or capillaries damaged as a result of head trauma. Acute subdural haematoma develops within 48 hours of the initial injury, however subacute subdural haematoma may develop slowly and present up to two weeks after initial injury. A few cases of chronic subdural haematoma may even present after some months. The haematoma may need to be identified using CT or MRI scanning and surgically removed.

Intracerebral haematoma

These develop in the cerebrum as a result of damage to small blood vessels within the substance of the brain. Penetrating injury or shearing forces damage the vessel walls resulting in haemorrhage. An intracerebral haematoma may expand resulting in an increase in ICP with compression of surrounding brain tissues.

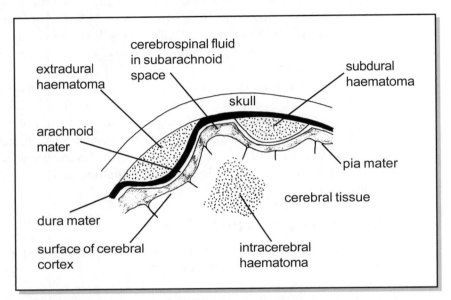

Diagram 14.2
The position of possible intracranial haemorrhages. Once blood has left the blood vessels it forms a haematoma and will clot over time. Any haematoma will take space within the cranial cavity and so constitutes a space occupying lesion.

Raised ICP

Intracranial pressure describes the pressure within the cranial cavity; this is normally about 10 mmHg when a subject is lying flat. Providing there is free circulation of cerebrospinal fluid this will be the same as the CSF pressure. As ICP rises there is a corresponding reduction in the Glasgow coma scale (GCS) score. Lumbar puncture is contraindicated in cases of raised intracranial pressure (RICP) as it will cause a sudden release of pressure below the level of the foramen magnum. If the ICP is raised sufficiently this will push brain tissues down into the foramen magnum causing coning.

Space occupying lesions (SOLs)

The skull is a rigid bone forming a closed intracranial cavity. Normally the cranial cavity is already filled to capacity with essential components including blood in blood vessels, cerebrospinal fluid and brain tissue. This means that if anything develops in addition to these essential components, the volumes of the existing components must decrease or intracranial pressure will rise. This is why any pathological inclusion within the cranial cavity is referred to as a space occupying lesion (SOL); it takes up space within the cranium. In cases of trauma, space may be taken up with inflammatory fluid causing cerebral oedema or haematoma.

As a haematoma develops it will start to displace cerebrospinal fluid (CSF) down into the spinal area of the subarachnoid space within the spinal dural sac. This displacement of CSF is a compensatory mechanism; it means that a haematoma may expand without a significant initial increase in ICP. However, after a time no more CSF can be displaced into the spinal dural sac and at this point even a small increase in the size of a haematoma will increase ICP. As ICP rises it compresses brain tissue and cerebral blood vessels leading to cerebral ischaemia. These effects will reduce the function of the cerebral neurones and so will compromise the ability of the cortex to generate consciousness. This will be seen as a reduction in the GCS explaining why a reduction of one point on the GCS is clinically significant and must be explained.

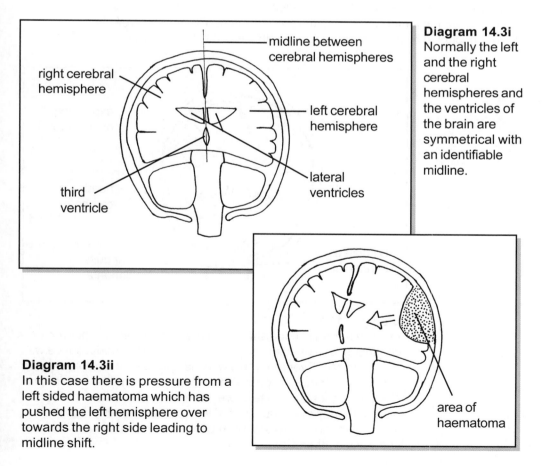

right cerebral hemisphere

midline between cerebral hemispheres

left cerebral hemisphere

lateral ventricles

third ventricle

Diagram 14.3i
Normally the left and the right cerebral hemispheres and the ventricles of the brain are symmetrical with an identifiable midline.

Diagram 14.3ii
In this case there is pressure from a left sided haematoma which has pushed the left hemisphere over towards the right side leading to midline shift.

area of haematoma

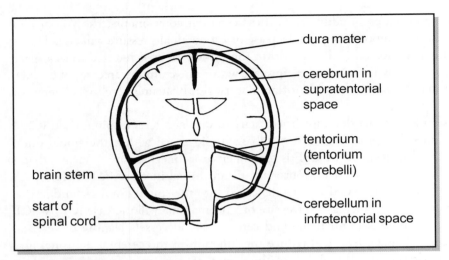

Diagram 14.4

The tentorium is an infolding of the dura mater which is composed of tough, supportive fibrous tissue. It supports the delicate lobes of the cerebrum above and covers the cerebellum below. The area of the cranial cavity above the tentorium is described as supratentorial and the area below, occupied by the cerebellum and brain stem, as infratentorial.

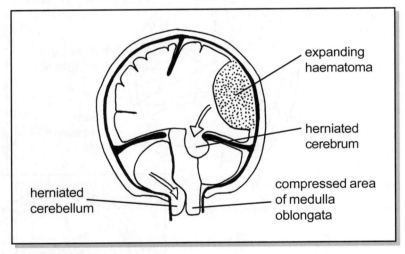

Diagram 14.5

In this diagram midline shift has already occurred. If a haematoma continues to expand the pressure in the supratentorial space will also increase. Eventually this will push part of the cerebrum down into the infratentorial space. This is termed a tentorial herniation. The consequent increase in pressure below the level of the tentorium may then push part of the cerebellum down into the foramen magnum. This will compress the brain stem and the vital centres it contains.

An increase in the pressure within one cerebral hemisphere will compress the oculomotor (III cranial) nerve on the effected side. This will lead to a reduction in the ability of the oculomotor nerve to carry nerve impulses from the brain to the intrinsic eye muscles. This explains why the pupil on the same side will become sluggish and eventually fixed and dilated.

Complications of raised intracranial pressure (RICP)

If intracranial bleeding persists the intracranial pressure will start to rise. Pressure from a haematoma will push and compress surrounding brain tissues. Initially a supratentorial haematoma will lead to midline shift. This means that the normal midline between the left and right cerebral hemispheres is distorted as a result of the pressure generated by the expanding haematoma.

Coning

The tentorium is an infold of the dura mater which separates the cerebrum from the cerebellum and supports the posterior part of the cerebrum. If the intracranial pressure above the tentorium increases, eventually the tentorium will fail to retain the cerebrum and part of the temporal lobe will be forced through to the infratentorial area normally occupied by the cerebellum and brain stem. This in turn will increase the pressure on the cerebellum and may force part of the cerebellum down through the foramen magnum which will compress the medulla oblongata. This part of the brain stem contains vital centres such as the cardiac, respiratory and vasomotor centres, as well as part of the reticular activating system. Compression of the brain stem therefore rapidly leads to brain stem death. The part of the cerebellum which is forced into the foramen magnum is the cerebellar tonsils, so this phenomenon is sometimes called tonsillar herniation. When the cerebellar tonsils herniate through the foramen magnum they compress vital centres in the medulla oblongata. This is termed 'coning' because the herniating brain tissues are forced into a cone shape. This complication again highlights the importance of early recognition and treatment of developing intracranial compression. Coning may often be prevented but once it has occurred is completely irreversible.

Infection

This is a risk when there is a depressed or base of skull fracture. Both of these may lead to tearing of the dura mater, allowing a route for infection into the meninges. Meningitis is uncommon in the first 2 days after the initial injury and may present months later. Another complication of infection following a dural tear is possible cerebral abscess. Antibiotic cover will be indicated if this is considered to be a potential risk.

CHAPTER 15

Endocrine Disorders

Endocrine disorders

In normal physiology the amounts of the various endocrine hormones present in the blood are precisely and homeostatically regulated. However, if a disease process affects an endocrine gland this can result in too much or too little of a particular hormone being secreted into the blood. If too much of a particular endocrine hormone is present in the blood, the target tissue will be over-stimulated giving rise to clinical features of hormone toxicity. If however, not enough of a hormone is secreted, the target tissue will be inadequately stimulated giving rise to features of hormone deficiency. For example, if the pituitary gland secreted too much growth hormone during childhood there will be excessive growth, resulting in a giant. Conversely, if not enough growth hormone is produced; the child will fail to grow normally, resulting in a dwarf. Endocrine disorders can affect any of the endocrine glands, but the more common examples discussed in this chapter are those effecting the thyroid and adrenal glands.

Thyroid disorders

After diabetes mellitus, thyroid disorders are the most common presentation of endocrine disease. There are two forms of thyroid hormone; these are T_4 and T_3 which is triiodothyronine. More T_4 is produced but T_3 is more active in stimulating metabolic processes. When the levels of thyroid hormone in the blood are too high this presents as hyperthyroidism, when the levels are too low, hypothyroidism presents.

Goitre

This term describes a chronic enlargement of the thyroid gland. An increase in the size of the thyroid gland causes swelling in the front of the neck. Goitre may occur in hypo or hyperthyroidism. Many goitres are non-toxic, that is not associated with the features of hyperthyroidism. A non-toxic goitre which is not associated with inflammation or neoplasm is termed a simple goitre. Simple goitre is about eight times more common in women than men. Any significant goitre may cause complications as a result of swelling in the neck; these problems include dysphagia as a result of compression of the oesophagus and inspiratory stridor from tracheal compression. Venous congestion of the head and neck may also occur. If there is compression of the recurrent laryngeal nerve the voice will become hoarse.

Hypothyroidism

Aetiology of hypothyroidism

In some parts of the world there is a deficiency of iodine in the diet, this is most likely to occur inland, as much iodine in the diet comes from sea food and sea salt. This deficiency disorder used to be common in areas such as Switzerland, central Africa, inland China, the Himalayas and in Derbyshire in the UK. The problem is less common today as iodine is usually added to salt supplies; however it is still occurs in some poorly developed areas.

Iodine is an essential component of T_3 and T_4, so if it is deficient, thyroid hormones cannot be synthesized by the thyroid gland. Iodine deficiency causes a simple goitre with an overall smooth enlargement of the thyroid gland. As the levels of thyroid hormone in the blood drop, the anterior lobe of the pituitary gland produces more thyroid stimulating hormone (TSH). Increased plasma concentration of TSH stimulates the growth of the thyroid gland to generate the goitre. As this used to be common in certain localities, it is called endemic goitre. Once an adult is given adequate iodine in the diet the goitre, and any clinical features of hypothyroidism subside. Hypothyroidism during pregnancy or childhood has serious consequences for the child, as discussed below.

Even when there are normal levels of iodine in the diet, primary hypothyroidism can still occur. This is more common in women and often presents during late middle age. In the majority of cases antibodies to thyroid tissues may be found in the blood. This indicates the disease has an autoimmune basis and the condition is termed Hashimoto's thyroiditis. In autoimmune hypothyroidism there may or may not be a goitre. Secondary hypothyroidism is much less common than this primary form and is caused by disorder of the pituitary gland resulting in a lack of TSH, or reduced secretion of TSH releasing hormone from the hypothalamus.

Pathophysiology and clinical features in hypothyroidism

Features develop slowly with an insidious onset. The patient complains of weight gain, lethargy and tiredness, they have difficulty concentrating and often feel cold. Generalised physical and mental slowness is sometimes called psychomotor retardation. These features are caused by a lowered metabolic rate; this means the rate at which the body can produce energy from metabolic processes is reduced, adversely affecting the brain and muscles. As reduced metabolism occurs, less heat is produced giving the patient increased sensitivity to the cold. Patients who complain of feeling tired all of the time can be screened for blood levels of thyroid hormones.

In the skin there is a change to the matrix or ground substance which occupies the intercellular spaces (this ground substance is composed of proteoglycans). Changes in the chemical nature of the ground substance mean it retains more water and the patient develops a form of oedema called myxoedema. This gives rise to a 'puffy' boggy appearance. Low levels of thyroid hormone also reduce secretions of sweat and sebum, leaving the skin dry and coarse. Vasoconstriction results in a pale coloured skin surface, this probably occurs because thyroid hormones have a role in dilating peripheral blood vessels. Hair becomes thin and dry.

Hypothyroidism can also affect the adult brain leading to memory loss, slowed mental processes, depression and paranoid ideas. There can be severe agitation, a condition sometimes called 'myxoedema madness'. As the metabolic rate of the myocardium is reduced, hypothyroidism reduces heart rate and stroke volume. Longer term oedema and swelling of myocardial muscle cells can lead to a 'flabby' dilated, enlarged heart. Hypothyroidism is also a factor in the development of atheroma, leading to coronary heart, cerebrovascular and peripheral vascular disease. Decreased metabolic activity in the GI tract reduces motility, leading to constipation and possibly serious faecal impaction, this is called myxoedema megacolon. Sexual dysfunction and reduced fertility are also probable. Serious untreated hypothyroidism will eventually result in a myxoedema coma. Clinical features of this end stage condition include unconsciousness, hypoventilation, cardiovascular collapse and hypothermia.

During pregnancy, thyroid hormones from the mother pass across the placenta into the fetal circulation. Maternal thyroid hormones are essential for the normal development of the babies brain, if the mother is hypothyroid during pregnancy the child will be born with potentially serious learning difficulties, (this really means mental retardation and sub normality of intelligence so it is very important to prevent). A hypothyroid woman who becomes pregnant typically needs an increased dose of thyroxine for the duration of the pregnancy. Also thyroid hormones are essential for normal development and maturation of the brain after birth. As there is rapid brain development during the first 6 months of life this early period is especially important. If a child has hypothyroidism during childhood they will also develop learning difficulties. A child who has low levels of thyroid hormone develops a condition called cretinism. This condition is not reversible once it has developed. A cretin will have stunted physical growth, learning difficulties, a large head, dwarfism, a pug nose, short neck, dry skin and little hair. If cretinism is caused by iodine deficiency it is termed endemic cretinism. Other cases may develop as a result of developmental defects of the thyroid gland, a condition termed thyroid dysgenesis. Cretinism can be avoided by replacement of appropriate levels of maternal or child thyroxine, simple iodine deficiency can be treated with supplementation.

Treatment principles

Hypothyroidism can be readily treated by giving oral thyroxine, which is T_4. Some patients may require a small initial daily dose of about 25-50 micrograms, which can then be increased. A typical maintenance dose is about 100-150 micrograms per day. Thyroxine therapy gives profound improvements which usually begin after about 2 weeks of therapy. Treatment is usually for life.

Hyperthyroidism

Hyperthyroidism refers to the clinical condition caused by an excess of circulating thyroid hormone and is about 5 times more common in women compared to men, it is commonly seen between the ages of 20-40 years. Hyperthyroidism is also referred to as thyrotoxicosis.

Aetiology of Graves' disease

Graves' disease (after Robert Graves, 1797-1853) is the most common cause of hyperthyroidism and has an autoimmune aetiology. In normal physiology, growth of the thyroid gland and increased secretions of thyroid hormone are stimulated by TSH, released from the anterior pituitary gland in response to low levels of circulating thyroid hormone. However in Graves' disease for autoimmune reasons, a group of B lymphocytes secrete an IgG (immunoglobulin type G) which fits into, and stimulates the TSH receptors naturally present on the cell membrane of the thyrocytes which synthesize thyroid hormone. These abnormal antibodies therefore have an agonist effect on TSH receptors. (An agonist describes a drug or other agent which interacts with a receptor to generate a positive response.) While the precise underlying aetiology of this disorder is still unclear it does tend to run in families and several genes have been associated with increased risk. Environmental factors may include smoking, emotional stress, trauma to the thyroid gland and some infections.

Clinical features in Graves' disease

The classical picture in Graves' disease is hyperthyroidism, diffuse goitre and exophthalmos which describes abnormal protrusion of the eyeballs. While goitre and hyperthyroidism occur in other forms of hyperthyroidism, exophthalmos is only seen in Graves' disease. This highly characteristic sign is caused by inflammation in the tissue lining the inside of the orbit and of the extraocular

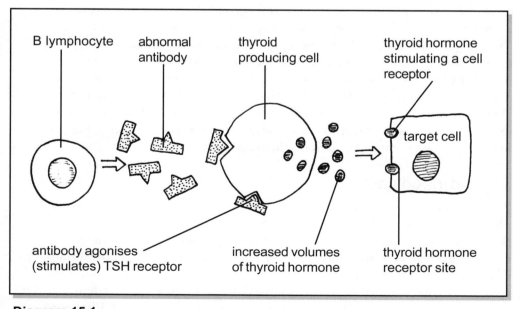

Diagram 15.1
Graves' disease is caused by abnormal antibodies which stimulate TSH receptors and therefore increase thyroid hormone production.

muscles which move the eyeball. Inflammation, oedema and swelling may eventually result in fibrosis. It is thought that this inflammation and fibrosis is caused by the stimulation of local fibroblasts by abnormal thyroid stimulating antibodies.

Clinical features of hyperthyroidism

Increased levels of thyroid hormone stimulate the overall metabolic rate of the body, this results in weight loss despite a usually increased appetite. As heat is produced as the end product of metabolic processes, the patient feels hot and will sweat a lot. As metabolic rate is increased, oxygen consumption also rises and the person may feel short of breath. There is increased stimulation of the sympathetic nervous system resulting in irritability, nervousness and restlessness. Increased metabolic activity in the heart will lead to tachycardia and palpitations may be reported, atrial fibrillation is a possible complication. Adverse effects on skeletal muscles cause tremor. Over activity in the GI tract may lead to diarrhoea. In women there may be scanty and infrequent menstruation (oligomenorrhoea). All forms of hyperthyroidism can cause lid lag where there is a delay in moving the eye lid as the eye moves downwards. This feature is caused by increased sympathetic stimulation of the muscle in the eye lid. Blood tests show increased plasma concentrations of T_3 and T_4 with T_3 being the more sensitive marker.

Treatment principles

Hyperthyroidism may be treated using anti thyroid drugs such as carbimazole, or methimazole. These drugs inhibit the formation of thyroid hormones. Treatment usually starts to have a beneficial effect after 2-3 weeks. Beta blockers are useful for short term symptom control, but should not be used long term. Radioactive iodine is another possible treatment; this involves giving iodine-131 which is radioactive. This radioactive iodine is taken up by the thyroid gland and emits radiation which progressively destroys thyroid tissue; this reduces the ability of the gland to secrete excess volumes of thyroid hormones. Surgery may be used by performing subtotal thyroidectomy.

Thyroid neoplasia

Benign neoplasms may develop in the thyroid gland; there may be a single nodule or multiple nodules. These overgrowths of thyroid tissue usually cause the gland to secrete increased volumes of thyroid hormones and are therefore a possible cause of hyperthyroidism. When nodules are associated with features of hyperthyroidism they are referred to as toxic nodules. As the nodules are adenomas, the condition is also referred to as toxic thyroid adenoma. Hyperthyroidism caused by toxic nodules, does not cause exophthalmos, presumably because there are not abnormal thyroid stimulating antibodies present, as in Graves' disease.

Thyroid cancer is relatively uncommon but is still the most common malignant tumour of the endocrine system. Most tumours derive from thyroid epithelium and secrete thyroglobulin, the detection of which can aid diagnosis. In most cases the cause is not known, although some have a familiar tendency and others are associated with radiation exposure. After the Chernobyl disaster in 1986, a lot of radioactive iodine was released into the environment. Radioactive iodine which enters the body is taken up by, and therefore concentrated in, the thyroid gland. This release of radioactive iodine therefore caused many cases of thyroid cancer. Thyroid cancer is usually treated by surgical resection.

Disorders of the adrenal gland

Addison's disease

This term (after Thomas Addison, 1795-1860) is used to describe primary hypoadrenalism. In this rare disorder the patient does not produce enough of the adrenal cortical hormones. These hormones include hydrocortisone and aldosterone. Most cases in Western countries are caused by autoimmune destruction of the adrenal cortex; however tuberculosis is another possible cause. Clinical features may include skin pigmentation, anorexia, weight loss, postural hypotension and weakness. Treatment is with lifelong replacement therapy. Hydrocortisone is used to replace the steroid hormones normally produced by the adrenal cortex. Fludrocortisone is given to replace the absent or reduced aldosterone.

Cushing's syndrome

Cushing's disease (after Harvey Cushing, 1869-1939) describes an increase in the volumes of glucocorticoids (mostly hydrocortisone) in the blood. While this endocrine disorder is rare, it is well known because the syndrome is commonly seen after giving therapeutic corticosteroid drugs. In other words it is seen as an iatrogenic disorder. Excess alcohol consumption can generate a Cushing's like appearance but is not actually Cushing's disease.

Most medical (non-iatrogenic) cases are caused by increased secretion of adrenocorticotropic hormone (ACTH) from the pituitary gland as a result of a pituitary adenoma. Rarer cases may be caused by a hormone secreting tumour in the adrenal cortex. Clinical features include weight gain with central obesity, thinning of the skin, development of a rounded moon face, change in facial appearance, hypertension and striae (red or purple streaks on the skin). In the longer term Cushing's disease can lead to infections, chronic hypertension, heart failure and myocardial infarction. Treatment of Cushing's disease involves controlling the disorder with drugs such as metyrapone and ketoconazole. Once the disorder is controlled surgery may be performed to remove the adenoma from the pituitary gland or to remove adrenal cortical tumours.

Disorder of the adrenal medulla

Occasionally a tumour may develop in the adrenal medulla, in the cells which produce adrenaline and noradrenaline, i.e the catecholamines. This tumour is called a phaeochromocytoma. Increased amounts of the catecholamines in the blood tends to occur from time to time giving rise to paroxysmal clinical features. The patient suffers from hypertension as a result of increased stimulation of the sympathetic nervous system. Increased blood pressure in the kidneys leads to increased excretion of sodium in the urine, which may in turn lead to features of postural hypotension. Sufferers also experience paroxysms of pallor, palpitations, sweating, headache, abdominal pain, weight loss and extreme anxiety. Drugs are usually given to control the clinical features and the plasma volume should be restored to normal before surgery to remove the adrenal medullary tumour.

CHAPTER 16

Diabetes Mellitus

Diabetes

The route of the word diabetes relates to large volumes of urine, (dia means 'through' and betes means 'to go', meaning lots of water goes through the body). For example, in diabetes insipidus, large volumes of watery (or insipid) urine are passed as a result of reduced antidiuretic hormone production. It is important to realise diabetes insipidus is a completely different disease from diabetes mellitus. 'Mellitus' means sweet, so in diabetes mellitus large volumes of sweet urine are produced. Diabetes mellitus is sometimes called sugar diabetes.

Diabetes mellitus

This is a common disorder affecting approximately 4-5% of the population in the UK. Everyone working in any clinical field will come across cases of diabetes mellitus in their patients and so needs to understand this disorder.

Background physiology

Insulin is produced by beta cells in the pancreatic islets of Langerhans.

Insulin

when blood glucose levels rise the beta cells detect this. Granules of insulin emerge from the cells.

Insulin is produced by the beta cells in the pancreatic islets (of Langerhans). Insulin lowers blood glucose levels. When blood glucose levels rise this is detected by the beta cells and secretory granules of insulin emerge from the surface of the cell membrane. This insulin then travels in the hepatic portal vein to the liver and then on to all tissues of the body via the systemic circulation. Insulin is eventually removed from the blood by being broken down by the liver and kidneys. The genetic information to synthesize insulin is carried on chromosome 11. This gene codes for the synthesis of the hormone insulin which is a small protein, composed of 51 amino acids.

Insulin then travels the hepa portal v to the li

Chromosome 11 carries the info to create insulin

Insulin and glucose

Insulin lowers blood glucose levels by converting soluble glucose into insoluble glycogen for storage in the liver and muscles. In addition insulin is needed to facilitate the transfer of glucose from tissue fluids into cells. Most cell membranes are impervious to glucose unless insulin stimulates and opens the cell membrane bound 'gate'. Glucose is then able to pass through the gate, from the tissue fluids into the cytosol of the cells. As glucose is transported into the cells the amounts in the blood and tissue fluid fall. Without this action of insulin, glucose will not be able to enter the cells and so cannot be used by mitochondria in energy production. This is the irony of diabetes mellitus; the blood and tissue fluid have far too much glucose, while the intracellular mitochondria do not have enough. The necessity for insulin to transport glucose into cells explains why people with insulin dependent diabetes need some insulin in the system at all times.

Insulin and proteins

Insulin stimulates protein metabolism. Insulin increases the transport of amino acids into cells and stimulates their synthesis into proteins. The presence of insulin also prevents the breakdown (i.e. catabolism) of proteins.

Insulin and fats

In addition to the effects insulin has on glucose and protein, it affects fat metabolism. Insulin promotes the synthesis of fatty acids which are then transported via blood lipoproteins to adipocytes for storage. This will happen when more carbohydrate is consumed than is needed as carbohydrates can be converted to fatty acids in the liver cells.

If blood glucose levels fall, insulin levels will also fall. This lack of insulin allows fat to be released from adipocytes and returned to the blood. Once in the blood these fatty acids and glycerol may be used by most of the body cells as an energy source. This is a useful physiological mechanism as it allows fat reserves to be used to maintain metabolic processes during times of food shortage. However, in poorly controlled diabetes mellitus where there is insulin lack, patients will have chronically high levels of fatty acids and glycerol in the blood causing hyperlipidaemia. This partly explains why insulin lack leads to the accelerated development of atheroma in poorly controlled diabetes mellitus.

Insulin receptors

Like all endocrine hormones, insulin is a signal molecule. Signal molecules circulate in the blood until they bind to a specific receptor molecule. Insulin can only exert a physiological effect when it is combined with this specific receptor. Insulin receptors are proteins, located in the external cell membrane of many cells. As they are transmembrane proteins they lie across the cell membrane, so part of the receptor molecule is outside and part inside the cell. When insulin binds with the external component of the receptor it induces a change in the receptor which then initiates further secondary responses inside the cell. After activating secondary mechanisms the insulin-receptor complex is taken into the cell where the insulin is broken down before the renewed receptor is returned to the cell surface for reuse.

Glucose physiology

It is essential that blood glucose concentrations are maintained at relatively constant levels. Glucose is the only form of sugar found in the blood. If other sugars, such as fructose or galactose, are absorbed from the gut, the liver quickly converts them into glucose. If there is too much glucose in the blood this will damage several body tissues, however if there is not enough, cells will not be able to use glucose as a fuel in the mitochondria. High blood glucose levels are referred to as hyperglycaemia and low levels as hypoglycaemia. All living cells need a constant supply of metabolic substrate to act as fuel, they also need

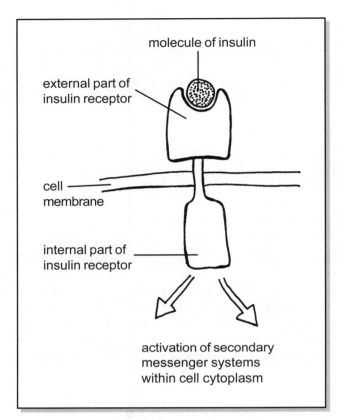

Diagram 16.1
A molecule of insulin binds with an insulin receptor on the surface of a cell membrane. This triggers a change in the receptor which then initiates further changes within the cell. For example the glucose-gating molecule is stimulated to migrate to the cell surface to transfer glucose from the tissue fluid into the cell cytoplasm.
Glucose will then diffuse through the cytosol to the mitochondria where it is oxidised to produce energy.

molecule of insulin

external part of insulin receptor

cell membrane

internal part of insulin receptor

activation of secondary messenger systems within cell cytoplasm

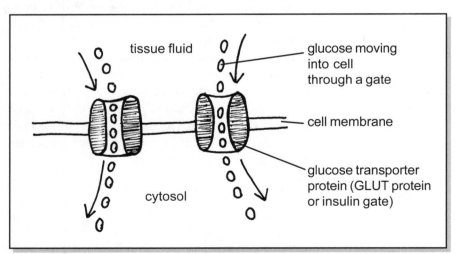

tissue fluid

glucose moving into cell through a gate

cell membrane

glucose transporter protein (GLUT protein or insulin gate)

cytosol

Diagram 16.2
Glucose enters most cells via specialised transporting 'gates'. These gates are actually specialised transmembrane structures called glucose-transporter proteins, (GLUT proteins). These only come to the surface of the cell if insulin first binds to insulin receptors.

oxygen. Neurones in particular need a constant supply of glucose in order to produce energy. In health, blood glucose levels are usually within the range of 3.5-8 mmol L. The normal fasting range for blood glucose is usually quoted as 3.6-5.8. When blood glucose levels rise they are lowered by insulin and when they fall they are maintained, at least for some time, by the action of glucagon. Glucagon is produced in the alpha cells of the pancreatic islets.

If there is not enough carbohydrate in the diet, the liver is capable of synthesising essential glucose by the process of gluconeogenesis. This process involves the chemical rearrangement of molecules derived from fat and protein. In an adult the brain consumes about 100g of glucose per day. Unlike other metabolically active tissues, such as muscles and liver, the brain is not able to use other fuels such as fatty acids; it can only function on glucose. In other words the brain is an obligatory glucose user. This physiology explains why acute hypoglycaemia is life threatening, if blood glucose drops very low the brain will no longer be able to generate energy and so brain cells will rapidly die. In order to protect the glucose supply to the brain, neurones are able to absorb glucose directly, without the gateing effect of insulin.

Pathophysiology

The key feature of diabetes mellitus is a raised blood glucose level. There is a chronic hyperglycaemia which may be caused by a lack of insulin. Alternatively there may be a reduced ability of body cells to use the insulin which is present in the blood; this is called insulin resistance.

Types of diabetes mellitus (DM)

Two forms of diabetes mellitus are currently recognised, simply referred to as types 1 and 2.

Type 1

Type 1 DM is associated with complete destruction of the beta cells and an absolute insulin deficiency. Type 1 diabetics are always insulin dependent; it is an IDDM (insulin dependent diabetes mellitus).

Type 2

In established cases of type 2 DM there is a reduced level of beta cell function. However, the disease process starts with the insulin receptors; these do not work properly or are reduced in numbers. This means that even though insulin is produced, the receptors are unable to make use of it. This situation is described as insulin resistance. These patients can often be managed without using insulin i.e. type 2 diabetes may be a NIDDM (non insulin dependent diabetes mellitus). However type 2 diabetes may progress to become insulin dependent, and so may become an IDDM. Type 2 disease is the most common form of diabetes mellitus.

Secondary diabetes

DM may develop secondary to a primary underlying condition, for example diabetes may occur after destruction of islet tissue in chronic pancreatitis or cystic fibrosis. DM may also occur as a side effect of steroid or thiazide diuretic treatment. Certain other endocrine disorders may lead to diabetes, such as thyrotoxicosis or Cushing's syndrome. Secondary diabetes mellitus only accounts for 1-2 % of cases of DM.

Diabetes as a complication of pregnancy

This is gestational diabetes which sometimes occurs in pregnancy. Glucose from the mother's blood passes into the fetal blood leading to fetal hyperglycaemia. This is detected by the fetal beta cells which respond by increasing the production of insulin. As mentioned, insulin promotes growth by stimulating protein synthesis. This means that if the mother's blood glucose levels are not controlled the baby will increase in size. These large babies make delivery more difficult and may necessitate a Caesarean section. Also, poor maternal glycaemic control, especially in early pregnancy, increases the probability of major developmental abnormalities including abnormalities of the large blood vessels, heart and nervous system. While gestational diabetes usually resolves after delivery, such women have an increased risk of developing type 2 diabetes in later life. Risk of developing permanent type 2 DM is probably increased with repeated pregnancies, especially if the woman is overweight. Overall, about 80% of women suffering from gestational diabetes go on to develop type 2 DM.

Type 1 diabetes mellitus

Aetiology

Type 1 DM is a progressive autoimmune disorder mediated through T lymphocytes (i.e. a type IV hypersensitivity reaction). Pancreatic biopsy, shortly after diagnosis, typically shows the presence of lymphocytes, natural killer (NK) cells and activated macrophages with inflammatory oedema in the pancreatic islets. These features illustrate how the body's own immune system is mistakenly activated against it's own beta cells. The efficiency of the immune system means that the total beta cell mass is progressively but completely destroyed. This pathological autoimmune process is probably initially triggered by a viral infection acting on predisposing factors. Additional evidence for the autoimmune nature of type 1 DM comes from autoantibodies which have been detected in the blood of 90% of newly diagnosed patients. Studies have recently demonstrated the presence of autoantibodies in children during the first few years of life; these children go on to develop DM type 1 several years later. Further support for the autoimmune explanation of the pathogenesis comes from observations that beta cell survival is prolonged if patients are given immunosuppressant drugs.

The incidence of type 1 DM is increasing in Europe by as much as 3-4% per year. Much of the increase is in very young children. Currently, approximately 10% of diabetics have type 1 DM. There is also a genetic predisposition to type 1 DM which increases susceptibility to the disorder. Siblings of a type 1 diabetic child have approximately a 16% chance of developing the disease. Predisposition also increases with a diabetic parent; if a father is type 1 diabetic the chances of a child developing DM by the age of 20 years is about 9%, while a type 1 diabetic mother is associated with a risk of 3%. Monozygotic twins who are genetically identical have a concordance rate of 30-50%.

Environmental factors also interact with the genetic susceptibility to the immune dysfunction seen in type 1 DM. The hygiene hypothesis suggests that because children are kept in very clean environments their immune systems fail to learn the difference between foreign antigens (such as bacteria or viruses) and the body's own tissue. However, children exposed to soil bacteria experience a healthy immune challenge which improves the future performance of the immune system making type 1 DM less likely to develop. If babies are exposed to cow's milk, some of the bovine serum albumin (cow protein) may be directly absorbed into the baby's blood leading to increased susceptibility. This is because the gut is partly permeable to non-digested proteins in the first year of life. Once in the blood these bovine (i.e. cow) proteins can trigger the production of antibodies which may go on to attack the beta cells. Circumstantial evidence also suggests young children should not be fed cured and smoked meats or coffee. Subclinical deficiency of vitamin D (i.e. a deficiency which is not severe enough to cause rickets) also seems to significantly increase the risk of a child developing type 1 DM. An understanding of these environmental risk factors clearly indicates areas for health education and promotion.

Because type 1 DM is an autoimmune disease, patients with the condition are at increased risk of developing other autoimmune pathologies. This explains the increased incidence of coeliac disease, pernicious anaemia, adrenal or thyroid insufficiency, and vitiligo. Vitiligo describes white areas of the skin where the melanocytes are lost, presumably as a result of autoimmune destruction.

Pathophysiology

In type 1 DM the insulin receptors are completely normal; the pathology is restricted to the beta cells. Loss of these cells means insulin is not produced. Destruction of the beta cells takes place over a period of time, probably years. When 70-90% of the beta cells have been eradicated there will no longer be sufficient insulin producing capacity to prevent hyperglycaemia and the other presenting clinical features of type 1 DM. Initially there will be impaired glucose tolerance and then overt symptomatic diabetes mellitus.

Presentation in type 1 diabetes mellitus

Classic triad

Type 1 DM typically has a juvenile onset, often around the time of puberty, although it may start at any time of life. The classic triad of presenting features are polyuria (producing large volumes of urine), thirst and weight loss. In an acute presentation there is normally a clinical history of about 2-6 weeks. On examination there will be glucosuria and elevated serum glucose.

Polyuria and glucosuria

Polyuria occurs as a result of an osmotic diuresis. This is a diuresis that occurs for osmotic reasons. Diuresis means an abnormally large volume of urine is produced. When the level of glucose in the blood increases there is an equivalent increase in the concentration of glucose in glomerular filtrate. The quantity of glucose the renal tubules are able to reabsorb is limited. In health, when blood glucose levels are normal, all of the glucose in the filtrate is reabsorbed; this means physiologically there is no glucose at all in urine. However, when glucose glomerular filtrate levels are abnormally high it cannot all be reabsorbed. This will result in glucose passing straight through the tubule into the urine.

When glucose is found in urine, the renal threshold for glucose has been exceeded. For most people the renal threshold is 11 mmol L (millimoles of glucose per litre of blood). This means that plasma concentrations greater than 11 mmol L will result in the appearance of glucose in the urine; below these levels it will not. In fact about 1% of the population may have glucosuria with normal serum levels of glucose; these individuals have a genetically low renal threshold for glucose. You can always check for this by comparing blood glucose levels with urine levels.

When abnormally large amounts of glucose are present in glomerular filtrate the osmotic potential of this fluid is increased. This happens because glucose is an osmotic molecule; it attracts water through a semi-permeable membrane. Glucose present in filtrate therefore osmotically attracts water, increasing the volume of the glomerular filtrate. As any filtrate which is not reabsorbed from the nephrons becomes urine, the urine volumes increase. The result of these processes is an osmotic diuresis of sweet urine.

Thirst

Thirst can be excessive in an acute presentation, leading to excessive drinking (sometimes called polydipsia). This is simply explained by systemic dehydration caused by the osmotic diuresis and subsequent polyuria. Despite excessive drinking, some patients presenting with type 1 DM are hypovolaemic, with consequent tachycardia and hypotension.

Weight loss

Weight loss may partly be as a result of dehydration. However, insulin promotes protein synthesis, therefore if it is absent, less protein will be built up into muscle. Insulin also prevents protein breakdown, so if insulin is absent more protein will be broken down. This will reduce the amount of protein present in the body and so reduce weight. Also, as glucose is not transported across cell membranes, cells are obliged to use fatty aids as a fuel rather than glucose; this will progressively deplete fat reserves, again resulting in weight loss. Stored fatty acids are also converted to ketone bodies which can also be used by mitochondria to produce energy.

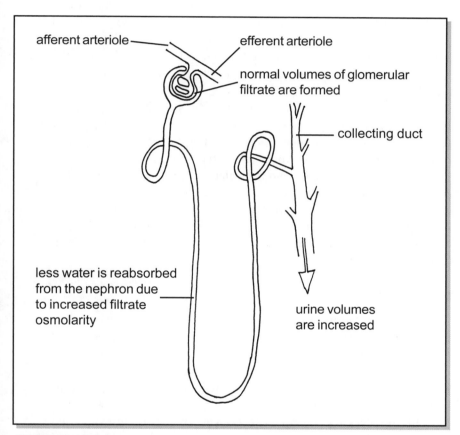

Diagram 16.3
The nephron in hyperglycaemia. Glucose in glomerular filtrate increases osmotic potential within the nephron; this attracts and retains more water resulting in increased urine volumes.

Ketosis

Ketosis refers to abnormally high levels of ketone bodies in the blood. 'Ketone bodies' is a collective term used to describe acetone and 2 organic keto type acidic compounds which are produced as a result of excessive fat metabolism. As the body cells are unable to utilise glucose, stored fatty acids are converted into ketone bodies, which are used as a fuel by the mitochondria, in place of the glucose they would prefer. (Ketosis is normal in starvation, when the body is obliged to use stored fats as an energy source.)

In addition to occurring in previously undiagnosed patients, ketosis may occur if insulin therapy is interrupted. This is another good reason why insulin therapy should never be stopped in type 1 DM. If no insulin is available, most tissues will switch to fat metabolism as they are unable to metabolise carbohydrates. It is this fat metabolism by the mitochondria, mostly in the liver, which generates the ketone bodies. Increased levels of acetone are formed in ketosis and accumulate in the blood. Acetone is a volatile substance and some of it is blown off in the expired air from the lungs. This causes the breath to smell of acetone; a smell usually described as being like 'pear drops'. Like most smells, once you have experienced it the first time you will immediately recognise it again.

If diabetes is not treated for a period of time the ketosis will worsen. As two of the ketone bodies produced by excessive fat metabolism are acids, the acidity of the patient's blood will progressively increase as the pH falls. This gives rise to the condition called ketoacidosis. In order to try and compensate for the acidosis the respiratory centre initiates hyperventilation. This will have the effect of somewhat lowering blood acidity by reducing levels of carbonic acid as a result of exhaling more carbon dioxide. This effect gives rise to the classical feature of 'air hunger' (Kussmaul respirations). This is an example of an attempted compensatory mechanism; in this case an attempted respiratory compensation for a metabolic acidosis.

Diagnosis

The World Health Organisation has suggested that diabetes is diagnosed when fasting plasma glucose is greater than 7.0 mmol L or when random levels exceed 11.1 mmol L. (These relatively low diagnostic levels illustrate how finely homeostatically controlled blood glucose levels are in normal physiology). In a patient without symptoms the test should be repeated to confirm the diagnosis. To diagnose gestational diabetes or borderline cases a glucose tolerance test may be used. This involves testing for fasting levels of plasma glucose then giving 75g of glucose in 300 mls of water and retesting after 2 hours. In normal patients the levels will have dropped to less than 7.8 mmol L, whereas in diabetes they will remain at 11.1 mmol L or more. Another method of diagnosis is to simply take blood and examine how much glucose has been absorbed into the haemoglobin in the red blood cells. The higher the average levels of blood glucose the more will absorb into the haemoglobin. This is called glycosylated haemoglobin and is tested for with the HbA_{1C} test. A value of greater that 6.5% indicates probable diabetes mellitus.

It is important to realise there is no such thing as 'mild' diabetes mellitus. Any individual who has blood glucose levels at or above these diagnostic criteria is at risk of developing long term complications.

Type 2 diabetes mellitus

Aetiology

This disorder typically develops in middle life and so is sometimes referred to as maturity onset diabetes. It is caused by the interaction of environmental (life style) and genetic factors. Environmentally, the incidence of the disorder increases with the degree of obesity (in the UK 80% of type 2 diabetics are obese), with abdominal fat being a significant risk factor. The risk of developing type 2 disease increases 10 fold with a body mass index (BMI) of 30 or over. Overeating increases risk. Increasing age and lack of exercise are also risk factors. Consumption of sugary foods increases risk by increasing the demand for insulin secretion. This increases the amount of insulin in the blood which then contributes to the overuse of the insulin receptors. Fatty foods are also a risk. This is because fats are metabolized by the body cells, meaning they require less glucose, which is then left to accumulate in the blood. Lack of physical exercise is a risk factor. If a person is physically active their muscles will use up sugar in the blood, lowering levels. As blood sugar levels are lowered so is the demand for insulin. These points are important to understand as people at risk of developing type 2 DM can change their lifestyle to eat less, lose weight and exercise more. People who do a lot of physical work and have limited access to calorie rich food develop significantly less type 2 DM than those who live a typical affluent western lifestyle. In some genetically predisposed individuals this may prevent the development of the condition. Even if the disease is not prevented, taking plenty of exercise and keeping slim will delay the onset of the disease, probably by many years.

Like type 1 DM there is a genetic component in the aetiology. Type 2 DM is much more common in people of African, Arab and South Asian extraction who live a western lifestyle than it is in equivalent white people. Further evidence for a genetic component in type 2 aetiology is a very high (often approaching 100%) concordance rate between identical monozygotic twins. Even between siblings the chances of a person developing type 2, if a brother or sister is affected, is 15-20%. While no single gene is responsible for causing type 2 DM, it seems that three principle genes each increase the risk of developing the disease by about 20% each. However, several other genes may also play a smaller role in causing type 2 disease making the aetiology polygenic (caused by many genes).

Babies who have low birth weight and children with a low weight at one year of age also seem more likely to develop type 2 DM in later life, this is sometimes called the 'bad start hypothesis'. Risk for such people is increased if they later become overweight. This illustrates the importance of giving mothers good nutrition during pregnancy and feeding young children well.

Pathophysiology

In type 1 disease the pathophysiology begins with the beta cells. Conversely, in type 2 DM the pathophysiology begins with the insulin receptors located on the cell surfaces, mostly on liver and skeletal muscle cells. As the insulin receptors are over-used over many years they begin to fail. It is useful to think of the insulin receptors as 'wearing out'. In addition to the insulin receptors it may be that the intracellular secondary messenger systems, which are normally activated by the insulin-receptor complex, do not work properly, partly for genetic reasons. This abnormality contributes to insulin resistance, in other words a given dose of insulin has less effect than it would if the receptors and cells were healthy. This means a particular dose of insulin will have a reduced hypoglycaemic effect.

In the early stages of developing type 2 DM blood glucose levels will start to rise slightly. However, in this early stage, the beta cells detect the increase in blood glucose levels and are able to increase insulin production to compensate. This means more use is made of any healthy insulin receptors which remain. For a period of time this relative hyperinsulinaemia will maintain essentially normal blood glucose levels, i.e. a euglycaemia will be maintained. However, over time this obligatory high insulin output wears out the beta cells resulting in a progressive decline in beta cell function and mass. Once the disease process has been developing over several years the total number of beta cells might be reduced by 30%. These factors mean that the levels of insulin in the blood progressively drop. This results in a combination of reduced insulin secretion and reduced insulin sensitivity. This reduction in blood insulin levels, in combination with the increased insulin resistance caused by defective insulin receptor function, means that blood glucose levels will progressively rise. Firstly there will be impaired glucose tolerance, followed by overt diabetes mellitus.

Presentation

The presenting features in type 2 DM are similar to those in type 1, but the onset may be over months or even years. However, as some insulin is still produced, some glucose is still transported into the cells for the mitochondria to use. This means that fats are not metabolized in the absence of carbohydrates so production of ketones is uncommon. This explains why ketoacidosis is unlikely in type 2 disease, but will occur in the absolute insulin deficiency found in untreated type 1 DM. Even the reduced amounts of insulin in type 2 DM are usually enough to suppress the metabolism of fats and proteins by the mitochondria, explaining why weight loss is uncommon in early type 2 DM. As the condition progresses and insulin production falls there may be increased metabolism of fats and proteins resulting in weight loss. Also over time the kidneys increase the amount of glucose they are able to reabsorb meaning that dehydration and thirst are less pronounced than in a type 1 presentation. Often the main feature which patients complain of is fatigue.

One of the problems with type 2 DM is that the patient may develop the disease and not be aware of any symptoms. Frequently, the condition is detected by the presence of glucose in urine (glycosuria) or elevated serum glucose, often while the patient is being investigated for some other complaint. This is one reason why urinalysis should be part of any routine health check. Despite an undiagnosed patient having no symptoms the chronic hyperglycaemia can be damaging several body tissues and organs, contributing to the development of the long term complications of diabetes. Part of this is that any insulin lack will lead to accelerated development of atheroma.

Metabolic syndrome

Type 2 DM is often associated with a group of other medical conditions. There may be dyslipidaemia with low levels of protective HDL and increased levels of LDL cholesterol and triglycerides. Hypertension and central obesity are also frequently present. This cluster of conditions is sometimes called metabolic or insulin resistance syndrome. These features all contribute to the formation of atheroma, leading to atherosclerosis of the large arteries. Each of the features of metabolic syndrome should be treated. Weight loss by diet and exercise is vital. Statins are needed to lower LDL cholesterol and hypotensive medications such as ACE inhibitors are needed to lower blood pressure.

Maturity onset diabetes of the young (MODY)

This condition sounds like a contradiction in terms but actually describes an uncommon variant of type 2 diabetes mellitus which presents in young people. The aetiology of this disorder is an autosomal dominant gene which gives a genetic predisposition. This is then acted on by poor life style factors such as over eating, obesity and lack of exercise.

Long term complications

Improvements in short term treatments of diabetes mean that patients should no longer die from hyperglycaemia or ketoacidotic coma. However, over time long term complications of diabetes may develop in type 1 and type 2 DM. The likelihood that long term complications occur largely depends on the degree of glycaemic control that can be achieved. In addition, it is important to control other risk factors such as obesity, dyslipidaemia and hypertension. With good control and life style the development of long term complications can be delayed or even prevented.

Macrovascular disease

Macrovascular disease affects the large arteries. It has been suggested that atheroma formation in diabetes is triggered by glucose levels in the blood being raised over a period of time. This allows glucose to migrate into the inner lining of arterial walls. Harmful low density lipoproteins seem to adhere to tissues which contain higher than normal levels of glucose, resulting in fatty accumulations in the vessel lumens. This process is then developed by higher levels of fatty material in the blood caused by the insulin lack mechanism already discussed.

The presence of fatty deposits in turn leads to the deposition of fibrous collagen and the development of atheromatous plaques.

Whatever the precise reasons, diabetics often develop more advanced atheroma than other people of the same age and sex. The development of atherosclerosis is accelerated in diabetes. Atherosclerosis affects the coronary arteries leading to angina and myocardial infarction. Coronary heart disease is the leading cause of morbidity in people with DM, accounting for up to 70% of deaths. Atheroma in the vessels supplying the brain leads to cerebral ischaemia and possible cerebrovascular accident. In the peripheral vessels atheroma will result in peripheral vascular disease. This leads to ischaemia and possible gangrene (areas of necrosis) in more advanced cases, explaining why lower limb amputations are significantly more common in diabetics compared to non-diabetics. Renal arterial involvement contributes to chronic nephron ischaemia.

Smoking will potentiate the development of macrovascular atheroma so it is particularly important that diabetics do not smoke. Serum cholesterol should be kept at low levels using statins as required. Blood pressure should also be closely monitored and lowered as necessary.

Microvascular complications

Smaller blood vessels such as arterioles and capillaries are also affected in diabetes mellitus. In these small vessels there is a progressive thickening and increase in rigidity of the basement membranes; this results in a narrowed lumen and loss of elasticity. These complications in turn lead to localised tissue ischaemia and hypoxia. When this ischaemia is compounded by macrovascular ischaemia the viability of tissues can be seriously compromised. Microvascular disease leads to complications affecting the kidneys, eyes and peripheral nerves. It is known that good glycaemic control, with a HbA$_{1C}$ of 7% or less significantly reduces the development of the microvascular complications.

Renal failure (diabetic nephropathy)

In the glomeruli of the kidneys there is microvascular basement membrane thickening and hardening (glomerulosclerosis). Despite the basement membrane of the glomerular capillaries being thicker, it is of reduced quality and becomes progressively more permeable to proteins. This leads to proteins passing from the blood into the glomerular filtrate. (In health protein molecules are much too large to be filtered into the glomerular filtrate). Initially this results in very small amounts of albumin passing into the glomerular filtrate and the development of microalbuminuria. This term describes the loss of very small volumes of albumin in urine not detectable by ward based 'dip stick' testing. However, even loss of such small amounts of protein is a predictor of subsequent more serious renal involvement. As the basement membrane thickening progresses there is loss of increasing volumes of albumin in the urine which may reach the nephrotic range. (In nephrotic syndrome substantial amounts of protein are lost in the urine resulting in a lowered osmotic potential of the blood plasma which can lead to oedema formation.) As the glomerulosclerosis develops the glomeruli are progressively lost leading to decreased renal function and eventual end stage renal failure (ESRF). In most western countries diabetic nephropathy is the most common cause of ESRF.

This pathology affecting the capillaries of the glomerulus can be complicated by hardening of the afferent and efferent arterioles. Other factors such as ischaemia caused by macrovascular atheroma and repeated urinary tract infections may also contribute to development of chronic irreversible renal failure. Hypertension is another risk factor for the development of diabetic nephropathy. Vigorous efforts should be made to prevent progression of nephropathy in patients presenting with microalbuminuria. Glycaemic control should be very good and there should be aggressive reduction in blood pressure, probably using ACE inhibitors.

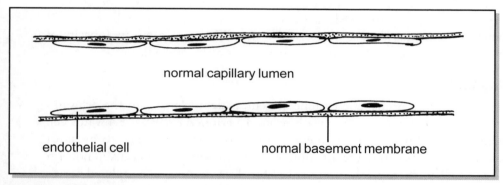

Diagram 16.4i
Normal capillaries and arterioles have a thin external basement membrane.

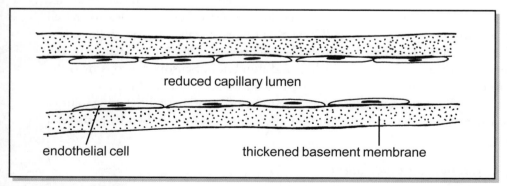

Diagram 16.4ii
In poorly controlled diabetes the basement membrane thickens and becomes rigid. Loss of elasticity in arterioles and capillaries means the blood flow is not smoothed out by the expansion and relaxation of elastic walls. In addition the volume of blood perfusing the tissues is lowered as vessel lumen diameter is reduced.

Blindness

Microvascular disease of the retina occurs as a result of basement membrane thickening. Retinal arterioles narrow and may become completely occluded. These changes lead to hypoxia in ischaemic areas of the retina. Chronic retinal hypoxia results in the release of growth factors including a factor which stimulates the rapid generation of new blood vessels. More blood vessels could carry more blood to the area and so counter the hypoxia. However there is a problem. In the retina the excessive growth of new small blood vessels is called proliferate retinopathy. These new vessels have fragile walls which can rupture and bleed; this will cause retinal haemorrhages which cause progressive damage to the light sensitive cells. Regular retinal examination and possible photocoagulation can cauterise new vessels before they have time to haemorrhage, this can prevent or delay the development of blindness. Poor glycaemic control, with hyperglycaemia is a definite risk factor for diabetic retinopathy. From this it is clear that good levels of glycaemic control reduce the probability of this complication developing. Hypertension is another risk factor for diabetic retinopathy which should therefore be managed. Diabetics are also more prone to cataracts (opacity of the lens) and glaucoma (increased pressure within the eyeball).

Neuropathy

Part of the cause of diabetic peripheral neuropathy is damage to the Schwann cells which form the myelin sheath around peripheral nerves. Schwann cell damage probably occurs for metabolic reasons and can lead to areas of demyelination. As part of the function of Schwann cells is to protect and nourish the nerve fibres there will be progressive fibre degeneration. In peripheral nerves the microvascular changes already described are likely to be an additional factor in the development of peripheral neuropathy. Ischaemia of peripheral nerves will lead to hypoxic damage as neurones are very sensitive to oxygen lack. Evidence for this comes from the fact that unmyelinated nerve fibres are affected as well as the myelinated fibres. Initially there will be shrinkage of axons followed by fragmentation. Neuropathy can lead to sensory and motor deficiency in the legs and often presents with tingling and numbness. Sensory neuropathy is the most common presentation resulting is reduced sensation and pain awareness from the feet. This can result in the patient being unaware of developing injuries to the feet. Bladder problems and impotence may also be caused by peripheral nerve defects.

Congestive cardiac failure

Poor glycaemic control is likely to be a risk factor for the development of congestive heart failure. Heart failure may be directly caused by glycosylation of heart muscle proteins. Glycosylation describes the addition of sugar molecules to proteins and lipids. Macro and microvascular disease will also contribute to congestive cardiac failure.

Predisposition to infections

Bacterial and fungal infections are more likely to occur in diabetics with high levels of blood glucose. These are likely to affect the skin, mucous membranes and urinary tract. For example, they are prone to develop staphylococcal skin lesions such as boils. Cellulitis is also a risk. Mucous membrane infections, affecting the mouth or genitals may be caused by the fungal infection Candida.

Increased problems with infections may simply be caused by higher levels of glucose in the tissue fluids which provide potential infecting bacteria and fungi with a ready supply of nutrition. In addition migration of phagocytes is inhibited by high levels of glucose in tissue fluids. This reduces the efficiency of this important part of the immune process. It also seems that microvascular basement membrane thickening decreases blood and oxygen supplies to areas of injury and infection, reducing the efficiency of the immune response. Increased rigidity of microvascular basement membranes also inhibits a normal inflammatory vasodilatory response. As the inflammatory response is necessary to combat infection and start the healing process, both of these are inhibited.

It is therefore important to monitor diabetics for the early signs and symptoms of infection so these can receive prompt treatment; this will prevent infections becoming more severe. Early infection is often more difficult to detect in diabetics as the normal inflammatory response to the presence of microorganisms is inhibited as just described. Internal infections may also occur; a urinary tract infection may develop into a potentially serious pyelonephritis (infection of the kidney tissue). Pneumonia is also a risk in poorly controlled patients.

Foot and leg problems

Macro and microvascular disease can lead to distal ischaemia eventually resulting in gangrene. As sensory neuropathy can lead to foot desensitisation, patients may not be aware of pressure effects from shoes, this can result in callous

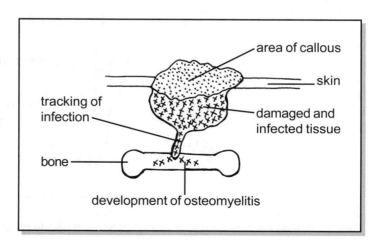

Diagram 16.5
Callous formation has led to an ulcerated area of tissue necrosis and infection. This infection has tracked down into underlying bone leading to osteomyelitis.

area of callous

skin

tracking of infection

damaged and infected tissue

bone

development of osteomyelitis

formation. Further pressure on hard areas of callous can lead to necrotic damage of underlying tissue. This occurs largely as a result of pressure from overlying callous impeding the blood supply, essentially leading to a pressure ulcer. These ulcers which develop under callous are prone to infection which may migrate down into the bone. This is why diabetic feet should be regularly inspected and areas of callous removed. Care must be taken when removing callous not to damage healthy underlying tissue as such injuries are prone to infection. If an ulcer does form under an area of callous there should be sharp debridement and the ulcer encouraged to heal by secondary intention.

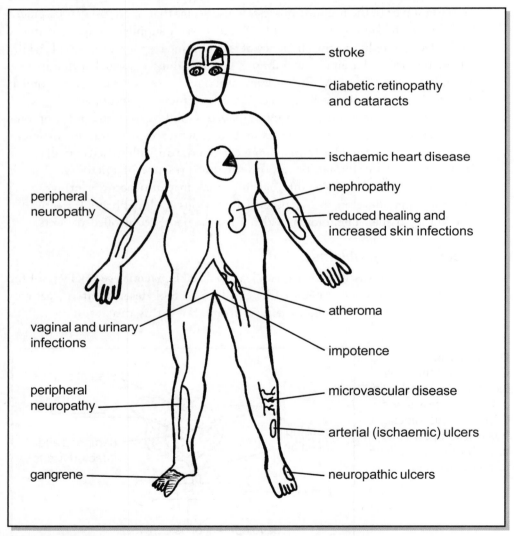

Diagram 16.6
Review of the possible long term complications of poorly controlled diabetes mellitus.

Hypoglycaemia

All of the complications mentioned above take time to develop, but hypoglycaemia can have an onset of just a few minutes and is potentially fatal. As hypoglycaemia is the most common complication of insulin therapy all practitioners need to be able to recognise and treat it.

Causes

By far the most common cause of hypoglycaemia is over administration of insulin. Occasionally it may also occur in patients taking oral hypoglycaemic medication. In this sense hypoglycaemia is an iatrogenic disorder (i.e. one caused by medical treatment). Sometimes a patient will take their insulin, but then fail to eat afterwards for some reason. Exercise and alcohol also lower blood glucose levels. Hypoglycaemia is also more likely to occur when patients have systemic infections, partly due to the increased metabolic requirements of fever generation. Hypoglycaemic attacks are most likely to occur before meals and at night.

Clinical features

The risk of developing hypoglycaemia is the main factor which makes it difficult to manage diabetic patients within normal ranges of blood glucose levels. In non-diabetic people symptoms of hypoglycaemia typically develop when blood glucose levels drop to 3 mmol L or below. However, in some diabetic patients, who are used to higher levels of blood glucose, clinical features may present at higher blood glucose levels. Onset of symptoms at particular glycaemic levels also varies between individuals. Patients who have been on insulin therapy for 20 years or more are more likely to develop hypoglycaemia which does not generate the usual clinical features. There is also an increased risk during sleep as patients may not be aware of the development of hypoglycaemia. This can lead to the so called 'death in bed syndrome'. When blood glucose levels drop, some clinical features are generated due to the release of adrenalin. Adrenalin is a counter-regulatory hormone, which has the effect of increasing blood glucose levels. As adrenalin stimulates the activity of the sympathetic nervous system it causes sweating, tremor, pallor and tachycardia. These are sometimes collectively referred to as adrenergic features.

A second group of features develop as a direct result of the hypoglycaemia reducing metabolic activity in the brain leading to possible confusion, behavioural change (which may resemble alcohol intoxication), slurred speech and drowsiness. If the condition is untreated there will be coma, and death is a possibility. In addition to the effects on the brain, it also seems likely that severe hypoglycaemia can lead to life threatening cardiac dysrhythmias and respiratory arrest. It is vital to understand that hypoglycaemia is an acute life-threatening condition.

Treatment principles in hypoglycaemia

Patients should be advised to eat some sugar or other form of carbohydrate if they feel they are becoming hypoglycaemic. Even drowsy patients should be able to swallow a drink containing some form of carbohydrate. Friends and relatives should be taught to recognise the clinical features and help the sufferer to eat or drink something. If the patient is unconscious no food or drinks may be given as these will be aspirated into the lungs. Unconscious patients should be given 30-50 mls of 20-50% dextrose solution intravenously. Alternatively they may be given an intramuscular injection of 1 mg of glucagon. This will mobilise stored glycogen from the liver and muscles and convert it into soluble glucose. Clearly, all doses would need to be adjusted for children. As a first aid measure syrup, honey or 'glucoGel' may be smeared on the mucous membranes of the mouth as some sugar will be absorbed. Once the patient is awake they should then be given something orally. If the hypoglycaemia has been caused by a long acting insulin the patient will need to be monitored and managed over time until fully recovered. Once the patient is fully recovered the normal food and insulin regime should be resumed and an increase in food, or reduction in insulin dose considered. Diabetic patients should carry a card or wear a medalert bracelet or necklace stating they are a diabetic on insulin. Insulin overdose is very dangerous but easy to treat if you think of it quickly enough.

General principles of diabetes management

It is now generally agreed that good glycaemic control is desirable in DM and will delay or prevent the development of many long term complications. Adequate amounts of insulin need to be taken in type 1 disease to prevent lipolysis (mobilization of stored fats) which will increase the amounts of fats and cholesterol in the blood.

Diet

People with diabetes should eat what would constitute a healthy diet for anyone. Unrefined, complex carbohydrates should be eaten as opposed to sugars. Complex carbohydrate will be slowly and progressively absorbed and will prevent sudden rises in plasma glucose. Over 50% of the total energy requirement should be taken in the form of carbohydrates. Plenty of fruit and vegetables should be eaten. Fat should make up less that 35% of the total energy intake, but should include adequate amounts of essential polyunsaturated and monosaturated fats. Protein should comprise about 10-15% of energy intake. Alcohol may be consumed up to the usual weekly recommendations. However, the calorie content of alcohol may contribute to obesity and alcohol will also lower blood sugar levels. The number of calories in the diet should be tailored to the activity level of the individual patient. Salt intake should be below 6 g per day.

General life-style

All diabetic patients should take plenty of exercise. If a patient is unfit an exercise programme should be followed to build up fitness. All patients should remain lean and overweight patients should be calorie restricted until excessive weight is lost. Smoking is unthinkable.

Type 2 DM

Diet and exercise are essential to successful management. Oral medication may also be used but it must be stressed this is 'as well as' not 'instead of' diet and exercise. Sulphonylureas stimulate insulin secretion from the remaining beta cells. Metformin type drugs (biguanides) have a hypoglycaemic effect by reducing the amount of glucose generated and released from the liver by inhibiting the process of gluconeogenesis. They may also increase insulin sensitivity. Over time type 2 diabetes usually gets worse and insulin eventually becomes necessary. Some recent thinking suggests that taking insulin at a relatively early stage in the progression of type 2 disease is associated with an improved prognosis. This is because by giving insulin, the patients own beta cells are allowed to rest and so may be physiologically active for longer.

Type 1 DM

Insulin is essential. As insulin is a protein it must be injected as it would be broken down by digestive enzymes if taken orally. The rate of insulin absorption after subcutaneous administration is increased by heat induced vasodilation, exercise and rubbing of the injection site. Several insulin preparations are available with variable durations of action. Typically, more rapid acting soluble insulin may be used during the day with an intermediate acting insulin used to cover the night. In theory, the lower blood glucose levels can be maintained the better as this will reduce the likelihood of developing long term complications related to chronic hyperglycaemia. However, low blood glucose levels carry the risk of hypoglycaemic attacks. For this reason it is usually advised to keep blood glucose levels above 4 mmol L (four is the floor). Before meals glucose levels should be below 7 and below 10 mmol L after meals.

Hopefully in the future it will be possible to harvest a patient's bone marrow and stimulate some stem cells to become beta cells which may then be injected into the liver. Here these cells could produce insulin in a physiological way and cure type 1 diabetes mellitus.

CHAPTER 17

Disorders of the Blood

Anaemia

Anaemia is normally defined as a reduced level of haemoglobin in the blood. Normal blood levels of haemoglobin are 13.5-18g/dL (grams per decilitre i.e. per 100mls of blood) for men and 11.5-16.5g/dL for women. The common feature in all forms of anaemia is a reduced oxygen carrying capacity of the blood. It is important to realise that anaemia is not a diagnosis; the underlying cause of the condition should be identified and treated.

Clinical features

Patients with anaemia often complain of non-specific symptoms such as tiredness, headache, feeling faint and shortness of breath on exercise. Tiredness may be explained by a reduction in the volumes of oxygen which are supplied to the brain and muscles. This will restrict the amount of energy these tissues can generate. Faintness may be caused by hypoxia of the brain; this is because neurones require a continuous supply of energy in order to function normally and to generate consciousness. Shortness of breath can be explained by low levels of oxygen in the blood stimulating the chemoreceptors in the aorta and carotid bodies which increase activity in the respiratory centre of the medulla oblongata. The consequent increased ventilation will increase blood oxygenation.

When the proportions of oxygen in the blood are low, there is stimulation of the sympathetic nervous system. This is a compensatory mechanism which increases the rate at which red cells circulate around the body. Increasing the speed at which red cells circulate will generate a corresponding increase in oxygen delivery to the tissues. This increased sympathetic activity is seen as a tachycardia with increased cardiac output. In severe and ongoing anaemia, this increased cardiac output will cause ventricular hypertrophy and eventually cardiac failure. Increased rates of red cell production are another attempted compensatory mechanism; this may cause bone pain, often affecting the sternum. As it is the red cells which transport oxygen, an increased number will result in more oxygen delivery from the lungs to the tissues.

Physical signs of anaemia usually include pallor of the skin, nail beds, conjunctiva and mucous membranes. This pallor is caused by a lack of haemoglobin in the blood near these body surfaces. The normal pink colour in these areas reflects adequate amounts of oxyhaemoglobin in the small blood vessels which perfuse the tissues.

If patients have any underlying ischaemic conditions, such as angina, cerebrovascular insufficiency or peripheral vascular disease, these will be exacerbated by anaemia. When the volume of blood supplying an area of tissue is reduced, the volumes of oxygen reaching the area will be correspondingly reduced. If the amount of oxygen carried in an already reduced blood supply is low, then the hypoxia will be even worse. This is why treatment of anaemia can often improve the clinical picture in ischaemic conditions.

Aetiology

Anaemia is caused by abnormal production, destruction or loss of haemoglobin or red cells. Iron deficiency, pernicious and aplastic anaemias are caused by reduced or abnormal production of red cells and haemoglobin. Haemolytic anaemias are caused by increased destruction of red cells by the reticuloendothelial (monocyte-macrophage) system, mostly in the spleen. Ongoing blood loss from chronic haemorrhage also depletes the amount of circulating haemoglobin and so reduces the oxygen carrying capacity of the blood. Individual forms of anaemia will now be considered.

Iron deficiency anaemia

This condition is globally very common and is endemic in many underdeveloped areas. Over a quarter of the world's population suffers from iron deficiency anaemia. Almost all of the oxygen carried by the blood is transported in the red cells by haemoglobin molecules. Iron is an essential component of haemoglobin; therefore if the body does not have adequate supplies of iron, haemoglobin cannot be synthesized in adequate amounts.

Aetiology

Iron deficiency anaemia may be caused by reduced intake or excessive loss of iron from the body. Poor diets, which contain inadequate amounts of iron are one cause. This is particularly a problem if no meat or other animal products such as eggs are eaten. Iron from meat is in the form of haem iron, which is readily absorbed from the GI tract, so is ideal for people with iron deficiency. Iron from other sources such as cereals and vegetables is not absorbed as efficiently. This partly explains why iron deficiency anaemia is more common in poor communities. Interestingly, when the body has low stores of iron, cells which line the duodenum are able to increase the amount they absorb, conversely when iron levels in the body are adequate, less iron is absorbed.

Iron requirement is increased during pregnancy as iron from the mother is needed for the developing baby. During growth, more iron is also needed as the growing child must increase blood and muscle volumes. These times of increased demand explain why iron deficiency is more commonly seen in pregnancy and childhood, if the diet is inadequate. The other obvious cause of increased iron demand is menstruation, when normal blood loss is about 30-40 mls per month.

Iron deficiency is also likely to develop in conditions where there is chronic blood loss. If blood loss during menstruation exceeds 100mls per month, the GI tract is unable to increase absorption sufficiently to compensate. Increased blood loss during menstruation is termed menorrhagia and is commonly seen with uterine fibroids and other gynaecological disorders.

Other causes of chronic blood loss include peptic ulceration, haemorrhoids, inflammatory gastrointestinal disorders and carcinoma of the colon. Ongoing use of non-steroidal anti-inflammatory drugs can also lead to chronic bleeding into the GI tract. In conditions where there is bleeding into the lumen of the GI tract, altered blood may be detected in the faeces which may be seen as melaena if the blood loss is large. Smaller losses can be detected using faecal occult blood tests. Frequent injuries with associated blood loss are another possible cause. Globally, the most common cause of iron deficiency anaemia caused by chronic blood loss is hookworm infection. Hookworms bite into the lining of the GI tract and drink the blood. This infection can be readily treated with oral mebendazole.

Iron in the body can be stored in combination with a protein called ferritin. This means that when blood loss is increased, or the diet becomes deficient, iron deficiency will take time to develop as reserves are used up. Blood testing for plasma ferritin levels is a specific test for iron deficiency as ferritin levels will also be low.

Pathophysiology

Iron deficiency anaemia results in red cells which are microcytic (small) and hypochromic (pale). As the red cells are small with reduced amounts of haemoglobin, the volumes of oxygen they are able to carry is reduced. Reduction in the physical size of the red cells can be detected using the mean corpuscular (cell) volume blood test when the MCV will be below 80fl (fentolitres are a small unit of volume). The pale, hypochromic colour, is caused by the reduced amount of haemoglobin in the red cells. This observation is supported by a mean corpuscular haemoglobin (MCH) of less than 27pg per red cell (picograms are a small unit of mass). With iron deficiency anaemia, there is also more variation in the shape and size of the red cells, when compared to normal erythrocytes. With experience, all of these changes can be seen by direct microscopic examination of blood films. Microcytic anaemia is also seen in sideroblastic anaemia, anaemia of chronic disease and in thalassaemia.

Clinical features

In addition to the general features of anaemia there may be other signs of iron deficiency. These include brittle or spoon shaped nails, brittle hair, inflammation of the tongue (glossitis) and small sores at the corner of the mouth (angular stomatitis).

Treatment

A careful history is taken and the underlying cause of iron deficiency anaemia should be identified and then corrected. Oral iron in the form of ferrous sulphate is the standard treatment; this may be given in 200mg tablets 3 times per day and is absorbed best on an empty stomach. Patients should be warned that these tablets will cause their faeces to become dark coloured. Iron therapy should be given until the haemoglobin and red cells have returned to normal and ferritin reserves are built up. This may mean giving the iron supplement for up to 6 months. Occasionally iron may be given by intramuscular injection, this should be 'Z tracked' to prevent skin staining.

Megaloblastic anaemia

A megaloblast is a large (MCV>100fl), immature red blood cell. Red blood cells normally develop and mature within the red bone marrow. During early erythrocyte development, the immature red cells have a nucleus to control the processes needed. As they mature, prior to release into the circulation, the nucleus is lost and the cell becomes physically smaller. In order for red cells to mature there must be activity of the DNA within the nucleus to control cellular development. If DNA synthesis is impaired, then normal development cannot proceed and results in large immature erythrocytes being released into the circulating blood. Normal DNA synthesis depends on a supply of the nutrients vitamin B_{12} (cyanocobalamin) and folic acid, so if either of these are deficient, normal DNA synthesis and cell maturation will not occur. In addition to the red cells being immature, fewer are released from the bone marrow. This is because abnormal large cells are destroyed within the bone marrow prior to release into the circulating blood.

Folic acid is found in green leafy vegetables, fruits, eggs and meat. Folic acid deficiency is usually caused by a low intake, so can be corrected by improving the diet. Demand for folic acid is raised during rapid growth in childhood, pregnancy and lactation when increased intake is needed.

Vitamin B_{12} is found mostly in foods from animal sources although some is synthesised by bacteria in the colon. Before dietary vitamin B_{12} can be absorbed, it must first form a complex with intrinsic factor (in this context B_{12} is the extrinsic factor). Intrinsic factor is produced by the gastric parietal cells (sometimes called oxyntic cells) which also produce hydrochloric acid (HCl). Specific receptors in the distal ileum absorb the complex of B_{12} and intrinsic factor. Lack of vitamin B_{12} in the diet is uncommon but is seen in strict vegetarians or vegans. More commonly there is a lack of vitamin B_{12} because of lack of intrinsic factor which may occur if portions of the stomach are surgically removed. However, the most common cause of reduced levels of intrinsic factor is pernicious anaemia.

Pernicious anaemia

Aetiology

In this autoimmune disorder, the immune system produces antibodies to the gastric parietal cells and often to the intrinsic factor. These autoantibodies therefore reduce the volumes of available intrinsic factor which in turn means that vitamin B_{12} cannot combine in order to be absorbed. The end result is

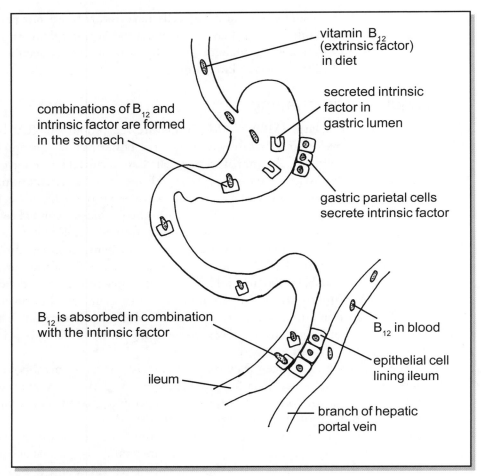

vitamin B$_{12}$
(extrinsic factor)
in diet

secreted intrinsic
factor in
gastric lumen

combinations of B$_{12}$ and
intrinsic factor are formed
in the stomach

gastric parietal cells
secrete intrinsic factor

B$_{12}$ is absorbed in combination
with the intrinsic factor

B$_{12}$ in blood

epithelial cell
lining ileum

ileum

branch of hepatic
portal vein

Diagram 17.1
Vitamin B$_{12}$ is not absorbed unless it is in combination with intrinsic factor. A
combination of B$_{12}$ and intrinsic factor is absorbed into the cells lining the
ileum. Here the intrinsic and extrinsic factors are separated and the B$_{12}$ is
systemically absorbed into the hepatic portal vein.

that the GI tract is unable to absorb orally ingested B$_{12}$. As it is the parietal cells
which produce hydrochloric acid, the concentration of this in the stomach is
also reduced, often termed achlorhydria (this literally means no HCl). Prevalence
of pernicious anaemia increases with age.

Pathophysiology

The presentation of anaemia caused by lack of B$_{12}$ or folic acid is the same; both
present with a macrocytosis, meaning that the red cells are larger than normal.
Red cells may also have an oval appearance and neutrophils may have more
lobes in their nucleus than normal (more than 5 lobes). Many of the abnormal

red cells are destroyed in the red bone marrow before they are released into the blood, therefore the total number of red cells which enter the circulation is reduced. This reduced cell number, in combination with the immature nature of the red cells, decreases the oxygen carrying capacity of the blood.

Clinical features

In pernicious anaemia the onset of clinical features is gradual, but the condition can become severe if not treated. In addition to anaemia, neurones need B_{12} to function normally. If there is a deficiency of vitamin B_{12} the peripheral nerves are usually affected first and then the spinal cord (a condition called subacute combined degeneration of the spinal cord). Eventually this will develop into paraplegia (paralysis of the lower half of the body). Dementia can also develop as a result of the brain cells being affected. If such neurological features are not treated by giving adequate amounts of B_{12} they can become irreversible.

Patients with pernicious anaemia are also more likely to suffer from other autoimmune diseases compared with the general population. These conditions include thyroid disorders, type I diabetes mellitus, ulcerative colitis and Addison's disease.

Treatment

As B_{12} is not effectively absorbed via the GI tract it is necessary to bypass this route with parenteral administration. Hydroxocobalamin is given via intramuscular injection. Once the disorder is corrected the patient will need 1 mg (1000 micrograms) every 12 weeks for life.

Aplastic anaemia

Aetiology

About two thirds of cases of aplastic anaemia are idiopathically acquired. This means the condition is acquired and develops without any known trigger. In these cases it seems likely that the blood producing stem cells in the bone marrow are attacked by the body's own cytotoxic T lymphocytes. This means that these cases are autoimmune. In addition to these idiopathic cases, several secondary causes of aplastic anaemia are known. Exposure to ionizing radiation, such as from X-rays or nuclear waste and fall out, has the potential to affect all fast dividing cells, such as those found in bone marrow. Certain chemicals such as benzene and some insecticides are a known risk, as are some drugs such as chloramphenicol. Often the risk of aplastic changes increases with the exposure dose of a causative agent. However, sometimes small doses can trigger the condition in idiosyncratic reactions. This means that for some reason which was not predicted, an individual seems to have a particular sensitivity to a causative agent, even in very small doses. Some viral infections and tuberculosis are other possible triggers.

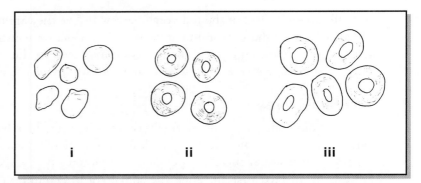

Diagram 17.2
Red blood cells (erythrocytes) in iron deficiency and pernicious anaemia.
i.   Red cells as seen in iron deficiency anaemia are of irregular shapes, hypochromic and microcytic.
ii. Normal red cells are 6 to 8 microns across, they are biconcaved disks and have a pale coloured central area which is equal to or less than a third of the cell diameter.
iii. Red cells in pernicious anaemia are large and often oval shaped; this is an example of megaloblastic anaemia.

Pathophysiology

In the bone marrow there is a group of stem cells which are pluripotent. This means they have the ability to differentiate into all of the types of blood cells (i.e. red cells and the various forms of white cell). In aplastic anaemia these stem cells fail to function resulting in bone marrow failure and a consequent reduced production of the whole range of blood cells. This means there are less red and white cells in the blood, a condition referred to as pancytopenia. (Pan-all, cyto-cell, penia-deficiency.) When the bone marrow is examined there is a hypocellularity (fewer cells than normal). Plastic in this context means a tendency to build up or regenerate tissue, so aplastic means without this tendency. Blood forming haemopoietic tissue is found in the bone marrow which is not built up and regenerated, so the blood cells are not replenished.

Clinical features

This disorder is serious, but fortunately rare. Bone marrow failure gives rise to anaemia, bleeding and infections. Lack of red cells reduces the oxygen carrying capacity of the blood causing anaemia. A lack of white cells is termed a leucopenia and, as these are needed for the functioning of the immune system, a deficiency leads to immunodeficiency and subsequent infection. Lack of platelets (thrombocytes) causes thrombocytopenia. As these are essential to the process of blood clotting their lack will lead to haemorrhagic complications such as bleeding. Aplastic anaemia often presents with this haemorrhagic complication.

Gums may bleed after brushing teeth, mouth blood blisters, nose bleeds (epistaxis), bleeding under the skin (ecchymosis) and bruising after slight knocks are other presentations.

Treatment principles

Stringent measures should be taken to prevent infections and, if any are suspected, aggressive antibiotic therapy should be given early. Red cell and platelet infusions may be given as indicated. Some cases have an apparently spontaneous remission while others become more severe, with death occurring as a complication of haemorrhage or infection. In younger patients bone marrow transplantation is the treatment of choice, if a suitable donor (often a sibling) is available. In older patients, or when no suitable donor is available, immunosuppressive therapy is helpful. This works by inhibiting autoimmune processes which attack the blood stem cells in the bone marrow.

Haemolytic anaemias

Haemolysis means the breaking up of blood cells. In haemolytic anaemias adequate numbers of red cells are manufactured by the bone marrow, but too many are broken down prematurely.

Pathophysiology

In order to compensate for the increased destruction of red cells the bone marrow increases production which results in an increased number of reticulocytes in the circulation. A reticulocyte is a young circulating red cell which still contains fragments of the nucleus which was present during cell development (mature red cells do not have a nucleus). An increase in the proportion of reticulocytes is termed a reticulocytosis.

As more red cells are destroyed there is an increase in the amount of the haemoglobin breakdown product bilirubin in the blood. This pigment may give rise to a slightly jaundiced appearance. Causes of haemolytic anaemia include spherocytosis, G6PD deficiency, thalassaemia, mechanical haemolysis, haemolytic disease of the newborn and sickle cell disease.

Hereditary spherocytosis

In this autosomal dominant disorder there is a genetic abnormality of a protein which forms the cytoskeleton of the red cells. (A cytoskeleton is a network of intracellular proteins which support a cell and give it shape.) An abnormal cytoskeleton has the effect of allowing the red cells to become more spherical, as opposed to the normal biconcaved shape. The spherocytes are also abnormally rigid and are destroyed at an accelerated rate by macrophages in the spleen. This increased activity in the spleen causes the splenic tissue to develop, leading to enlargement, a condition termed splenomegaly. The anaemia tends to be mild, but may become worse as a result of some infections. There may be mild jaundice and there is an increased risk of cholelithiasis (gallstones). These stones contain a lot of bilirubin and form as a result of the increased secretion of this product of haemoglobin breakdown, present as a consequence of the increased haemolysis.

G6PD deficiency

G6PD stands for the enzyme glucose-6-phosphate dehydrogenase. Deficiency is an X linked genetic disorder; this usually means that females carry the disorder and males suffer from it. These patients are normal for much of the time but a haemolytic episode can be triggered by infections, some drugs and certain food stuffs, particularly fava beans. This disorder is more common in black Africans and peoples from around the Mediterranean.

Thalassaemia

There are many forms of thalassaemia, but they all cause anaemia as a result of the production of abnormal haemoglobin. The main classifications of the disease are alpha and beta thalassaemia, after the particular structural globin molecular chains affected. The disorder is genetic with the alpha form being most prevalent in Mediterranean areas whereas the beta form is most common in Southeast Asia. The anaemia is caused by reduced haemoglobin synthesis, the presence of abnormal haemoglobin and increased destruction of red cells in the spleen and liver. This increased activity gives rise to a splenomegaly and hepatomegaly. Supportive measures may include folic acid and regular blood transfusions to maintain adequate haemoglobin levels. Bone marrow transplantation has been successfully used.

Mechanical haemolytic anaemia

Sometimes red cells may be physically broken up by mechanical forces. One cause is prolonged marching or running. When the foot hits the ground, some red cells in the pressure bearing surfaces under the foot, are crushed. This will give rise to an increase in free haemoglobin in the blood resulting in haemoglobinaemia. As the free haemoglobin is excreted in urine there will be a haemoglobinuria. The urine will be dark or even reddish in colour, due to the presence of the haemoglobin. A similar mechanical haemolysis is seen in patients who have undergone heart valve replacement. The mechanical action of the valve will crush red cells as it closes.

Haemolytic disease of the newborn

The most serious form of this disorder is caused by rhesus (Rh) factor incompatibility. This problem arises when a mother is Rh negative and the father is Rh positive. As the Rh positive gene is dominant, this will usually result in a Rh positive baby. During the birth, some of the baby's red cells will enter the mother's circulation. As these cells contain the Rh factor antigens, the mother's immune system will be stimulated to produce Rh factor antibodies.

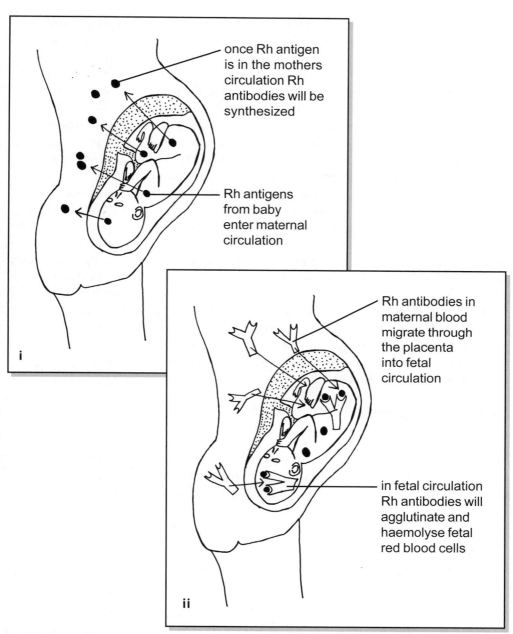

once Rh antigen is in the mothers circulation Rh antibodies will be synthesized

Rh antigens from baby enter maternal circulation

i

Rh antibodies in maternal blood migrate through the placenta into fetal circulation

in fetal circulation Rh antibodies will agglutinate and haemolyse fetal red blood cells

ii

Diagram 17.3

Rhesus factor incompatibility is a problem in a Rh negative mother with a Rh positive baby.

i. At the end of the first pregnancy, some Rh positive cells from the baby enter the mother's circulation during the process of birth.
ii. In a second pregnancy the mother has produced Rh factor antibodies which pass into the fetal circulation through the placenta and umbilical cord. They then attack his or her red cells.

This sensitization will take place during the first few days after delivery so will not affect the child which has already been born. However, if the mother becomes pregnant a second time, some of her Rh factor antibodies will migrate across the placenta into the fetal circulation. Maternal Rh antibodies will lead to agglutination and haemolysis of fetal red blood cells, leading to severe fetal anaemia and hyperbilirubinaemia. In an attempt to produce more red cells the fetal spleen and liver enlarge. Hepatic enlargement leads to reduced liver function. As albumin is synthesised in the liver, levels of this osmotic protein in the blood drop. This reduces the osmotic potential of the plasma and so tissue fluids are not effectively reabsorbed. Accumulation of fluid, in the tissue spaces, leads to severe generalised oedema. Affected babies are also jaundiced due to the presence of red cell breakdown products such as bilirubin. Without treatment about 20% of these babies will die in utero.

These babies may need intrauterine or post delivery blood exchange transfusions. However, the whole problem can usually be prevented by giving Rh negative mothers a Rhesus immune globulin. This contains antibodies to the Rh factor. If given shortly after birth, this will result in an agglutination of the Rh positive fetal cells within the mother's circulation, before they have had enough time to sensitise her immune system. This prevents the formation of maternal Rh antibodies so there should be no problems with the next pregnancy. In practise, the preparation injected is anti-D. The D factor is the most antigenic component of the Rh factor.

Sickle cell disease

Pathophysiology

This disorder causes a form of haemolytic anaemia and is associated with numerous other problems; this is why the more general term sickle cell disease is used. In this autosomal recessive condition there is an abnormal form of haemoglobin, called haemoglobin S present in the red cells. When this abnormal haemoglobin deoxygenates, it transforms the erythrocyte into a sickle shape. Initially the sickle shaped cells return to being biconcave discs when they are reoxygenated, but after a few cycles they become rigid and fixed in the sickle position.

In normal physiology, red cells are readily able to deform and squash down in order to fit through small capillaries. However, these rigid sickle cells are unable to pass through small capillaries. Sickle cells are also more adherent to the endothelial lining of small blood vessels, increasing the development of occlusive complications. These abnormalities result in obstruction of the microcirculation through organs, leading in turn to loss of organ function with acute painful swelling. Plugging of small vessels in the bone marrow also leads to acute, very severe pain in some bones. As the abnormal sickle cells pass through the spleen they are destroyed at an increased rate by macrophages, resulting in increased haemolysis and subsequent haemolytic anaemia.

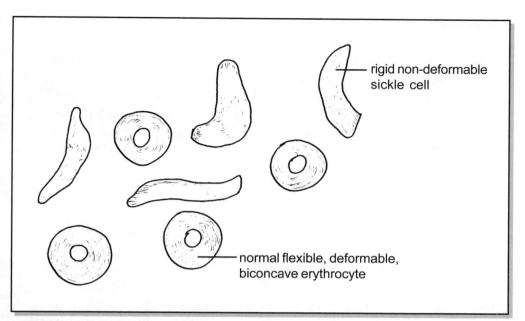

rigid non-deformable
sickle cell

normal flexible, deformable,
biconcave erythrocyte

Diagram 17.4
A comparison between normal and sickled red blood cells.

Clinical features

While most patients are able to adapt to the anaemia, capillary occlusion leads to impaired function of most tissue and organ systems. Anaemia generates obligatory high cardiac output, leading in turn to cardiomegaly and heart failure. These cardiac effects can be complicated by obstruction of the coronary microcirculation; other organs which are affected by occlusive pathology include the liver, spleen, lungs, kidneys and brain. Progressive destruction of the spleen leads to reduced immunity leaving the patients vulnerable to infections, a particular risk being Streptococcus pneumoniae, leading to pneumonia or meningitis. Obstruction of dermal capillaries may lead to leg ulcer formation.

When people with sickle cell disease become dehydrated or suffer an infection, the severity of the disease may worsen into a sickle cell crisis. In a crisis, the occlusion of small blood vessels leads to severe pain in the bones, chest and abdomen. Children with sickle cell disease are prone to a condition termed sequestration crisis. This is caused by a sudden pooling of red cells, particularly in the spleen and liver. As blood is pooled, there is less left for the systemic circulation and death may occur as a result of acute hypovolaemia. The most common cause of death is acute sickle chest syndrome. This may be caused by occlusion of the pulmonary circulation, infection or fat embolism arising from infarcted necrotic bone. Patients suffer from shortness of breath, hypoxia, chest pain and areas of pulmonary consolidation.

Epidemiology

Sickle cell disease is most common in African populations; this is because the presence of the gene in heterozygous form gives some protection against falciparum malaria, which may cause cerebral malaria. Sickle cell disease is also seen in some Indians, Middle Eastern and Mediterranean populations. People who are homozygous for the abnormal sickle cell gene show the full clinical features of sickle cell disease. Heterozygous carriers are said to have sickle cell trait; they normally do not develop red cell sickling and are asymptomatic with normal life expectancy.

Treatment principles

Factors known to cause exacerbations, such as hypoxia, dehydration and infection, should be avoided and treated promptly if they do occur. Daily folic acid is helpful to promote the compensatory increased red cell production. Prophylactic penicillin V reduces the likelihood of pneumococcal infection. Acute episodes should be supported with analgesics, oxygen, antibiotics and aggressive rehydration. Blood transfusions may be needed. The oral cytotoxic agent hydroxycarbamide has been shown to reduce the occurrence of acute chest syndrome and episodes of pain.

Other forms of anaemia

Sideroblastic anaemia

A sideroblast is an immature red blood cell found in the bone marrow. In sideroblastic anaemia these cells accumulate an abnormal ring of iron around the nucleus. This occurs because there is ineffective haem synthesis, leaving excess iron in the sideroblast. The abnormal sideroblasts are seen in bone marrow samples. The end result is that mature red cells lack haemoglobin, giving rise to microcytic hypochromic red cells, as seen in iron deficiency. The condition may be genetic, primary or acquired. Acquired causes include lead poisoning, alcohol abuse or myeloid leukaemia.

Anaemia in renal disease

Many renal diseases are associated with reduced production of erythropoietin (EPO). This hormone is normally produced by the kidneys in response to oxygen lack. It then stimulates the production of erythrocytes by the process of erythropoiesis in red bone marrow. If adequate quantities of EPO are not released, there will be reduced stimulation of red cell production in the red bone marrow. This condition can now be treated by giving injections of EPO. Endurance athletes have given themselves injections of EPO to artificially increase the proportion of red cells in their blood. This has the effect of increasing aerobic capacity and improves performance in endurance events. However, this is not a safe procedure and is of course cheating.

Anaemia of chronic disease

This mild form of anaemia is frequently seen in patients who have chronic infections, malignant or inflammatory diseases, such as rheumatoid arthritis. Chronic infective conditions include tuberculosis, endocarditis or osteomyelitis. The anaemia is caused by abnormalities of iron metabolism and storage with reduced levels of erythropoietin. This means that despite there being normal or even increased reserves of iron in the form of ferritin there is a functional deficiency. These pathophysiological changes are probably caused by cytokines. As a result of inflammation or malignancy, cytokines are released by tissue cells and white blood cells. These cytokines then have an inhibitory effect on iron metabolism and erythropoiesis (red cell formation). The MCV is usually normal with red cells of normal size and colour. If a trial course of oral iron is given anaemia of chronic disease will not improve. Treatments to reduce the severity of the underlying chronic condition will be helpful.

Cigarette smoking

Smoking is not often recognised as a cause of anaemia, but it does result in a reduced oxygen carrying capacity of the blood. Carbon monoxide (CO) in tobacco smoke combines with haemoglobin in red blood cells to form a relatively stable compound called carboxyhaemoglobin. Carboxyhaemoglobin does not readily dissociate, as haemoglobin and oxygen do, so it remains in the blood. When the oxygen carrying sites in the haemoglobin molecule are occupied by CO, the haemoglobin is no longer able to transport oxygen. This means the more carboxyhaemoglobin present in the blood, the less oxygen can be carried. This is one reason why smokers become short of breath with exercise. If a person stops smoking, the CO attached to haemoglobin will dissociate after a few days which frees up more haemoglobin to transport oxygen again.

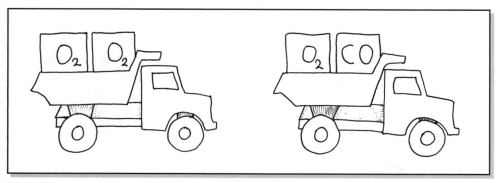

Diagram 17.5
Haemoglobin is an oxygen carrier molecule. If some of the carrier sites are occupied by CO, less oxygen can be transported to the tissues. The first truck has a full load of oxygen, however the second one has half of the carrier sites occupied by firmly bonded CO, halving the volumes of oxygen it is able to transport.

This means as long as smoking is stopped before lung and heart damage occurs, the smoker can rapidly increase their exercise tolerance. Large doses of inhaled carbon monoxide can be fatal, as high levels of carboxyhaemoglobin mean that tissues will not receive enough oxygen to sustain life essential metabolism. This may occur when exhaust fumes collect in a confined space, as a result of fires, or poorly maintained gas appliances. It is important to remember that oxygen saturation probes cannot differentiate between oxyhaemoglobin and carboxyhaemoglobin, so in carbon monoxide poisoning, oxygen pulse oximetry saturations may appear falsely normal.

Polycythaemia

In a sense this is the opposite of anaemia. In polycythaemia there are too many cells in the blood causing an erythrocytosis. This will cause an increased red cell count and packed cell volume (PCV); haemoglobin is also usually raised. In addition to an increase in red cell mass, there are usually increased numbers of white cells and platelets. The primary form of the disease is called polycythaemia ruba vera (PRV) and is a disorder of the blood stem cells in bone marrow. Normally a proportion of newly formed blood cells undergo apoptosis (programmed cell death). However, in PRV this does not happen, resulting in too many new blood cells being produced.

As the blood is thicker, due to the increased numbers of blood cells, thrombosis is more likely to occur. This problem is made worse by an increased number of platelets (thrombocytosis). Thrombus formation can lead to life threatening thromboembolic disease. Polycythaemia is often controlled by regular bleeding (venesection) of the patient to reduce the numbers of cells in circulation.

The secondary form is caused by an increase in erythropoietin stimulation of the red bone marrow. Whenever there is a generalised hypoxia, the kidneys are stimulated to release more EPO. Generalised hypoxia may be caused by reduced oxygen uptake in any form of chronic lung disease such as COPD or lung cancer. Another common cause of polycythaemia is cigarette smoking. An EPO response is also stimulated as part of an adaptation to living at altitude. While blood letting (venesection) may be appropriate to manage the symptoms in some cases of secondary polycythaemia, the underlying cause should be identified and treated.

Thrombocytopenia

Pathophysiology

This refers to a reduced number of thrombocytes (platelets) in the blood. As platelets are essential for the process of blood clotting, a reduction leads to haemorrhagic problems. Reduced production of platelets by the bone marrow may lead to thrombocytopenia, as seen in aplastic anaemia. However, there may also be increased destruction of platelets after their release into the blood.

Acute autoimmune idiopathic thrombocytopenic purpura (AITP) is most commonly seen in children, often after a viral infection. The immune system develops autoantibodies which attach to platelets leading to their premature destruction by the monocyte-macrophage system. As platelets are phagocytosed in this way, less will be left in circulation, reducing the ability of the blood to clot. Fortunately acute AITP usually remits spontaneously. A chronic form of idiopathic thrombocytopenia is also seen, most commonly in adult females.

Clinical features

Purpura and bleeding from mucous membranes are the common features seen in thrombocytopenia. Purpura is a physical sign, seen as a result of the collection of blood cells in the tissue spaces. There is spontaneous extravasation of blood from capillaries into the skin. This blood is seen as red spots called petechiae which may remain small or enlarge. Over time they turn purple, as the red cells become deoxygenated in the tissues. On superficial examination purpura looks similar to bruising. Rare cases of severe thrombocytopenia may lead to oral and nasal bleeding, gastrointestinal or retinal haemorrhage and even intracranial haemorrhage.

Treatment principles

The corticosteroid drug prednisolone may be used to reduce the production of autoantibodies. This works because corticosteroids reduce the immune response in general. Another possible treatment is intravenous infusions of immunoglobulin. These immune proteins work by blocking the receptors on macrophages which recognise the autoantibodies which become attached to platelets. This means macrophages are not stimulated to phagocytose the autoantibody labelled platelets. If the platelet count is very low, or haemorrhage is an actual or potential problem, concentrated platelets should be intravenously infused. Splenectomy may become indicated in ongoing cases which do not respond to other measures. As always, splenectomy is not a desirable treatment as it results in immunocompromise.

Haemophilia

Haemophilia A is an X chromosome linked, recessive genetic disorder, affecting about 1 in 5000 males in the UK. A mother who is a carrier of the abnormal gene has a 50% chance of having an affected male child with a further 50% chance of a daughter who may carry the disorder on to the next generation. Queen Victoria (reigned 1837-1901) was a well known example of a female carrier. The disorder is caused by a mutation of the normal gene which codes for factor VIII on the X chromosome. Factor VIII is one of the 12 essential clotting factors present in the blood. Some cases of haemophilia can be traced back through a family for generations while others seem to mutate spontaneously, giving rise to new cases.

Clinically there may be spontaneous bleeding into muscles, internal organs and joints, which swell up and become painful. Permanent damage to joints may occur without correct management. Without treatment, bleeding into the brain is probably the most common form of death. Effective blood clotting in wounds does not occur and bruising develops even with mild trauma. Haematuria may present as a result of renal bleeding. Obstruction of the respiratory and gastrointestinal lumens may also occur as a result of bleeding. Disease severity varies considerably between individual sufferers, depending on the amount of factor VIII they are still able to synthesise.

Treatment consists of giving infusions of factor VIII to compensate for the deficiency. As the half life of this clotting factor is only 12 hours, it may need to be given on a regular basis or via infusion to cover surgery. In mild cases the levels of factor VIII may be stimulated by giving synthetic vasopressin. Unfortunately, between 1979 and 1985, many patients were given coagulation factors contaminated with HIV and hepatitis C. This arose because many blood donations need to be pooled to have enough factor VIII to effectively treat an individual, which of course greatly increases the risk of infection. As it is now possible to clone the gene for factor VIII, recombinant factor VIII is being produced; however if this is not available it is still sometimes necessary to use plasma derived product. Clearly, all patients should be vaccinated against hepatitis A and B and carry a 'med alert' card or bracelet.

Other less common clotting factor deficiencies are haemophilia B (also called Christmas disease) caused by lack of factor IX and von Willebrand's disease caused by lack of a type of factor VIII and defective platelet function.

Other causes of impaired coagulation

Liver disease

Several of the 12 coagulation factors are proteins which are synthesised and secreted by the liver. When the liver has extensive damage, it is no longer able to synthesise adequate levels of these essential proteins. In severe liver disease the coagulation time is extended in proportion to the deficiency of clotting factors. This can lead to potentially severe haemorrhagic problems.

Vitamin K deficiency

Vitamin K, like many other vitamins, works as a cofactor or coenzyme. This means that vitamins are essential to facilitate specific biochemical reactions. Vitamin K is an essential cofactor for the synthesis of 4 of the clotting factors which are produced by the liver. In the absence of vitamin K, the liver is not able to synthesise factors II, VII, IX and X. Deficiency of these factors will delay blood coagulation. Neonates do not have much vitamin K so are usually given some shortly after birth. In adults the form of vitamin K which is most efficiently absorbed is synthesised by bacteria living in the colon. Some antibiotic treatments can kill many of these friendly bacteria and result in deficiency. Dietary deficiency is also possible. The treatment in both situations is to give vitamin K.

Disseminated intravascular coagulation

This disorder complicates conditions such as severe sepsis, major trauma, widespread cancer and other serious disorders. Extensive tissue injury or damage to the vascular endothelial lining triggers off the clotting cascade. This results in the generation of large amounts of fibrin within the blood vessels. This pathological formation of fibrin in the intravascular compartment causes two basic problems. Firstly, it leads to the formation of widespread fibrin thrombi which occlude numerous small blood vessels. This leads to ischaemia of many organs including the brain, skin, kidneys, GI tract and lungs. Secondly, the formation of large amounts of fibrin uses up all of the clotting factors and platelets, leading to a deficiency. This in turn leads to haemorrhagic complications. Haemorrhage into the GI tract or brain may be fatal. Treatment consists of correction of the underlying pathology if possible with maintenance of blood volume and tissue perfusion. Transfusions of platelets and other plasma clotting factors will help to restore the ability of the blood to clot. Whole blood or red cell transfusions may be necessary if there has been a lot of haemorrhage.

Alterations in white cell numbers

Lymphocytes

An increase in the number of circulating lymphocytes is called a lymphocytosis and may be seen in viral infections and chronic bacterial infections such as tuberculosis. Lymphocytes produce antibodies which act against viral infections. They also synthesise and secrete chemical messengers called cytokines which stimulate the activity of other components of the immune system including neutrophils, monocytes and cytotoxic lymphocytes. Lymphoma and lymphocytic leukaemia are possible pathological causes of lymphocytosis.

Neutrophils

Neutrophils are the most abundant form of granulocytes and an increase in circulating neutrophils is termed a neutrophil leucocytosis or neutrophilia. This may occur in response to bacterial or fungal infections and tissue damage caused by trauma, surgery, burns or infarction. This is why there is an increase in circulating neutrophils after myocardial infarction. Other causes are inflammatory conditions, solid tumours and Hodgkin's lymphoma. Neutrophilia is also seen after giving corticosteroids, during exercise and in pregnancy.

Neutrophils are able to phagocytose bacteria and dead tissue cells. If dead tissue cells are not removed they may act as a habitat and food source for bacterial infection. A reduction in circulating neutrophils is called a neutropenia. When neutrophils are almost absent it is termed agranulocytosis. Reduction in neutrophils may be caused by viral infections and some severe bacterial infections. Chemotherapy and idiosyncratic drug reactions are other possible causes of neutropenia. As the numbers of neutrophils in the blood fall, there is a corresponding increased risk of infection. Life threatening infections such as pneumonia and complicated sepsis are possible with very low neutrophil counts. Antibiotics may be given as infection prophylaxis while the neutropenia persists.

Eosinophils

Eosinophilia means an increase in the number of eosinophils. As these granulocytic cells are involved in generating allergic responses and in combatting infection with parasites (e.g. worms and protozoa), their numbers are increased in these conditions.

Basophils

Normal blood contains very low numbers of basophils. A basophilia may be seen in allergies, some infections, malignant and inflammatory conditions.

Monocytes

Monocytes migrate into the tissues of the body where they are termed macrophages. An increase in circulating monocytes is termed a monocytosis and is seen in chronic bacterial infections, solid cancers and inflammatory conditions.

Leukaemia

Aetiology

Leukaemias are relatively uncommon malignancies in the UK with an incidence of about 10 per 100,000 per year. In some forms of leukaemia there is an inherited predisposition to the disease, which may explain why leukaemia has an increased incidence in people with Down's syndrome. Incidence is increased in the identical twin of a patient with leukaemia. There are also some racial differences with chronic lymphocytic leukaemia being rare in Chinese and related peoples.

Radiation exposure has increased the incidence of leukaemia in survivors of nuclear explosions and accidents. Other forms of radiation, such as X-rays, are a risk factor. Fetal exposure to X-rays carries a significant risk of subsequent leukaemia development, explaining why we should always ask about possible pregnancy before women are X-rayed. Chemical carcinogens including benzene may also cause the disease. Iatrogenic risk factors include long term immunosuppressive therapy or previous treatments with cytotoxic drugs. Immunodeficiency is a risk factor and one rare form of T-cell leukaemia is associated with a retroviral infection.

While leukaemia can present at any age, acute lymphoblastic leukaemia is the main form seen in children. Acute myeloid and the chronic forms are the more common presentations in older adults with the incidence increasing after the age of 50 years.

Background physiology

Blood cells differentiate from stem cells, which ultimately derive from pluripotent cells in the bone marrow. However, a lot of leucocytes (white cells) are also found in lymph nodes, liver, spleen and lymphoid tissue. Haemopoiesis is the name given to the process that forms the different blood cells. All adult blood cells ultimately derive from a pluripotent, blood forming stem cell, found in the bone marrow. These pluripotent stem cells are a form of 'master' cell which have the potential to differentiate into all of the different types of blood cells. As a result of mitosis and differentiation, pluripotent cells divide into myeloid or lymphoid stem cells. Lymphoid stem cells differentiate, via the blast cell stage, to form natural killer, B or T lymphocytes. B lymphocytes mature in the bone and T lymphocytes in the thymus gland. Myeloid stem cells have the potential to differentiate into all of the other types of blood components including granulocytes, monocytes, platelets and erythrocytes.

Pathophysiology

Leukaemia is a malignant neoplasm of the blood forming cells, i.e. there is a hyperplasia of haematopoietic cells. Normal bone marrow is replaced with many actively dividing immature neoplastic cells; these cells spill out and are seen in the blood. Leukaemia literally means 'white blood' this is because large numbers of malignant white cells are seen when the blood is examined. Malignant leukaemic cells may also infiltrate the liver, spleen, lymph nodes and the central nervous system.

Different forms of leukaemias occur depending on the cell types involved. In lymphocytic leukaemias, there is a proliferation of immature cells from the lymphoid stem cell lineage; these include lymphoblastic stem cells and immature lymphocytes. Myeloid leukaemias derive from the myeloid stem cell line so result in the production of numerous immature granulocytes, erythrocytes or thrombocytes.

Leukaemias may be acute or chronic, so there may be acute myeloid leukaemia (AML), acute lymphoblastic leukaemia (ALL), chronic myeloid leukaemia (CML) or chronic lymphocytic leukaemia (CLL). Myeloid is sometimes referred to as myelogenous. Diagnosis is made by examination of the blood and bone marrow.

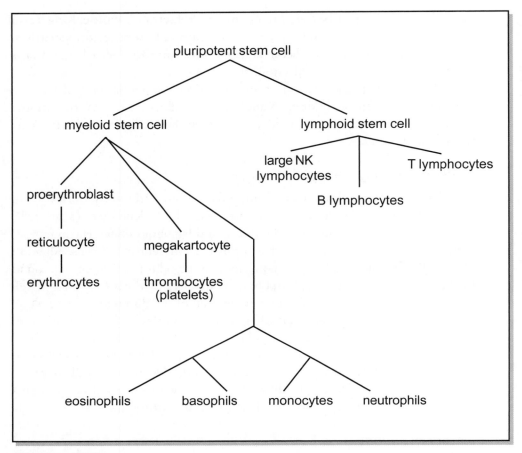

Diagram 17.6
Pluripotent stem cells from the bone marrow are capable of differentiating into all of the cellular components of the blood. These 'master' cells divide into lymphoid or myeloid stem cells which undergo further divisions and differentiations to form blast cells. Blast cells then go on to mature into the finished cellular components of the blood, (many intermediate cellular stages have been omitted).

Clinical features in acute leukaemias

Clinical features in acute leukaemias can be explained in terms of failure of the bone marrow to produce red and white blood cells. As leukaemic cells pack the bone marrow, the production of all blood cells will be adversely affected.

Acute leukaemia may present with symptoms of anaemia due to the disruption of normal red cell production. The individual will feel tired and weak with shortness of breath especially on exertion and there may be pallor.

Although the blood, bone marrow and other organs may be packed with a proliferation of white cells, these leucocytes are malignant and immature. This means they do not perform the normal immunological function of white cells.

In addition, there may be a reduced number of functional white cells as a result of generalised bone marrow failure; this will result in a neutropenia, again decreasing the efficiency of the immune system. As a consequence the patient may suffer from numerous infections, abscesses and fevers. There is a risk of overwhelming life threatening infections.

Failure to produce normal megakaryocytes will result in disruption to platelet (i.e. thrombocyte) production. This means the normal blood clotting mechanisms will be defective. As a result the individual may suffer from haemorrhagic features such as bleeding from the mouth or nose, excessive bruising and purpura. Blood clotting will be delayed if the patient cuts themselves or after venepuncture.

As the liver, spleen and lymph nodes will be infiltrated with large numbers of malignant leukaemic cells, clinical features may result from enlargement and swelling of these structures. If leukaemic cells cross the blood brain barrier they will also infiltrate the CNS giving rise to features such as headache, nausea, vomiting and papilloedema (swelling of the optic discs).

Weight loss may present as a result of the rapid proliferation and metabolism of leukaemic cells. Bone pain may occur as a result of bone marrow expansion caused by the medullary cavity being packed with leukaemic cells.

Chronic myeloid leukaemia (CML)

This usually starts with insidious onset of anaemia, fevers and weight loss with abdominal discomfort as a result of an enlarging spleen. During this initial chronic phase there is a proliferation of fairly well differentiated myeloid cells such as the granulocytes. This chronic phase usually lasts for 3 to 4 years. After this there is an accelerated phase where symptoms worsen with increased splenomegaly, worsening anaemia, thrombocytopenia, low grade fevers, night sweats, weight loss and bone pain. Thirdly, there is a terminal blast cell crisis phase. This represents the evolution of the condition into acute leukaemia. During this phase increasing numbers of immature and blast myeloid cells are found in the blood.

Chronic lymphocytic leukaemia (CLL)

In this disorder there is usually a proliferation of B lymphocytes although in a rarer form of the condition there is proliferation of T lymphocytes. Increase in the number of lymphocytes is termed a lymphocytosis. Anaemia, bleeding and infections occur as a result of bone marrow failure. Infection risk is further increased as the B cells no longer produce antibodies normally which results in a hypogammaglobulinaemia. Life threatening infections may develop which should be detected at an early stage and aggressive antibiotic therapy given. There will also be painless lymph node enlargement and an enlarged spleen. Overall the prognosis of CLL is much better than for CML.

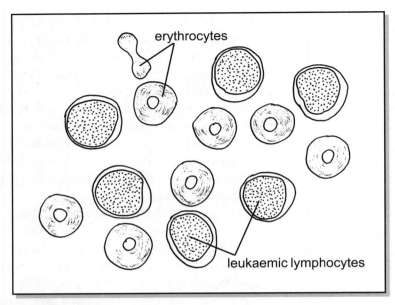

Diagram 17.7
Peripheral blood in chronic lymphocytic leukaemia. Numerous
small to medium sized malignant lymphocytes are seen.

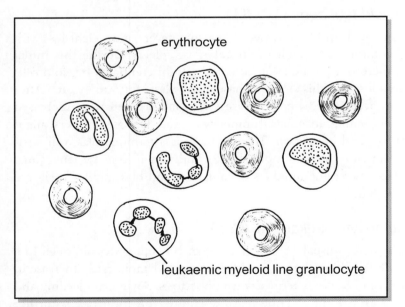

Diagram 17.8
Peripheral blood in chronic myeloid leukaemia. Numerous
malignant granulocytes are seen at various stages of
development. (Remember, in normal blood there are about 700
times more red cells than white cells, so in both of these
leukaemias the numbers of white cells are massively increased.)

Management principles

A range of supportive treatments can help. For example, blood transfusion will counter anaemia and infusions of platelets can treat haemorrhagic problems. Infections should be identified and aggressively treated at an early stage. A central venous catheter (Hickman line) may be inserted for the delivery of chemotherapy. A range of chemotherapeutic drugs are available to treat leukaemias, which are given in combinations over cycles. The aim of chemotherapy is to destroy the leukaemic clone of cells while preserving the normal blood forming stem cells. Chemotherapy causes some bone marrow suppression and a consequent pancytopenia (reduced production of all blood cells). This carries a significant risk of the patient acquiring a fatal infection so it is vital to provide adequate protection from this complication.

Some patients may be suitable for bone marrow transplantation. Firstly however, a compatible bone marrow donor needs to be found. The best chance of finding a donor is from the patient's first order relatives. There are also some databases of possible marrow donors which can be scanned for a possible tissue type match. If a suitable donor is found, the existing bone marrow must be killed using high doses of radiation or medication which will also kill all of the leukaemic cells. After this the donor bone marrow can be infused to seed the recipient's bone marrow with new haemopoietic stem cells. This is clearly a risky and technically difficult procedure but may be curative. Another biological approach is to harvest and store some of the patients own stem cells from peripheral blood. These can then be reintroduced after the patient has received conditioning therapy to prepare them for the procedure.

CHAPTER 18

Gastrointestinal Disorders

Useful terms and concepts

The abdomen

The surface of the abdomen is divided into areas to allow for precise description of particular regions.

Diagram 18.1
Regions of the abdomen.

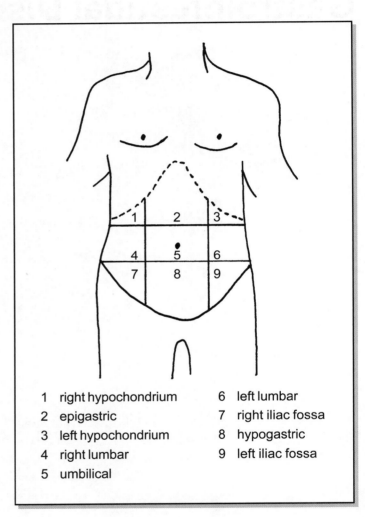

1	right hypochondrium	6	left lumbar
2	epigastric	7	right iliac fossa
3	left hypochondrium	8	hypogastric
4	right lumbar	9	left iliac fossa
5	umbilical		

Anorexia

This term describes a loss of appetite. Most conditions which cause nausea and vomiting first cause anorexia. In addition, a wide range of physical disorders can cause loss of appetite, as can emotions such as depression, fear and anxiety. This is a common experience; if we do not feel well we are often 'off our food'.

In common speech the term 'anorexia' is often used as an abbreviated version of the disorder called anorexia nervosa. This is a psychological eating disorder.

Aetiology of this condition is a complex interaction between a possible genetic susceptibility with psychological and familial factors. Sufferers lose weight and are in danger of starving themselves to death. 'Anorexia' is in fact a misnomer in this particular disorder as the sufferers often feel very hungry, yet do not eat.

Dysphagia

This means difficulty in swallowing. Normal swallowing requires the coordination of several muscle groups under precise nervous coordination. Therefore if the function of muscles or nerves is impaired, as in a stroke, swallowing becomes difficult. Dysphagia may also occur as a result of physical obstruction in the mouth, pharynx or oesophagus. For example, there may be an accumulation of fibrous tissue in the lower oesophagus as a result of peptic acid regurgitation. More ominously, dysphagia may be caused by carcinoma of the oesophagus, obstructing the lumen and preventing the normal passage of food into the stomach.

Nausea

This is a general feeling of 'sickness'. The unpleasant feeling is probably generated by neurones which are near, or part of, the vomiting centre in the medulla oblongata of the brain stem. Nausea usually precedes vomiting. Conditions affecting the upper GI tract commonly cause nausea. Numerous other disorders can also produce such 'sickly' feelings. Other features of nausea and pre-vomiting include effects generated by the autonomic nervous system such as increased salivation, pallor, sweating and tachycardia.

Vomiting

Vomiting can be seen as a useful defence mechanism. If food contains any toxins these can be ejected from the body before substantial doses have been absorbed. Prior to vomiting, excessive distension or irritation of the upper GI tract will cause antiperistalsis to occur. This is waves of peristalsis, propelling gut contents from the small intestine, back up into the stomach. These antiperistaltic waves are in the opposite direction to normal and may return GI contents from as far down as the ileum.

If there is sufficient upper GI irritation, there will be stimulation of the two vomiting centres in the medulla oblongata. These medullary areas in turn will activate the vomiting reflex. Vomiting may also be stimulated by another separate area of the medulla called the chemoreceptive trigger zone. This area responds to the presence of toxins in the blood to initiate vomiting. Many drugs, such as morphine and digoxin, may stimulate this area causing vomiting. Motion sickness may also cause vomiting. In this case, impulses from the inner ear are transmitted to the chemoreceptive zone, which again may stimulate vomiting.

Vomiting is largely an autonomic process. First the patient takes a deep breath. Next the upper oesophageal sphincter is opened and the epiglottis closes off the entrance to the airway. This is important to prevent aspiration of vomit into the trachea and bronchial passages. There is a strong downward contraction of the diaphragm and contraction of the abdominal wall muscles to compress gastric contents. Contraction of the stomach and relaxation of the lower oesophageal sphincter ejects material into the oesophagus. Gastric contents are then propelled up the oesophagus by waves of antiperistalsis.

Diarrhoea

In diarrhoea the faeces is soft or watery, ('rhoea' means to flow). Like vomiting, this is often part of a natural way of rapidly expelling unwanted contents from the body. Common causes of diarrhoea are bacterial and viral infections. If these are not flushed out then they will be able to multiply, making the infection worse. Patients with diarrhoea need to be given plenty of fluids and electrolytes to compensate for the losses incurred. If antiemetics and antidiarrhoeals are given in infectious gastroenteritis, this will prevent the normal clearance of the infectious agents.

Steatorrhoea

This term describes the presence of excessive fat in the stools ('stear' means fat). The condition arises from any disorder in which fat is not properly digested or absorbed from the GI tract. The faeces is foul smelling and as fat is lighter than water the stools will float.

Haematemesis and melaena

'Haem' means to do with blood and 'emesis' is vomiting, haematemesis therefore refers to the presence of blood in vomit. Melaena describes dark tarry stools caused by the presence of altered blood, usually from upper GI bleeds.

Dyspepsia

This term describes what most people call indigestion. Dyspepsia is a vague term used to describe any unpleasant sensation caused by eating. 'Heartburn' is a common presentation of dyspepsia which involves reflux of gastric contents into the oesophagus or mouth; in the mouth this generates a characteristic bitter taste. Reflux refers to movement in the opposite direction to the normal. Dyspepsia may be associated with so called 'alarm features', indicating the possible presence of serious pathology. These alarm features are dysphagia, palpable abdominal mass, haematemesis, melaena or anaemia (indicating bleeding), vomiting, or weight loss. Any of these features are indications for urgent further investigations.

Constipation

Constipation refers to incomplete, infrequent or difficult defecation. Defecation means passing of faeces out of the body. There is a wide spectrum of normal bowel activity. Opening of the bowels between three times per day to three times per week is considered to be normal. Individuals may be consistent in their bowel habits over many years.

Normal bowel function is aided by the presence of fibre in the diet. Fibre is material which passes through the bowel without being acted on by digestive processes, this means it goes out in the same form as it went in. There are basically two forms of fibre. Non-water soluble fibre is made of cellulose and found in cereals; water soluble fibre is found in fruit, vegetables and oats. Both forms of fibre aid normal bowel activity by adding bulk to faeces. This allows for efficient peristaltic movement of material along the lumen of the GI tract, especially through the colon.

Plenty of fluids also promote efficient bowel activity. Volumes of fluid required depend on activity levels and the weather. However, it is a good idea to drink enough water to produce 2 litres of urine per day. General mobility and exercise also aid normal bowel function.

Ascites

This is a collection of fluid in the peritoneal space. In other words, the potential space between the parietal and visceral peritoneal membranes becomes an actual fluid filled space. Ascites may develop as part of a generalised systemic cause of oedema, such as congestive cardiac failure or hypoproteinaemia. Alternatively there may be a localised cause within the abdominal cavity, for example inflammation or tumours of the peritoneum. Obstruction of the portal venous drainage system, secondary to liver cirrhosis, can cause profound ascites.

The mouth

Dental caries

Dental caries means decay of the teeth (caries is Latin for rotten). Caries will only occur in the presence of a type of bacteria called Streptococcus mutans and dietary sugar. If dietary sugar or S. mutans can be removed, dental caries should not develop.

Plaque refers to material which accumulates on the surface of teeth. S. mutans may colonise this plaque and therefore be in close proximity to the enamel surfaces. As these bacteria metabolise, they produce organic acids as waste products which are therefore also in close contact with enamel. Despite tooth enamel being the hardest substance in the body it can easily be dissolved by acid. Acids react with calcium in enamel leading to demineralisation and progressive destruction. Initially there will be pitting, followed by perforation of the enamel.

Streptococcus mutans probably colonise the mouth during early childhood. They may come from the mouths of parents or playmates. As saliva has a pH of 6-7 it is able to decrease the acidity of waste organic acids if it comes into contact with them. This will neutralise waste acids so they will no longer be capable of attacking enamel. The reason refined sugar increases the risk of caries is that sugar thickens the plaque and renders it impervious to saliva. This prevents saliva coming into contact with the tooth surfaces. This means that saliva is no longer able to buffer acids near the surface of the enamel. As a result of this, acids are not neutralised and are therefore free to cause caries.

Once enamel has been penetrated the underlying dentine is less resistant to acids resulting in cavity formation. If erosion continues, bacteria will reach the pulp and cause an inflammatory reaction with pain. Pain is explained by the exposure of sensory nerves present within dental pulp. If the process continues down the pulp, infection may reach under the tooth leading to very painful abscess formation.

Enamel is very much less prone to acid damage if it contains some fluorine. Therefore it would seem appropriate to ensure young children have adequate amounts of this trace element in their diet or drinking water. Keeping the teeth clean and eating less sugar will also help to prevent caries. Other preventative measures involve changing the profile of the oral bacterial flora.

Periodontitis

This is the most common cause of tooth loss in adults and describes inflammation of tissues surrounding the root of a tooth. Plaque can build up between the tooth and gum (gingiva) causing gingivitis (inflammation of the gums). This can cause bleeding of the gums and over time causes loss of gum tissue. Infection and inflammation can spread, causing a pocket to develop between the gums and teeth. Continued infection leads to progressive destruction of the ligaments which support the teeth. Eventually this may expose an unsupported root allowing the tooth to fall out. As gum tissue is lost the teeth appear to be longer than normal, giving rise to the expression 'long in the tooth'. Removal of plaque at an early stage can prevent progression of the condition.

Conditions affecting the oesophagus

Gastro-oesophageal reflux disease (GORD)

Everyone gets some degree of reflux of gastric contents into the oesophagus, most commonly after a large or fatty meal. However, in some people the cardiac sphincter, which regulates the passage of food from the oesophagus and prevents reflux, does not function normally allowing regurgitation. Acids and digestive enzymes from the stomach then cause inflammation in the lining of the oesophagus. Hiatus hernia is another possible contributing factor. In hiatus hernia part of the stomach herniates through the diaphragm into the

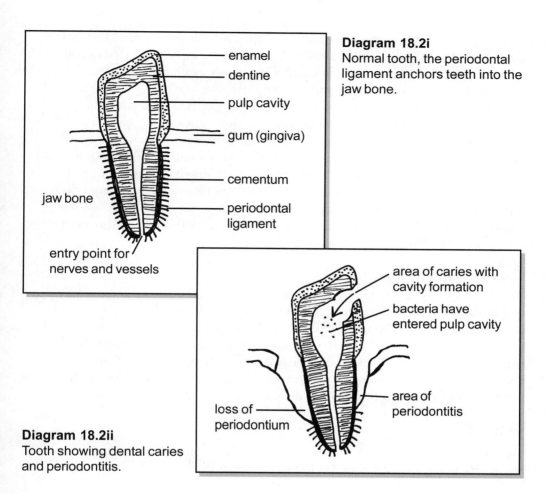

Diagram 18.2i
Normal tooth, the periodontal ligament anchors teeth into the jaw bone.

enamel
dentine
pulp cavity
gum (gingiva)
cementum
periodontal ligament
jaw bone
entry point for nerves and vessels

area of caries with cavity formation
bacteria have entered pulp cavity
area of periodontitis
loss of periodontium

Diagram 18.2ii
Tooth showing dental caries and periodontitis.

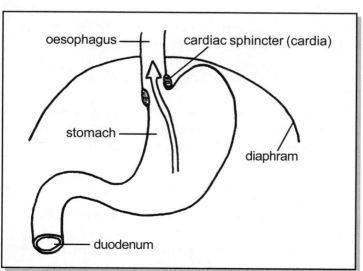

oesophagus
cardiac sphincter (cardia)
stomach
diaphram
duodenum

Diagram 18.3
Reflux of gastric contents through the cardia into the oesophagus. Normally the ring of muscle which forms the cardiac sphincter contracts to prevent reflux. If this does not happen efficiently acidic gastric contents reflux into the oesophagus.

thorax. Symptoms may include heartburn, epigastric or retrosternal (behind the sternum) pain and excessive burping. Symptoms are rapidly but temporarily relieved with antacids. Proton pump inhibitors such as omeprazole are often effective in healing oesophagitis and relieving symptoms.

Prolonged and repeated exposure of the oesophageal wall to gastric contents damages the epithelial lining. Such persistent reflux causes progressive damage to the lower oesophagus. This may lead to the formation of scar tissue and fibrous strictures. Prolonged reflux also produces a condition called Barrett's oesophagus. In Barrett's oesophagus the normal squamous epithelium is progressively replaced with columnar cells, similar to those which compose the lining of the stomach. Barrett's is an example of a metaplasia, 'meta' means change and 'plasia' relates to tissues. This is important as Barrett's is associated with a 30-40 fold increased risk of oesophageal cancer.

Cancer of the oesophagus

Basically there are two forms of cancer of the oesophagus, adenocarcinoma and squamous cell. Adenocarcinoma typically affects the lower, distal end of the oesophagus and usually arises from a Barrett's oesophagus. Squamous cell carcinoma usually affects the upper two thirds of the oesophagus and is associated with drinking very hot fluids, alcohol and tobacco consumption. Cancer of the oesophagus usually presents with dysphagia, first for bulky, then later for softer thinner foods, eventually even drinking becomes difficult.

Gastritis

Gastric means related to the stomach. Gastritis is caused by inflammation of the gastric mucosa which lines the lumen of the stomach.

Acute gastritis

This is a relatively common condition which usually resolves within a few days. The patient complains of stomach related pain and discomfort. In mild disease there may be moderate swelling and hyperaemia (increased volumes of blood present) of the gastric lining. More severe gastritis can cause acute ulceration and bleeding.

There are several possible causes of acute gastritis. Direct irritants such as alcohol, NSAIDs (non steroidal anti-inflammatory drugs, e.g. aspirin) and caffeine are common causes. Inflammation may also be caused by toxins released from the bacteria which cause food poisoning.

Chronic gastritis

Chronic gastritis may be caused by prolonged use of agents involved with acute inflammation. Cigarette smoking also contributes to the condition. However, 80% of cases of chronic gastritis are caused by infection with the bacteria Helicobacter pylori. Less common causes of chronic gastritis include autoimmunity, viral infection, reflux from the duodenum and Crohn's disease. Chronic gastritis leads to changes in the tissues lining the stomach. These may in turn lead to peptic ulcers and gastric carcinoma.

Peptic ulcer disease

This is a common disorder affecting more than 10% of individuals during their lifetime. The duodenum is the most common site for peptic ulceration, followed by the stomach and oesophagus. Peptic ulcer disease is a chronic condition with a natural pattern of relapses and remissions.

Aetiology

Peptic ulceration is caused by exposure of tissues to gastric acid and pepsin, the protein digesting enzyme produced by the stomach. Despite only infecting the stomach, Helicobacter pylori cause duodenal as well as gastric ulceration. About 90% of patients with duodenal ulcers (DU) are found to be infected with H. pylori. In gastric ulceration 70% of patients have the infection. It is believed that these bacteria cause the ulceration because eradication of the infection allows ulcers to heal without recurrence. However, only about 15% of people infected with H. pylori develop DU so other factors seem to be involved. These include, increased acid secretion, smoking and genetic predisposition, both duodenal and gastric ulceration are more common in men. NSAIDs are the second most common cause of gastric ulcers and also cause some DU. Interestingly, the risk of duodenal ulcers (but not gastric) is 30% higher in people with blood group O.

Clinical features

Epigastric pain is the common presenting feature. Pain is often well localised and the patient may point to the site of the pain. DU pain is often worse at

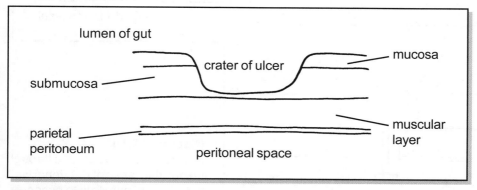

Diagram 18.4
Peptic ulcers are usually 2-3cm in diameter; a crater is formed as the acid and pepsin digest into the gut wall.

night and when the patient is hungry. Anorexia may lead to weight loss, especially in gastric ulcers. If peptic ulcers are not treated they tend to come and go with spontaneous relapses and remissions.

Complications

Bleeding may occur from granulation tissue causing chronic ongoing haemorrhage which may lead to progressive anaemia. Occult blood will be noted if the stools are tested, (occult means hidden, i.e. there is no obvious blood to see but it is present). Gastric acids and pepsin may digest the walls of an artery or vein in the gut wall. This may lead to large bleeds resulting in haematemesis and melaena. If a large blood vessel is involved significant volumes of blood may be lost into the lumen of the duodenum or stomach leading to vomiting of frank blood.

Ongoing injury and repair may lead to accumulation of fibrous scar tissue. Partial obstruction may be caused by swelling or the contraction of such scar tissue. This usually prevents the free movement of material through the pyloric sphincter between the stomach and duodenum. Such gastric outlet obstruction leads to nausea, vomiting and abdominal distension. If an ulcer eats into deeper tissues it may perforate all of the way through the wall of the gut allowing gastric or duodenal contents to enter the peritoneal cavity causing peritonitis. Peritonitis most often occurs from the duodenum, often without a history of epigastric pain and may present in acute or chronic ulceration.

Diagram 18.5i
Peptic ulceration has eroded the walls of a blood vessel in the gut wall leading to haemorrhage into the GI lumen.

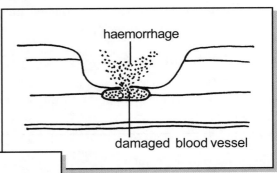

haemorrhage

damaged blood vessel

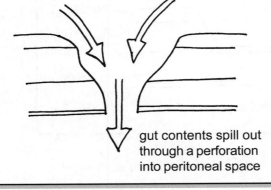

gut contents spill out through a perforation into peritoneal space

Diagram 18.5ii
Here the ulcer has eroded through the full thickness of duodenal wall allowing gut contents to escape into the peritoneum with serious consequences.

Treatment of peptic ulcers

Symptoms can usually be treated by reducing the levels of gastric acid. Traditionally this has been done by giving antacids. Today H2 blocking drugs (e.g. ranitidine) and proton pump inhibitors (e.g. omperazole) reduce the production of hydrochloric acid effectively. However, these treatments do not remove the cause of most cases of peptic ulceration which is gastric H. pylori. Curative treatment therefore involves eradication of the bacteria.

Stress ulcers

These are ulcers which develop in the GI tract as a result of major physiological stress. They occur in patients with burns, sepsis and trauma. They may also occur after major surgery or with various serious medical disorders. Stress ulcers probably result from ischaemia of the stomach and duodenum. This happens as part of the sympathetic response which reduces blood supply to the gut and redirects blood to the heart, lungs and essential organs. Traumatised patients are often given H2 blockers or proton pump inhibitors to prevent this complication.

Helicobacter pylori infection

H. pylori is a bacteria which may cause infection under the mucus layer in the stomach. The bacteria often enters the body as a result of person to person contact in childhood, however rates of overall infection increase with age, indicating ongoing cases of new infection. Initial infection leads to long term colonisation of the stomach. In western countries colonisation rates are usually more than 35% of the population. In many developing countries the rates may be as high as 90%. As discussed above H. pylori may lead to gastritis and duodenal ulceration and is a risk factor for gastric malignancy.

Eradication therapy

The good news is that H. pylori infection can be treated. There are various eradication therapy protocols available. These involve giving a triple therapy of drugs. A proton pump inhibitor or H2 blocker is given to reduce levels of gastric acid. The other two drugs are antibiotics to kill the bacteria. (Commonly used antibiotics include metronidazole, clarithromycin and amoxicillin; bismuth is also used in some eradication protocols.) Good compliance is essential for the therapy which is usually given for one week. Eradication therapy is successful in about 90% of cases on the first attempt.

Gastric cancer

This is the seventh most common form of cancer in the UK and is a common malignancy seen throughout the world. Adenocarcinoma is by far the most common pathology found arising from mucus secreting cells in the gastric crypts.

Aetiology

Helicobacter pylori is a major causative factor in cancer of the stomach. The infection leads to chronic gastritis and metaplasia, as in the oesophagus this metaplasia is a premalignant change. Diets high in salt, nitrates, smoked and pickled foods may contribute to malignant changes in the stomach, smoking and alcohol are also factors. Eating plenty of fruit and vegetables reduces the risk. As in many cancers there is also some genetic predisposition with some particular genes significantly increasing risk.

Clinical features

Early disease is asymptomatic but later patients often present with weight loss and epigastric pain. Pain from gastric carcinoma is similar to that caused by peptic ulceration; it is also relieved by reducing the levels of gastric acid and by food. A mass may sometimes be palpated in the epigastric area. Sometimes there may be a palpable lymph node just above the clavicle. This is called a Virchow's node and develops as lymphatic fluid carrying malignant cells drains via this lymphatic node before entering the venous circulation. Chronic bleeding may lead to anaemia and the stools are likely to be positive for occult blood. Common sites of metastases include the liver, peritoneum, lungs and bone marrow.

Treatments

Patients with ongoing, or new-onset dyspepsia should be considered for upper gastrointestinal endoscopy, especially if accompanied by vomiting, weight loss, anaemia, dysphagia, haematemesis, melaena or a palpable abdominal mass. If the condition is detected endoscopically, early surgical resection carries a good prognosis. Unfortunately gastric carcinoma usually presents at a relatively late stage. Gastric adenocarcinoma is an aggressive tumour and spreads by direct local invasion, via the lymphatics, and to the lymphatic site above the clavicle. Spread via blood to the liver is also likely. As a result patients who present with more advanced disease have a poor prognosis.

Inflammatory bowel disease (IBD)

There are two forms of inflammatory bowel disease not associated with infections; these are Crohn's disease and ulcerative colitis. The clinical features of both disorders result from inflammatory processes. Both diseases are also characterised by periods of remission and exacerbation.

Crohn's disease

Crohn's disease can affect any area of the GI tract however, most lesions are seen in the distal ileum and colon. Skip lesions may occur in any part of the GI tract, with sections of healthy tissue in between. Aetiology is unknown although the inflammation is produced by an environmental trigger acting on a genetic predisposition. The trigger is thought to be components of certain bacteria which are present in the gut. These factors cause activation of the bodies own immune cells such as macrophages, lymphocytes and neutrophils. As the immune system causes the inflammation it is reasonable to classify Crohn's as an autoimmune disease. The condition typically presents in young adult life with weight loss, colicky abdominal pain and diarrhoea.

Complications of Crohn's disease include perforation and obstruction. As inflammation may affect the whole thickness of the gut wall, the visceral peritoneum may be inflamed leading to adhesions. No specific curative treatment is available for Crohn's but symptoms are often treated using steroids to suppress inflammation. Surgery is indicated in cases of obstruction, perforation, abscess or fistula.

Ulcerative colitis

As the name implies, this condition only affects the rectum and colon. Aetiology of ulcerative colitis is not known but several factors have been identified. It has been suggested a transmissible agent is involved but none have been identified. A diet low in fibre and high in chemical food additives is another possible factor. As with many conditions there is an increased prevalence in families suggesting a genetic predisposition. The inflammatory changes seen in the colon probably have a similar autoimmune basis to those seen in Crohn's disease.

Inflammation of the inner lining of the colon leads to development of increased vascularity and haemorrhage. Ulcers and necrotic areas may also develop. Inflammation is often worst in the rectum (proctitis). In colitis the inflammation is limited to the inner mucosal layer, unlike Crohn's where the inflammation is transmural, i.e. it involves the deeper muscular layers of the gut wall.

Clinical features are similar to those caused by intestinal infections; there is diarrhoea, often with mucus, blood and pus. Sufferers typically pass very frequent diarrhoea stools, but some may pass pellety stools. Abdominal cramps may also present. Severity of the condition shows a wide spectrum from mild to possible acute fulminating disease. Clinical features are often made worse by psychological stress. Colitis is a recognised risk factor for adenocarcinoma of the rectum and colon. After 20 years of severe disease the risk of developing malignant change is almost 20%.

Some patients find that avoiding milk, very spicy foods, caffeine and gas forming foods relieves the symptoms. Eating plenty of fibre may help to reduce the amount of diarrhoea. Immunosuppressant drugs and corticosteroids help to reduce inflammation, but must be used carefully due to their side effects. Many drugs may be given via enema or suppositories; this gives high concentrations of drugs locally and reduces levels of systemic absorption. Surgical resection of part or the entire colon is the treatment of last resort. Clearly surgery becomes necessary if adenocarcinoma develops.

Diverticular disease

This disorder may affect any part of the colon but is most common in the sigmoid and descending colon regions.

Aetiology

Very occasionally congenital diverticular disease presents but most commonly the condition is acquired. Diverticular disease is common in developed western countries but rare in traditional African communities. In the UK it becomes more common with increasing age and the prevalence in the elderly may be as high as 50%. Association with developed countries has given rise to the idea that low fibre diets are a cause. Low faecal residue obliges the colon to generate high pressures within the lumen in order to propel small volumes of faeces along to the rectum. This idea is supported by the observation that symptoms usually improve with a high fibre diet which all patients should be given.

Pathophysiology

Reduced dietary fibre reduces the volume of residual material in the colon. This increases the workload of the muscular wall of the colon leading to muscular hypertrophy. However there are gaps in between the smooth muscle fibres in the wall of the colon to allow the entry of blood vessels. As the pressure in the lumen is high, mucosa is pushed out through these gaps, forming small blind-ended pouches. (A diverticulum is a blind-ended pouch which herniates through the wall of a hollow or tubular organ.) Faeces may collect in the pouches, resulting in accumulation of bacteria and subsequent inflammation. If diverticula are present but not causing any problems the condition is often referred to as diverticulosis. When the diverticula become inflamed the condition is referred to as diverticulitis.

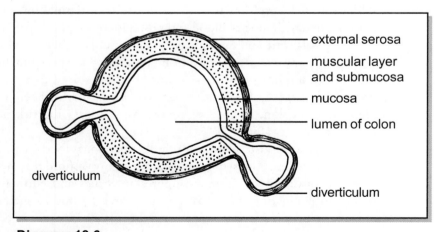

Diagram 18.6
Diverticula are blind ended pouches pushed out between muscle fibres.
The pouch wall consists of mucosa with surrounding serosa.

Clinical features

Commonly there are irregular bowel habits with episodes of diarrhoea and constipation. Stools often consist of hard pellets of faeces. Patients may complain of lower left or lower central abdominal pain. In acute inflammatory episodes there is local tenderness with guarding and rigidity (these symptoms have been referred to as a 'left sided appendicitis'). Diagnosis is usually confirmed with a barium enema and colonoscopy used to eliminate other possible pathologies.

Complications

Inflammation, caused by bacterial infection, may occur which spreads to a segment of bowel. This will produce severe abdominal pain and tenderness with possible pyrexia and rectal bleeding. Occasionally, there may be massive haemorrhage resulting in shock. A fistula may sometimes form with the bladder causing urinary infections, as bacteria from the gut migrate into the urinary system. Fistula formation may also occur into the vagina leading to passage of flatus and faeces PV (per vagina). (A fistula is a tube-like pathological communication which develops between two organs or an organ and the surface of the body.) If there is perforation of a diverticula this will allow colon contents into the peritoneal cavity causing abscess formation or peritonitis. Infective inflammatory episodes should be treated with antibacterial agents such as metronidazole and a cephalosporin. Supportive therapies may include intravenous fluids, nasogastric aspiration and analgesia. Surgery should be reserved for perforation or significant haemorrhage.

Cancer of the colon and rectum

This is the third most common site of malignant primary lesions in the UK, following after breast and bronchogenic carcinoma in incidence. The condition becomes more common with increasing age.

Aetiology

About 80% of cases of colorectal carcinoma are described as 'sporadic'. These cases are primarily caused by environmental (largely dietary) factors. Colorectal cancers are more common in countries with high levels of saturated animal fat and red meat in the diet. Processed red meat carries additional risk, probably because of carcinogenic amines formed during cooking. It is also believed that these foods promote the development of particular species of bacteria in the colonic flora. These bacteria then convert bile salts into chemicals which are carcinogenic. These carcinogens lie in contact with the mucosa leading to the development of malignant change. Long standing ulcerative colitis and Crohn's disease also increase the risk of developing colorectal malignancy.

Eating a high red meat and fat diet, in combination with inadequate fibre is particularly risky. If there is plenty of fibre and fluids in the diet the GI transit time will be reduced. This means that even if some carcinogens are produced they will not be in contact with the mucosa for prolonged periods; this will reduce their opportunity to induce malignancy. From this it can be seen that the best advice is to take plenty of fibre and fluids and restrict animal products. Eating plenty of green vegetables seems to be particularly protective as these foods contain flavonoids and other protective anticarcinogens. Again the importance of eating plenty of fruit and vegetables in the diet will provide fibre as well as these protective micronutrients.

Cancer Research UK have recently announced that regular physical exercise reduces the risk of colon cancer by an impressive 50%. It is currently unclear physiologically why exercise is so protective, but the finding is based on large scale epidemiological studies. Vitamin D, aspirin and HRT (female hormone replacement therapy) are also protective.

The remaining 20% of colorectal carcinomas have a strong genetic factor in the aetiology. Familial adenomatous polyposis (FAP) is a thankfully rare autosomal dominant condition but carries a 90% risk of the development of colorectal cancer by the age of 50. Up to 10% of cases are caused by another autosomal dominant condition called hereditary nonpolyposis colon cancer (HNPCC). A further 10% of cases will also have a well defined family history of the disease.

Pathophysiology

Most malignancies (about 98%) of the colon arise from glandular tissue located in the mucosa which lines the lumen; they are therefore classified as adenocarcinomas. Most of these cases arise from collections of neoplastic cells called adenomatous polyps. An adenoma is a benign (non-malignant) tumour which arises from a lining epithelium which contains glands. A polyp is any mass which protrudes into the lumen of the gut. Although adenomatous polyps are benign in themselves they have the potential to develop from adenomas into adenocarcinomas. This is described as the polyp adenoma-carcinoma sequence. Often the only clinical feature at the adenoma stage is blood or occult blood in the faeces. If polyps are removed during colonoscopy, before they turn malignant, the development of cancer can be prevented.

Colorectal cancer is staged using the Dukes' classification. In Duke's stage A, the tumour is limited to the mucosa and submucosa. When the tumour has penetrated through the muscle layers this is described as stage B. Stage C classification represents more advanced disease with malignant spread through the wall of the colon and lymphatic involvement. In stage D the condition is complicated by distant metastases to sites such as the liver. Clearly the prognosis worsens with each increasing stage. The rectum and sigmoid areas are the most common sites of colon cancer, but any area of the colon can be involved.

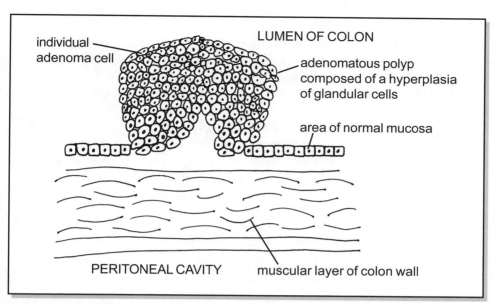

individual adenoma cell

LUMEN OF COLON

adenomatous polyp composed of a hyperplasia of glandular cells

area of normal mucosa

PERITONEAL CAVITY

muscular layer of colon wall

Diagram 18.7i
Neoplastic (new cells) have arisen from the glandular tissue of the epithelial lining of the colon and formed an adenomatous polyp. Adenoma is an example of a hyperplasia, as there is an abnormal increase in the numbers of cells present.

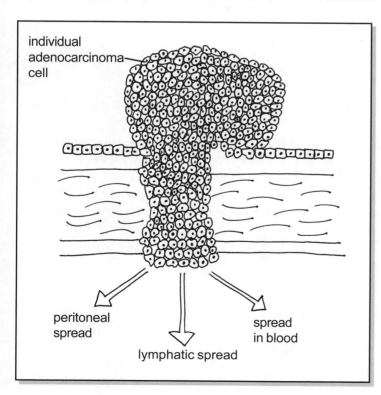

individual adenocarcinoma cell

peritoneal spread

lymphatic spread

spread in blood

Diagram 18.7ii
The adenoma has undergone malignant transformation and so has developed into an adenocarcinoma. The malignant cells start to invade down into the wall of the colon. This diagram illustrates at least Dukes' stage B as the full thickness of the colon wall has been penetrated. Once the wall has been fully penetrated malignant cells will go on to invade other sites.

Spread

Tumour cells which arise in the mucosa penetrate downwards through the submucosa and muscular layers of the colon wall. Once they penetrate through the wall they may spread into structures such as the uterus, bladder or other parts of the abdomen via the peritoneal space. Tumours in the peritoneal membranes cause ascites.

Tumour cells may also be carried to local lymph nodes in the lymphatic drainage; from here they can spread through other lymphatic vessels. Malignant cells may enter the blood capillaries of the colon and from here they are carried in the venous blood flow into the hepatic portal vein and on to the liver. This explains why secondary tumours of the liver frequently complicate primary bowel malignancies.

Clinical features

Clinical features depend on the area of colon involved but include alterations in bowel habit, rectal bleeding, passing mucus, a feeling of fullness in the rectum, unexplained weight loss and anaemia. Colicky lower abdominal pain is another possible presentation. Some cases present with intestinal obstruction or perforation. Early disease may be screened for by carrying out occult blood tests over the age of 50 years. If this is positive it may be followed up by colonoscopy, which is the investigation of choice in all suspicious presentations.

Treatment

Surgical resection is the usual treatment. This may be accompanied by adjunctive therapies such as radiotherapy and chemotherapy.

Acute peritonitis

Peritoneum

The peritoneum is a thin membrane which has many folds and covers the outer surface of the intestines and lines the abdominal cavity. The inner wall of the abdominal cavity is lined with the parietal peritoneal membrane while the visceral membrane covers the organs of the GI tract. Peritoneum is glistening and smooth and secretes serous fluid to act as a lubricant. Parietal peritoneum is very sensitive to mechanical causes of pain such as trauma, cutting or burning. Conversely the visceral peritoneum is not sensitive to mechanical injury but does generate pain when under tension, e.g. if the bowel is over distended.

Causes

Most commonly peritonitis is caused by a perforation of the GI tract, allowing gut contents to escape into the peritoneal cavity. For example, perforation may complicate an acute inflammatory appendicitis. Other possible causes of perforation include perforating peptic ulceration, Crohn's disease, ulcerative colitis, diverticulitis, ulcerating carcinomas and acute intestinal obstruction.

There can also be disruption of the intestinal wall, leading to perforation and leaking, as a result of abdominal trauma, penetrating injuries or as a post-operative complication. Gangrene of the gall bladder allows bile to leak into the peritoneal cavity. Bile causes significant inflammation and secondary bacterial infection.

Infarction or severe ischaemia of a segment of bowel can lead to gangrenous necrosis and perforation. Bacterial infection causing salpingitis may spread from the uterine tubes into the peritoneal cavity. Peritonitis may also complicate peritoneal dialysis and ascites where there is free stagnant fluid in the peritoneal space. Infection may also spread to the peritoneum via the blood as a complication of septicaemia or tuberculosis.

Pathophysiology

Peritonitis describes inflammation of the peritoneal membranes, usually caused by bacterial infection. If any part of the intestine is perforated enteric, aerobic and anaerobic bacteria, may enter the peritoneal cavity causing widespread inflammation. A large perforation can result in a generalised peritonitis as material may spread throughout the cavity.

A purulent inflammatory exudate will accumulate in the peritoneal cavity leading to a loss of fluid, electrolytes and protein from the blood. These losses will lead to developing dehydration and hypovolaemia, electrolyte imbalance and hypoproteinaemia. Free gases may also accumulate within the peritoneal cavity as a result of bacterial activity. Accumulation of fluid and gases in the peritoneal space leads to gross distension of the abdomen which will cause pressure on the diaphragm. There is therefore a risk that peritonitis may affect the lungs leading to lung collapse or pneumonia.

Bacterial toxins in the inflammatory exudate are toxic to the intrinsic nerves in the wall of the GI tract. This leads to paralysis of the muscular gut wall causing the bowel to become flaccid and dilated. When the bowel is paralysed the condition is termed paralytic ileus. Peritonitis causes inflammation over large internal surfaces allowing the absorption of toxins into the blood. If untreated systemic septicaemia is likely to rapidly develop. From these complications it is clear that acute peritonitis is an immediate life threatening condition.

A similar clinical picture may be produced by the presence of blood, bile, or pancreatic enzymes in the peritoneum. These will initially cause inflammation as a result of chemical irritation with bacterial infection as a common complication.

Clinical features of peritonitis

Often the onset is sudden, presenting with severe burning and continuous pain. The pain begins at the site of the underlying pathology but may rapidly spread over the whole abdomen. Patients lie still as movement makes the agonising pain worse. Breathing is shallow as large movements of the diaphragm move the inflamed peritoneum causing increased pain. Irritation of the diaphragm may also lead to referred pain in the shoulder tip. Abdominal muscles contract to guard the painful area giving rise to a tender, rigid abdomen with rebound tenderness. Patients experience nausea and usually vomit. Inflammation and infection will lead to pyrexia and the pulse rate will rise. A marked leucocytosis will rapidly develop.

After a time the bowel sounds will cease as paralytic ileus (paralysis of the gut resulting in loss of peristaltic movements) develops. Abdominal distension will develop over time as a result of the accumulation of inflammatory fluid and free gas in the peritoneal cavity. Untreated the patient will become shocked due to sepsis and hypovolaemia with a fast and feeble pulse, cold peripheries, moist, cold and cyanosed skin.

Principles of treatment

As soon as a diagnosis is made pain relief should be given, usually intravenous morphine. Intravenous fluids and electrolyte replacement, where possible based on blood biochemistry results, will help to stabilise the haemodynamic status. Nasogastric drainage should be used to decompress the bowel as far as possible; this will also reduce the risk of aspiration during anaesthesia. Intravenous antibiotics are needed to combat infection. Surgical correction of the underlying cause is life saving e.g. repair of perforation, resection of infarcted bowel or drainage and removal of an infective focus.

Acute appendicitis

This is the most common surgical emergency in the UK. It may occur at any age but is most common between the ages of 5 to 30 years.

Aetiology

Usually acute appendicitis is caused by a faecolith obstructing the lumen of the appendix. 'Faeco' relates to faeces and 'lith' means stone. A faecolith is therefore a hardened, 'stone' like concretion of faeces. Swelling around the neck of the appendix is another possible cause. Such swelling may be due to infection as the wall of the appendix contains lymphoid tissue. Viral infection may cause swelling of this immunological tissue leading to obstruction of the lumen. Intestinal worms or twisting of the appendix are other possible causes of obstruction.

Pathophysiology

The vermiform appendix is a blind ended tube, branching from the caecum in the first part of the large intestine. As it is blind ended, obstruction of the lumen means that the contents become trapped, isolated and static. As is usually the case, stasis leads to infection. Static bacteria, already present in the lumen, multiply leading to an inflammatory response and ulceration of the mucosal lining. Inflammation leads to swelling which interrupts the normal blood supply which can lead on to gangrene. Once an area of the appendix wall has necrosed, the integrity of the tissues will be lost allowing perforation. While an acute episode of appendicitis may spontaneously resolve, another attack is likely to develop. This ongoing problem is often describes as a 'grumbling appendix'.

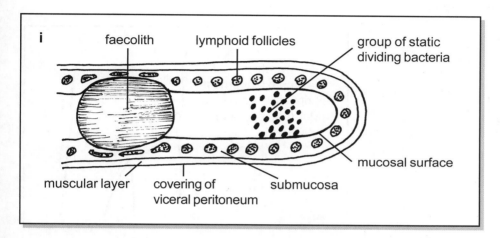

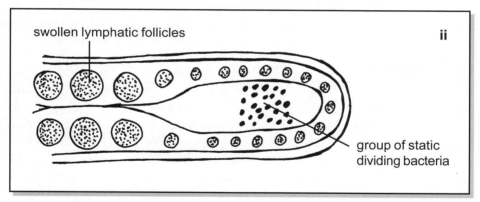

Diagram 18.8
Causes of appendicitis.
i. Impaction with a hardened faecal mass called a faecolith.
ii. Swollen lymphoid tissue secondary to infection.

Clinical features

Typically colicky pain starts abruptly in the centre of the abdomen around the umbilicus. After a few hours the pain usually becomes localised in the right iliac fossa (RIF). This area will be tender and there will be guarding due to localised peritonitis. Rebound tenderness is also present. Early pain comes from the stretching of the visceral peritoneum and later pain from inflammation of the parietal peritoneum. If the appendix is lying in an atypical position the area of pain will vary accordingly. Movement will usually aggravate the pain as it will cause movement of the inflamed peritoneal membranes. Patients prefer to lie still, often with the hips and knees flexed. Vomiting and anorexia are usually present and constipation is common. Pyrexia is usually low grade with a temperature around 37.8°C. White cell count will be raised as part of a systemic immune response.

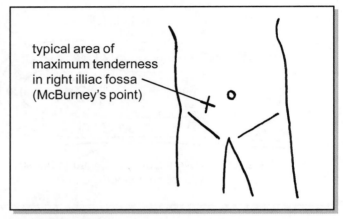

typical area of
maximum tenderness
in right illiac fossa
(McBurney's point)

Diagram 18.9
Pain begins around the area of the umbilicus and over a few hours localises in the right iliac fossa.

Complications

If the appendix is not surgically removed, there is a risk it will necrose and perforate. Perforation may lead to generalised peritonitis and toxaemia which are clearly life threatening. Spread of infection within the peritoneal cavity may lead to an abscess developing under the diaphragm (subphrenic) or in the pelvis. Alternatively, after perforation, the omentum may be able to contain the escaped gut contents leading to abscess formation in the RIF. Treatment is appendicectomy, which may be performed by laparoscopy.

Acute intestinal obstruction

In this condition material is no longer able to pass through the GI tract resulting in an obstruction to the normal flow.

Aetiology

Intestinal obstruction may have a mechanical or paralytic cause. Mechanical obstructions are subdivided into intraluminal, mural and extramural. Intraluminal obstruction arises from a physical obstruction within the gut lumen. Mural causes arise from the wall and extramural causes arise externally to the bowel.

Ileus is a state of gut paralysis. This means that obstruction occurs secondary to loss of normal forward propulsion of material along the GI tract. This means the cause is loss of motility rather than mechanical.

Causes of intraluminal obstruction

This is obstruction which occurs as a result of a direct blockage within the lumen of the gut. Such obstruction may be caused by a tumour or even intestinal worms. Some poorly chewed foods may also cause obstruction, e.g. segments of fibrous food such as oranges. Severe faecal impaction may progress on to a complete obstruction. Another classical cause of obstruction is a large gallstone which has passed into the lumen of the gut. These typically cause obstruction in the relatively narrow ileum.

Causes of mural obstruction

Intussusception occurs in young children, usually at the ileocaecal junction between the large and small intestine. Most commonly the cause is swelling of lymphoid tissue in response to a viral infection. A segment of small bowel is dragged, by peristaltic contraction, into the large bowel. This is analogous to closing up a telescope; there is a 'telescoping' of the bowel. The blood supply to the area of bowel which has been drawn in is interrupted leading to congestion, oedema and eventual necrosis. There may also be haemorrhage into the bowel lumen resulting in bleeding per rectum.

Inflammatory conditions such as tuberculosis, Crohn's disease and diverticulitis may lead to the development of fibrous tissue strictures which may also lead to mural obstructions.

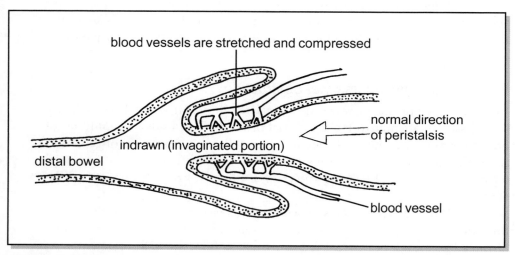

Diagram 18.10
Intussusception disrupts the normal blood supply to a length of bowel.

Causes of extramural obstruction

Peritoneal adhesions are bands of fibrous tissue which develop after inflammation or surgery. Inflammation leads to the release of fibrinogen leading to fibrin accumulation. Over time fibrous tissue replaces the fibrin resulting in portions of peritoneal membrane adhering to each other. This essentially adheres sections of bowel together interrupting the continuity of the lumen. Fibrous tissue accumulation around the outside of a section of bowel may contract and so directly constrict the bowel.

A hernia occurs when a loop of bowel protrudes through a weak point in the wall of the abdominal cavity. Small hernias may manually be pushed back into the abdominal cavity, if this is possible it is called a reducible hernia. Bowel protrusion is uncomfortable or painful and there is a risk that the loop of protruding bowel is squeezed by the abdominal wall which forms the edges of the hernia. This can 'nip off' a section of bowel, closing off the lumen, leading to obstruction. The pressure from the edges of the hernia will also cut off the blood supply to the herniated bowel. This is referred to as a strangulated hernia and will cause pain and eventual necrosis.

Sometimes a length of bowel may twist around on itself. This cause of obstruction is called a volvulus. The common site for this pathology to occur is the area of the sigmoid colon. A length of sigmoid colon may twist around on its own axis. This will cause complete obstruction. As was the case in intussusception, there is disruption of the normal blood supply and infarction, necrosis and peritonitis will ensue.

Paralytic ileus

This describes paralysis of the gastrointestinal tract as a result of neurogenic or muscular impairment. Transient paralytic ileus is seen most commonly after abdominal surgery but may also be caused by peritonitis. Thrombosis in the mesenteric artery supplying blood to the bowel can also lead to a paralysed segment.

Pathophysiology in intestinal obstruction

Normal peristaltic waves above (proximal to) the obstruction become more vigorous in an attempt to move material onwards. This leads to a build up of pressure within the lumen of the gut as a result of accumulation of gases and fluids. Intraluminal pressure leads to distension of the bowel before (proximal to) the obstruction. The area of bowel past (distal to) the obstruction will be empty.

As a result of increased pressure within the bowel lumen, veins in the wall of the intestine will be compressed and closed off. Blood supply may also be disrupted as a result of external pressure, such as from the walls of a hernia. As a result of venous compression, blood will not be able to leave an affected area of bowel leading to congestion and oedema. Venous obstruction will prevent

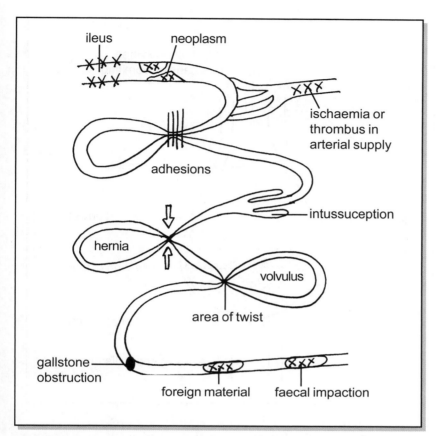

Diagram 18.11
Review of possible causes of intestinal obstruction.

blood flowing normally through the tissue resulting in arterial blood no longer being able to enter the area. This vascular interruption will lead to cell death and tissue necrosis.

Bacteria present in the gut are able to reproduce as they are not washed along in the normal flow of fluid and material from mouth to anus. Bacteria produce gases as a waste product, leading to further distension of the bowel. The combination of fluid and gas accumulation causes abdominal distension.

Eventually bacteria will leak through the necrotic segments of bowel causing peritonitis. Untreated, peritonitis will lead to overwhelming systemic infection and death. Even without perforation there may be significant systemic absorption of endotoxins from strangulated bowel segments leading to sepsis.

Clinical features

Vigorous peristalsis above the obstruction initially leads to increased bowel sounds and colicky pain. Colic refers to pain from a hollow structure such as the bowel. Increased peristalsis and reduced blood supply cause metabolism to

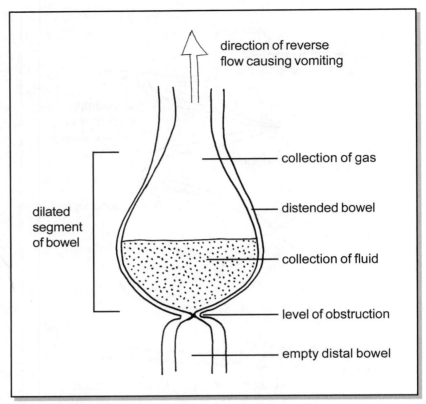

direction of reverse
flow causing vomiting

collection of gas

dilated
segment
of bowel

distended bowel

collection of fluid

level of obstruction

empty distal bowel

Diagram 18.12
The bowel above and below an intestinal obstruction.

change from aerobic to anaerobic. Anaerobic metabolism (in the absence of oxygen) causes the formation of lactic acid which accumulates in the tissues of the gut wall causing pain. Pain is also generated as a result of bowel distension stretching the covering visceral peritoneal membrane.

Vomiting is common as an early feature in high bowel obstruction but will occur later if the blockage is lower down in the GI tract. Retroperistalsis will propel material in the reverse direction, resulting in the accumulation of small bowel contents in the stomach. The vomit reflex will then cause this to be ejected.

Absolute constipation means a failure to pass either faeces or flatus. This is an early feature in large bowel obstruction as material cannot pass the obstructed area of colon. In small bowel obstruction the patient may pass some normal stools as the lower bowel empties after the onset of an obstruction.

Up to 8-10 litres of fluid are secreted into the bowel every day. In health all but 100 mls of this is reabsorbed. However, in obstruction stagnant fluid collects in bowel loops leading to distension. This stagnant fluid is lost to the circulatory system and so is an example of third spacing of body fluids. As a result dehydration and hypovolaemia will develop. This may be exacerbated by fluid loss from vomiting. Hypovolaemia can cause the patient to become shocked, resulting in oliguria or even anuria. (Oliguria means reduced volumes of urine are produced and anuria means none is produced.) Stagnation within the bowel and vomiting also lead to electrolyte disturbance.

Principles of treatment in obstruction

Acute intestinal obstruction is a surgical emergency. Intravenous fluid replacement can delay the onset of shock and help to stabilise the patient prior to surgery. Partial decompression of the bowel can be achieved using a nasogastric tube to aspirate stagnant fluids from the stomach. Surgically the obstruction can be relieved. If there has been delay in treatment, areas of bowel may have already necrosed and require resection, anastamosis or colostomy formation. Intravenous antibiotics are given to treat infection.

CHAPTER 19

Disorders of the Liver

Jaundice

Perhaps the best known expression of liver disease is jaundice, a clinical feature generated by raised bilirubin levels in the blood. The old name for jaundice is icterus.

Physiology

Red cells are naturally broken down (haemolysed) at the end of their life spans, mostly by macrophages located in the spleen. Haemoglobin from haemolysed red cells is converted into the yellow pigment bilirubin which is transferred to the liver in blood plasma. Hepatocytes (i.e. individual liver cells) take up bilirubin and join it to a chemical called glucuronic acid. This joining process is called conjugation and it increases the solubility of bilirubin to allow excretion in the bile. After bilirubin has been conjugated it enters the bile ducts and passes into the gall bladder to be stored and concentrated. Once in the bile ducts the bilirubin is oxidised and as a result turns green. This green bile pigment is called biliverdin. When it is needed, bile passes from the gall bladder down the common bile duct into the duodenum. In the lumen of the small bowel bile emulsifies fat and colours and partially deodorises faeces.

The yellow colour of bilirubin also explains why bruises (contusions) turn yellow as they fade. The dark coloured red cells, trapped in the tissue spaces as a result of the haemorrhage, are gradually phagocytosed by macrophages. First, the haemoglobin from the red cells is degraded into haem pigment and globin components. Then the haem molecules are destroyed by macrophages leaving the yellow pigment bilirubin.

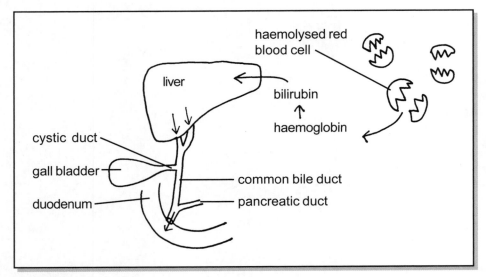

Diagram 19.1
Bilirubin derived from haemolysed red cells is conjugated in the liver and is incorporated into bile; from here it enters the duodenum.

Classification of jaundice

Prehepatic jaundice

Hepatic means to do with the liver. In prehepatic jaundice the abnormality occurs before bilirubin reaches the liver. If there is increased breakdown (that is haemolysis) of red blood cells, bilirubin may enter the blood more rapidly than the liver is able to incorporate it into bile. The result of this is an accumulation of bilirubin in blood and tissue fluids. In this disorder, the excess bilirubin found in the blood is unconjugated, as it has not yet passed through the liver cells. This form of jaundice is usually mild as a healthy liver can excrete up to six times the normal load of bilirubin before the pigment starts to accumulate in the blood.

Hepatic (or hepatocellular) jaundice

This describes jaundice which occurs as a result of disorders affecting the liver cells (i.e. the hepatocytes). Hepatocyte function can be reduced in viral hepatitis (A,B,C,D or E), primary liver cancer or as a result of poisons or drugs. Damaged liver cells are less able to conjugate and transfer bilirubin from the blood into bile. Due to reduced liver cell function conjugated and unconjugated bilirubin therefore accumulates in the blood. In addition to reduced uptake of bilirubin, swelling of the hepatocytes may partly occlude some of the small bile channels, leading to an obstructive component of the jaundice.

Post hepatic (cholestatic) jaundice

This form of jaundice occurs as a result of pathology affecting the bile ducts, i.e. after the bilirubin has passed through the hepatocytes. This has the effect of obstructing the normal flow of bile through the bile ducts into the duodenum. As the normal drainage of bile is obstructed, conjugated bile dams back into the liver. Damming back of bile allows this conjugated bilirubin to enter the blood. As conjugated bilirubin is highly soluble, some of it is excreted by the kidneys in urine. This gives the urine a dark colouration and the bilirubin is easily detected using ward-based dipsticks. As the obstruction of the ducts prevents bile entering the duodenum, bile is no longer able to colour faeces as normal, which results in pale coloured stools.

Obstruction may occur as a result of bile duct lumens being blocked at any level of the biliary tree. For example, any condition leading to swelling within the liver will compress the small bile ducts. Obstruction may occur because of blockage within the lumen of the bile ducts as a result of gallstones. Blockage may originate in the walls of bile ducts as a result of bile duct carcinoma or postoperative strictures. External compression of the larger bile ducts may also lead to obstruction of the normal flow of bile. This may occur as a result of swelling of the pancreas caused by pancreatitis or carcinoma of the head of the pancreas. Over time, the presence of dammed back bile in the liver can lead to progressive hepatic failure.

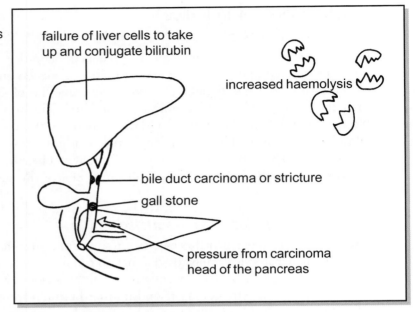

Diagram 19.2
Possible causes of jaundice; increased haemolysis, hepatocellular failure, post hepatic obstruction.

failure of liver cells to take up and conjugate bilirubin

increased haemolysis

bile duct carcinoma or stricture

gall stone

pressure from carcinoma head of the pancreas

Clinical features of jaundice

A patient is described as being jaundiced when raised levels of bilirubin lead to a yellowish discolouration of the conjunctiva and skin. This occurs because raised levels of bilirubin in the blood lead to raised levels in the tissue fluid, which gives tissues a characteristic yellow appearance. Itching (pruritus) is a common feature in jaundiced patients, probably caused by accumulation of bile salts which irritate sensory receptors in the dermis.

Treatment principles in jaundice

Treatments for prehepatic jaundice are the same as those for haemolytic anaemia as discussed in the chapter on blood disorders. Hepatic jaundice should be treated by addressing the underlying cause. Post hepatic jaundice can often be treated by surgical interventions such as removal of gallstones, relieving strictures or putting in a stent.

Liver tumours

These may be primary or metastatic (secondary) tumours.

Primary liver tumours

Primary liver tumours arise within the liver, the most common of which is hepatocellular carcinoma. This is relatively rare in developed countries but common in Africa and the Far East. Clinical features often include malaise, weight loss, anorexia, jaundice and abdominal discomfort.

People who have liver cirrhosis or hepatitis B or C infection are much more likely to develop hepatocellular carcinoma than people with previously healthy livers. There has been an increase in the incidence of hepatocellular carcinoma in recent years in Western countries which has been attributed to the increased prevalence of hepatitis C infection. This means that many cases could be prevented by controlling the transmission of hepatitis B and C. Clearly hepatitis B vaccination is a useful tool in prevention. Preventing alcoholic cirrhosis will also help to prevent tumour development.

Early surgical removal of a hepatocellular carcinoma provides the best prognosis. However, tumours may arise at several sites within the liver making this option difficult. Percutaneous ablation with ethanol is helpful for small tumours. Liver transplantation also carries a reasonable prognosis if available. If a tumour is suspected it can be identified using CT, MRI or ultrasound scanning. Clinically the disorder typically presents at a later stage when unfortunately surgery is no longer an option. This is why ultrasound screening every 3 to 6 months is ideal in high risk individuals. Primary liver cancer is likely to spread to the lymph nodes, but spread to the lungs or bones is less common.

Benign liver tumours such as haemangiomas are relatively common. These are usually asymptomatic and are often picked up as an incidental finding during ultrasound examinations. Less common benign liver masses include hepatic adenoma and focal nodular hyperplasia.

Metastatic liver tumours

Secondary liver tumours are seen frequently in cancer care. Commonly they arise from the stomach, colon, breast, pancreas or lung. Often the tumour deposits are multiple and give rise to weight loss, jaundice, right upper abdominal pain and ascites. Ascites refers to the accumulation of free serous fluid which collects in the peritoneal cavity. Sometimes hard masses may be felt in an enlarged liver. Surgical resection of single or localised liver metastases may sometimes be possible. Untreated liver metastasis usually leads to death within a few months.

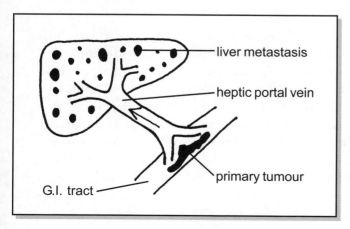

liver metastasis

heptic portal vein

primary tumour

G.I. tract

Diagram 19.3
Tumours in the colon and stomach frequently metastasise to the liver. Tumour cells are washed along in the normal blood flow from the GI tract to the liver via the hepatic portal vein. Arrow indicates normal direction of blood flow and path of tumour spread.

Liver trauma

Blunt trauma caused by a blow to the upper abdomen is the most common cause of liver injury. Frequently this presents with bleeding into the abdominal cavity. Sharp trauma to the liver may be caused by a stab wound; these usually stop bleeding by themselves if the patient remains still for a period of time. This is because movement may cause blood clots to be dislodged restarting bleeding. Surgery is indicated if the blood loss is leading to shock.

Viral hepatitis

Hepatitis refers to inflammation of the liver; this may be caused by viral infection, drugs or alcohol. The viruses which specifically infect liver cells are classified as hepatitis A, B, C, D, and E viruses. Individual hepatocytes swell and may degenerate as a result of the viral infection. Variable numbers of liver cells die leading to areas of necrosis. The extent of necrosis varies considerably between individuals infected with the same virus. Most only suffer small areas of hepatic necrosis but less commonly some patients may develop massive hepatic necrosis resulting in fulminating liver failure (FLF). Fulminating is a term used to describe a condition which develops quickly and is severe. FLF is life threatening and can occur as a complication of hepatitis regardless of the cause. Paracetamol overdose is a common cause in the UK but globally most cases are caused by one of the hepatitis viruses.

Clinical features in viral hepatitis

Even though there are five forms of hepatitis virus, and the incubation periods vary, the clinical presentations are usually similar. There is malaise, lethargy and fatigue with generalised flu-like symptoms. A low grade fever is typical although some patients may have a higher temperature. Anorexia and weight loss may develop. If the patient is a smoker they usually do not feel like smoking. Hepatic inflammation leads to a tender, swollen liver (liver enlargement is described as hepatomegaly).

As the liver cells are inflammed and not functioning as normal, the bilirubin is not taken from the blood and incorporated into the bile. In addition, the swelling of the liver will reduce the flow of bile through the small bile channels within the liver. These effects lead to increased levels of bilirubin in the blood, i.e. bilirubinaemia. In the kidneys the bilirubin from the blood is incorporated into urine, giving rise to dark coloured urine (like tea without milk). The same effects will result in less bile and bilirubin passing through the bile ducts into the lumen of the gut. This means there is less bile and bilirubin to colour and deodorise the faeces, resulting in pale and foul smelling stools. Bilirubinaemia is also likely to give rise to a degree of jaundice. Viral skin rashes may present.

Hepatitis A

This RNA based enterovirus is the most common agent causing viral hepatitis. The incubation period refers to the time between a person being infected and the onset of symptoms; with hepatitis A virus (HAV) the average time is 30 days (range 15-50 days). HAV replicates in the hepatocytes and is excreted in bile. Since bile passes into the intestine the virus is present in the stools of an infected person. Viral excretion in the faeces starts about 2 weeks before the patient develops symptoms and carries on for a further 2 weeks after. Once an infected person has passed this stage of viral excretion they do not go on to become carriers. A 'carrier' is a person who carries an infection but does not currently present any clinical features; they therefore do not suffer themselves, but may pass infection to others. If sanitation or hygiene is poor, viral particles from an infected person can contaminate the food or water of other people resulting in them becoming infected. This mode of transmission is called the faeco-oral route. Like other similar infections, HAV often occurs in outbreaks or epidemics.

Jaundice can be mild and usually develops 1 to 10 days after the onset of symptoms and approximately coincides with the patient starting to feel better. No specific treatment is available. The vast majority of patients make a full recovery after 3-6 weeks. Rarely (less than 0.2% of cases) fulminant hepatitis may develop. Hepatitis A vaccination is available and highly advisable for anyone who may be exposed to HAV.

Hepatitis B

This infection is caused by a specific DNA based hepatitis B virus (HBV) sometimes called the Dane particle. As hepatitis B virus is found in the blood of an infected person the virus is transmitted by what is described as the serum route. This is why infection can spread as a result of needle stick injuries or other wounds caused by infected sharps. Splashing infected blood into the eyes is also a risk. Serum spread puts clinical workers at particular risk of acquiring the infection during their work and is why we should all be vaccinated against the possibility. If we do accidentally stab ourselves with a used needle, we should make the wound bleed by squeezing out as much blood as possible and encourage further bleeding by running the wound under a hot tap. This is important as potentially infecting viral particles may be washed out with the flow of blood. If you feel you have been exposed to HBV then it is possible to reduce the risk of infection further by receiving specific hepatitis B immunoglobulin. This should be given as soon after exposure as possible. Serum transmission has also occurred as a result of poor aseptic technique from acupuncture, body piercing and tattooing. Sadly, poor standards of asepsis in medicine and dentistry have caused many cases worldwide. Infection can also be spread by blood and blood products which is why all donated blood in the UK is screened for hepatitis B, C and HIV. HBV has been found in saliva and the condition can be spread by sexual intercourse. Homosexual or heterosexual anal sex is of particularly high risk. Vertical transmission from an infected mother to child during birth is likely.

The clinical picture of hepatitis B is similar to that seen in hepatitis A, although HBV infection is often more severe and the patient may feel unwell for several months. The incubation period is typically around 2 to 3 months (range 1 to 6 months). Most patients make a full recovery with about 1% developing fulminant hepatitis. In a further 1-10% of cases, DNA from the HBV integrates itself into the host DNA of the hepatocytes. This causes chronic hepatitis B infection and most of these patients become long term carriers of the disease. Chronic hepatitis B infection also carries a significant risk of developing cirrhosis and hepatocellular carcinoma. There is no proven specific treatment for acute infection but in chronic infection interferon and lamivudine are both helpful.

Hepatitis C

This is caused by a serum transmission of the RNA based hepatitis C virus (HCV). Transmission may therefore occur via the serum route as it does with HBV. The incidence in intravenous drug users is particularly high and cross infection during tattooing has also been implicated. Vertical and sexual transmission are less likely than is the case with HBV but may occur. Incubation is usually between 6 to 7 weeks (range 2-26 weeks). Acute infection with HCV is often asymptomatic although some patients do have flu like illness with some jaundice. The big problem with HCV is about 80% of patients go on to develop chronic liver disease with increased risk of cirrhosis and hepatocellular carcinoma. Alcohol increases the risk of chronic problems in HCV infection and should be avoided. Treatment with interferon may be of benefit in acute infections to prevent chronic disease development.

Hepatitis D

This virus can only replicate in the presence of hepatitis B virus. This means a person will only get hepatitis D if they have or carry HBV. This is why hepatitis D virus is sometimes referred to as a 'piggy back' virus. Like HBV, transmission of HDV is via the serum or sexual route. If a person with HBV does contract hepatitis D this is referred to as co-infection and carries an increased risk of fulminant hepatitis.

Hepatitis E

This RNA virus produces an illness similar to HAV. Transmission is faeco-oral and large epidemics have occurred where sanitation is poor. The risk of fulminant hepatitis is about 1-2% unless the patient is pregnant when it is much higher. Chronic liver disease does not occur and there is no chronic carrier state. The incubation period for hepatitis E is about 40 days (range 15-60 days).

Alcohol

Alcoholic drinks are popular in most countries of the world as many people find the immediate effects on the mind pleasurable. In order to assess how much a person is drinking it is useful to use the units system. A unit of alcohol is approximately 8 grams, or 10 mls of pure alcohol. A litre of wine at 10% alcohol by volume would therefore contain 100 mls of ethanol (i.e. ethyl alcohol which is the form of alcohol in alcoholic drinks) representing 10 units. One unit is roughly the amount of alcohol in a single whisky, a small glass of sherry, a small glass of table wine, a quarter of a pint of strong lager or half a pint of beer. What is important for health is the total amount consumed; alcohol in beer is just as dangerous as alcohol in spirits. The advisable safe weekly maximum for men is probably 21 units and 14 for women; however some say it is 28 units for men and 21 for women. This should be spread over three or more occasions, with alcohol free days included in the week. Women can tolerate less because they are usually smaller than men and have a relatively greater proportion of adipose tissue. Regular heavy drinking is more harmful than occasional binges.

Even in small doses alcohol inhibits the function of the mind and muscular coordination. Consumption of about 4 units will result in a blood alcohol level of about 80 mg per 100 mls of blood and will reduce inhibitions and promote relaxation. Increasing to about 8 units, most drinkers slur speech a little and become clumsy. Emotional reactions vary a lot but often become highly exaggerated. Increased doses may cause agression, staggering, loss of balance, nausea and finally loss of consciousness with associated risk of inhalation of vomit causing choking and suffocation.

As physical and mental function is impaired, accidents of all forms are a common risk. Acute alcohol poisoning, a potentially fatal condition, is possible with a large intake over a short period of time. Young people are prone to this as they may not have learned how much alcohol their bodies can handle. Like any drug overdose, this is a tragic way for a young person to die. A severe 'hangover' can occur after a single episode of drinking. Unwanted pregnancies and sexually transmitted disease are possible consequences of disinhibition.

Prolonged 'heavy' drinking is associated with many pathological conditions, the level of risk increasing with consumption. Men drinking over 5 units per day have a slightly increased risk of developing alcohol related conditions. In men drinking 10 units a day (or 5 units for women) the risk is much increased. However, if a man drinks 20 units per day (10 units for women) for a period of time there is a high risk of developing alcohol related disease.

In chronic drinking, psychological and physical dependence may occur. Sudden withdrawal of alcohol in continuous drinkers results in delirium tremens. This is characterised by anxiety and tension, tremor of the hands, insomnia, seizures, hallucinations, tachycardia, hypotension, vomiting, diarrhoea and fever. Long term alcohol consumption increases the risk of cancer of the mouth, pharynx, oesophagus and larynx. The combination of smoking and drinking increases risk of these tumours still further. Liver cancer may complicate cirrhosis and there is some increased risk of breast cancer. In addition to liver disease alcohol may contribute to gastritis, peptic ulceration, pancreatitis, cardiac dysrhythmias, cardiomyopathy, high blood pressure, stroke, peripheral neuropathy, impotence, obesity, diabetes, gout, physical and psychological dependence and nutritional deficiencies.

Drinking in pregnancy may lead to reduced rates of fetal growth, CNS disorders, craniofacial malformations and other abnormalities such as disorders of the ears, eyes and CVS. Collectively these conditions may comprise fetal alcohol syndrome. Parents planning a family should ideally both stop drinking pre-conceptually.

Excessive or prolonged drinking can cause a range of psychological problems. These include insomnia, anxiety, depression, poor concentration, increase in suicide rates, hallucinations and periods of amnesia (memory loss). Alcoholic dementia (Korsakoff's psychosis) may occur and in addition to the usual features of dementia is characterised by confabulation. This means sufferers make up events for the periods of time they have no memory of.

There are many possible social consequences of drinking which vary with the circumstances of the individual. Associations exist between alcohol, family problems and divorce. Unemployment and financial problems are also possible consequences of excess drinking. Violence and inappropriate sexual behaviour are more likely during intoxication.

Moderate consumption of alcohol slightly raises levels of protective high density lipoproteins in the blood. This means small amounts of alcohol may be beneficial. However, there will always be a sector of the population who will drink to excess, so as professionals we should never advise a non-drinker to start drinking on health grounds.

Alcohol and the liver

In the presence of alcohol liver cells are able to take up fatty acids normally. However, they are unable to incorporate these into lipoproteins for export. This means fat accumulates within the hepatocytes. As the presence of fat in liver cells causes them to swell, the overall size of the liver also increases, resulting in a bulky, fatty liver. A 'fatty' liver is one cause of hepatomegaly (abnormal liver enlargement); such livers may be palpable below the right lower costal margin in the upper right quadrant of the abdomen. In heavy drinkers the liver often appears yellow due to the amount of fat it contains and may double or treble in weight. Steatosis is the term used to describe fatty infiltration of the liver. Despite the gross increase in liver bulk, the patient may not suffer any features of liver disease at this stage. This is one of the problems in alcoholic liver disease; by the time clinical features present the disease is already well advanced and may be irreversible. However, if a person stops drinking at the fatty liver stage, the liver cells will resume fat export, recover completely and return to normal size. If drinking continues, a fatty liver may develop irreversible cirrhosis. If cirrhosis progresses there will ultimately be liver failure and death.

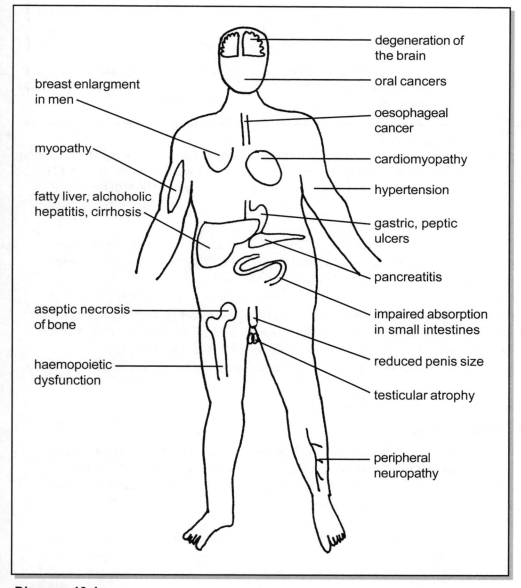

Diagram 19.4
Review of the possible adverse affects of drinking too much alcohol.

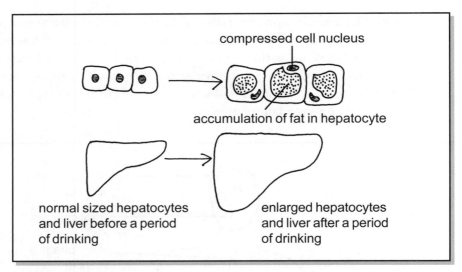

Diagram 19.5
Liver cells and liver before and after a period of heavy drinking. The presence of large volumes of fat within the hepatocytes will compress the cytoplasm; the nucleus will be squashed and pushed to the periphery of the cell.

Alcoholic hepatitis

This is a form of progressive liver inflammation which develops in heavy drinkers. Ongoing alcohol exposure causes inflammation leading to hepatocyte necrosis and progressive liver injury. There is a wide spectrum of severity in alcohol induced hepatitis from mild with no symptoms to severe with features of liver disease such as fever, hepatomegaly, jaundice, coagulopathy, ascites and hepatic encephalopathy. The liver is usually enlarged and a little tender. In patients that present with such acute features the mortality is about 30%. If cirrhosis is not already present it will develop if alcohol drinking continues.

Cirrhosis

Pathophysiology

Cirrhosis is the end stage of chronic liver disease with a fairly consistent clinical and pathological presentation regardless of underlying cause. In cirrhosis fibrous tissue accumulates within the liver, converting the normal hepatic architecture into structurally abnormal fibrous nodules. A nodule is usually described as a small, firm or knotty mass.

Normally around the liver sinusoids (i.e. the liver capillaries) stellate cells are present in the space of Disse. This is the tissue fluid filled space between the sinusoids and the hepatocytes. As a result of liver injury the hepatocytes and Kupffer cells (specialised liver macrophages) release cytokines which activate the stellate cells. Once activated the stellate cells proliferate and produce collagen which is the main component in fibrous tissue. Cirrhosis therefore occurs as a result of ongoing cell injury and inflammation which is followed by the formation of fibrous scar tissue.

The presence of fibrous areas or nodules within the liver obstructs the normal flow of blood and bile through the organ. In most affluent countries alcohol is the most common cause of cirrhosis, resulting in the development of numerous small fibrous nodules. Another cause associated with affluence and high fat diets is a form of non-alcoholic fatty liver disease (NAFLD) called non-alcoholic steatohepatitis (NASH). Recently in Europe and the US there has also been an increase in hepatitis C related cirrhosis. Worldwide, viral hepatitis is the most common cause of cirrhosis; this results in the presence of larger nodules of various sizes. Once cirrhotic damage has occurred, there are no treatments which will reverse the process. However, if the underlying cause is removed, e.g. the patient stops drinking, then further disease progression can be halted.

Complications of cirrhosis and liver failure

Liver failure

Liver failure is most commonly seen as the end stage of chronic cirrhosis. However, acute liver failure may present as a consequence of acute fulminant hepatitis or in patients who have suffered from previously unrecognized chronic liver disease who acutely decompensate. Clinical hepatic failure develops when 80-90% of liver function has been lost. As the liver normally carries out a range of chemical processes essential for life, hepatic failure is often a terminal condition if transplant is not available.

Jaundice

Reduced numbers of functional hepatocytes will reduce the ability of the liver to take up and conjugate bilirubin. Also cirrhotic fibrous tissue within the liver will compress and obstruct bile ducts. Therefore jaundice in cirrhosis has hepatic and cholestatic components.

Portal hypertension

Cirrhosis is the most common cause of portal hypertension. The presence of fibrous tissue within the liver obstructs blood flow through the organ. This in turn prevents the free entry of blood from the hepatic portal vein (HPV). As there is a backlog of blood within the HPV pressure is increased, resulting in hypertension of the portal system. This hypertension leads to an increase in pressure within the vessels draining the gastrointestinal tract and spleen. Portal hypertension in turn causes other complications associated with cirrhosis including oesophageal varices, ascites, hepatic encephalopathy, and hypersplenism.

Oesophageal varices

As the veins in the lower part of the oesophagus drain into the hepatic portal vein, portal hypertension will increase the pressure in these veins. This will cause lower oesophageal veins to engorge with blood, stretching and thinning their walls. These damaged and engorged veins are called oesophageal varices. If the walls of the varices rupture there can be profuse, life threatening haemorrhage into the oesophagus. This usually leads to vomiting of large volumes of frank or altered blood.

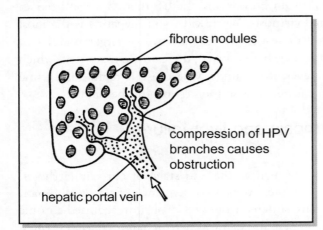

Diagram 19.6
Obstruction of branches of the hepatic portal vein in the liver will cause obstruction to blood entering the liver with consequent portal hypertension, (arrow indicates direction of blood flow from gut).

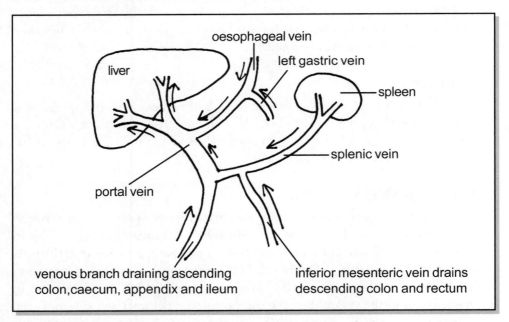

Diagram 19.7
As the portal system drains blood from the stomach, oesophagus, spleen and rectum; all of these structures can be involved and complicate portal hypertension.

Ascites

Ascites refers to an accumulation of fluid within the peritoneal cavity and is another common presentation in chronic liver disease. Three pathophysiological processes contributing to ascites in cirrhosis will be discussed here.

Firstly, pressure dams back in the veins of the hepatic portal system so reducing the ability of blood to drain from the mesenteric capillaries. This increases the blood (or hydrostatic) pressure within these capillaries. As pressure inside the capillaries is increased it becomes more difficult for tissue fluid to re-enter the capillaries so reabsorption of tissue fluid is reduced. As a result more fluid is left to accumulate in the peritoneal cavity. As the veins of the hepatic portal system drain a large area of capillaries within the peritoneal cavity, large volumes of fluid may accumulate.

Secondly, it is the liver which produces the plasma protein albumin. It is albumin which generates most of plasma osmotic pressure. In hepatic failure the liver is unable to synthesise normal volumes of albumin; this lowers the concentrations of albumin in the plasma and so lowers plasma osmotic pressure. As it is the osmotic pressure of the plasma which causes reabsorption of tissue fluid back into the capillaries, any reduction in plasma osmotic pressure will reduce reabsorption, again leaving more fluid outside the capillaries to accumulate in the peritoneal cavity.

Thirdly, in liver failure the kidneys excrete less sodium which increases the amount of sodium in the plasma. Increase in plasma sodium attracts more water into the blood increasing intravascular volume. This will increase venous pressures further, leading to less reabsorption of tissue fluid.

The first line of medical management in ascites is salt restriction. Eating less salt will reduce the amount of sodium in the plasma and therefore help to lower blood volume and so venous pressures. Second line management is to give diuretics which will reduce the total volume of water in the blood, therefore encouraging the reabsorption of fluid from the peritoneal cavity. Thirdly fluid may be drained directly using paracentesis where a needle is inserted into the fluid which is then allowed to drain out of the body.

In patients with ascites a high index of suspicion should be maintained for infection in the large volumes of static fluid present in the peritoneal cavity. This is called spontaneous bacterial peritonitis and is life threatening unless aggressively treated with antibiotics. In addition to cirrhosis it is important to remember that ascites may also present in malignant disease of the liver or peritoneum, cardiac failure, pancreatitis, hypoalbuminaemia and some gynaecological cancers.

Hepatic encephalopathy

Hepatic encephalopathy describes the neurological features which may arise as a result of liver failure. In normal physiology the majority of the blood draining from the GI tract passes directly through the liver via the hepatic portal circulation. This arrangement means the liver can detoxify products of bacterial metabolism which have been absorbed from the gut. These toxins are generated by the large numbers of bacteria present in the gut lumen. However, in portal hypertension, portal blood is diverted directly into the systemic venous drainage. This means blood containing bacterial waste products does not go directly to the liver for detoxification, but enters the blood allowing the toxins to circulate to the brain where they act as neurotoxins. Clinically, irritability may be an early feature but later there is lethargy, sleepiness and ultimately hepatic coma. If the encephalopathy affects the motor areas of the brain a 'liver flap' can be present. Liver flap describes a tremor of the wrists when the arms are held out with the wrists extended in dorsiflexion.

Levels of ammonia are increased in the blood and brain of patients with liver failure. Ammonia acts as a neurotoxin and is generated as a result of protein metabolism and the action of bacteria on proteins in the gut. As proteins contain nitrogen, metabolism of amino acids results in the production of some nitrogen as a metabolic waste product. Some of this waste nitrogen reacts with water to form ammonia which is NH_3. Ammonia is a very toxic molecule so normally the liver rapidly converts it into urea which is less toxic. Once formed the soluble urea is excreted by the kidneys. In liver failure the hepatocytes fail to convert ammonia into urea, resulting in an accumulation of toxic ammonia.

While hepatic encephalopathy may occur as part of terminal liver failure, it is more common for episodes of encephalopathy to be reversible. This can be done using lactulose and antibiotics such as neomycin. This antibiotic is poorly absorbed into the blood, so most of it remains in the lumen of the gut. Here it kills a lot of bacteria which means that less ammonia and other toxins are produced. As less toxins are produced the levels of ammonia and toxins in the blood are reduced. Lactulose works by reducing the pH of the contents of the colon. This acidity neutralises the ammonia, which is a strong alkaline. As the ammonia is neutralised, there is less to enter the blood. As the levels of ammonia and bacterial waste products are reduced the hepatic encephalopathy will be reversed. Low protein diets are no longer considered beneficial.

Hypersplenism

As the hepatic portal system also drains the spleen, portal hypertension will cause this organ to become congested with blood. As a result the spleen increases in size, a condition termed splenomegaly. It is the normal function of the spleen to remove old blood components such as red cells and platelets. However, in portal hypertension the spleen is congested and blood flows through very slowly. This gives the spleen more time to remove blood components than it does in normal physiology. This syndrome of splenetic over activity is called hypersplenism. The spleen removes too many red cells leading to anaemia and too many platelets causing thrombocytopenia and therefore reduced blood coagulation. Too many white cells are also removed leading to decreased resistance to infection.

Haemorrhage

In health, the liver synthesizes the blood clotting factors fibrinogen, prothrombin and factors V, VII, IX and X. In liver failure these are no longer produced in sufficient quantities resulting in a failure of normal blood clotting. As blood does not clot normally, numerous haemorrhagic complications may present such as bruises, purpura, epistaxis or menorrhagia. Lack of clotting factors is commonly complicated by thrombocytopenia (low levels of platelets in the blood) which may develop as a result of hypersplenism or bone marrow depression.

Hepatorenal syndrome

This describes renal failure which develops secondary to hepatic failure. In liver failure there is a reduction in renal blood flow with a consequent reduction in glomerular filtration rate. This results in the usual features of renal hypoperfusion which are oliguria, uraemia and increased plasma creatinine levels. Salt excretion will also be inhibited leading to possible hypernatraemia. Hepatorenal failure develops because vasoactive toxins which are produced (or not metabolised) by the failing liver, cause large and small renal arteries to constrict leading to renal hypoperfusion. Vasoconstricting substances which are raised in cirrhosis include angiotensin, antidiuretic hormone and norepinephrine (noradrenaline).

Hepatopulmonary syndrome

This describes the reduced pulmonary function which may present in cirrhosis. Ascites may directly lead to elevation of the diaphragm and so reduce ventilatory efficiency. There may also be pleural effusion, pulmonary oedema and blood may not fully perfuse the pulmonary capillaries. As this is a potentially life threatening complication, oxygen saturations should be monitored in patients with cirrhosis.

Hypoproteinaemia

It is a normal function of the liver to produce albumin which is the principle protein generating plasma osmotic pressure. In liver failure the synthesis of albumin is reduced resulting in a hypoalbuminaemia. This reduces plasma osmotic pressure and so results in generalised oedema.

Endocrine complications

As the liver normally metabolizes steroid hormones various endocrine effects are likely to present. There is an increase in the levels of circulating oestrogens as the liver normally breaks down (catabolises) these hormones into inactive metabolites. Some male hormones called weak androgens are also converted into oestrogen like molecules in peripheral tissues. As a result of raised oestrogen levels men develop breast enlargement (gynaecomastia), a female distribution of pubic hair and testicular atrophy. Women usually develop amenorrhea and sterility. Both sexes have a loss of libido (interest in sex).

Increased levels of oestrogen in the blood probably explain spider angiomas (also called spider nevi) which develop in the upper half of the body. Localised vasodilation caused by accumulation of endocrine hormones also causes the palms of the hands to appear red. This redness is described as palmar erythema or 'liver palms'.

Reduced hepatic metabolism of aldosterone will result in increased plasma levels of this hormone. As a consequence there will be increased salt and water retention by the kidneys with increased excretion of potassium. This will contribute to fluid and electrolyte imbalance characterised by fluid overload, hypernatraemia and hypokalaemia.

Fetor hepaticus

Fetor hepaticus may be noted in advanced liver failure. This refers to a characteristic smell of the breath, often described as sweetish or musty. The odour arises from the metabolic waste products of intestinal bacteria which are no longer broken down by the failing liver.

CHAPTER 20

Disorders of the Gall Bladder and Bile Ducts

Gallstones

Gallstones (or cholelithiasis) are very common. About 10% of women in their forties have gallstones and this rises to about 30% after the age of 60. The figures for men are about half those for women. Most gallstones (about 75%) are a mixture of cholesterol and bile pigments although pure cholesterol or bile pigment stones also occur.

Aetiology of gallstones

Pure cholesterol and mixed gallstones develop when crystals of cholesterol form in the gall bladder. Once these have formed, more cholesterol and bile salts may precipitate out of the bile and stick to the crystals. This leads to an increase in crystal size and eventual stone formation.

Bile consists of water, cholesterol, bile salts, bile acids and phospholipids (these are fats associated with phosphate). Normally cholesterol is soluble in bile due to the presence of the bile salts and phospholipids. However, if the proportions of cholesterol increase, or the amounts of bile salts and phospholipids decrease, cholesterol will become supersaturated and start to precipitate out, leading to crystal formation. This supersaturated bile is sometimes termed lithogenic (stone forming) bile. The proportion of cholesterol in bile may increase as a result of stimulation by oestrogen; the levels of this hormone in turn may be increased by oral contraceptives, pregnancy and obesity. Diets high in cholesterol and animal fat probably make gall stone formation more likely. A low fibre diet is a risk factor as some cholesterol in the gut will bind onto any fibre present and so be excreted in the stools, preventing cholesterol from being reabsorbed.

Stasis of bile is another risk factor. This may occur as a result of physical compression of the bile ducts during pregnancy, and multiple pregnancies increase overall risk. Stasis will also occur during fasting as bile is not stimulated to pass from the gall bladder into the duodenum because there is no fat to emulsify. There is also an increased incidence in diabetes mellitus and a family history of gallstone disease is not uncommon. It is also likely that low grade infection in the gall bladder may start off stone formation. Bacteria may form the nucleus on which crystals may develop.

The much less common bile pigment stones occur in haemolytic anaemia when too many red blood cells are broken down by the monocytes-macrophage system (mostly in the spleen). This will increase the amounts of bile pigments (mostly bilirubin) entering the biliary tract leading to precipitation.

Clinical features

Most gallstones remain within the gall bladder and are therefore 'silent', not generating any clinical features. This is why gallstones can often be diagnosed as an incidental finding, for example during ultrasound investigations. However, if they move out into the bile ducts symptoms are generated. In symptomatic disease pain caused by colic is often reported after eating food with a fatty content.

Complications of gall stones

Most of the complications of gallstones develop as a result of obstruction of the cystic duct or common bile duct. This is why gallstones may lead to biliary colic. Biliary refers to the bile ducts and colic is a pain generated in the walls of a hollow or tubular organ. As the smooth muscle in the wall of the bile ducts tries to push the obstructing stone along there is muscle spasm which generates severe pain.

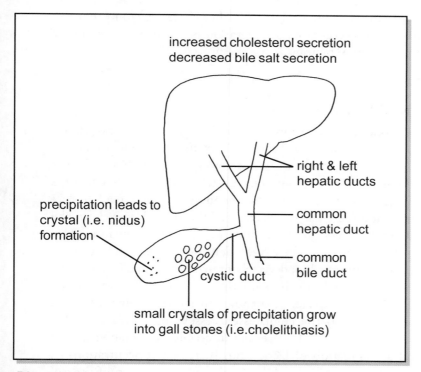

increased cholesterol secretion
decreased bile salt secretion

right & left hepatic ducts

precipitation leads to crystal (i.e. nidus) formation

common hepatic duct

common bile duct

cystic duct

small crystals of precipitation grow into gall stones (i.e.cholelithiasis)

Diagram 20.1
Most gallstones contain cholesterol and bile pigments but some only contain cholesterol. These two groups of stones are thought to start in the same way. Cholesterol is highly insoluble in bile and is only made soluble by the presence of bile salts. If the hepatocytes secrete more cholesterol or less bile salts this balance is disturbed and the cholesterol will no longer be kept in solution. This will result in supersaturation of bile with cholesterol and consequent precipitation. Once there is a solid crystal (or nidus) in the bile, stone formation will continue as a result of ongoing precipitation resulting in the accumulation of further material.

Secondary infections are also more likely including acute or chronic cholecystitis and acute cholangitis. Cholecystitis is inflammation of the gall bladder and cholangitis is inflammation of the bile ducts. Gallstones are the most common cause of pancreatitis and it seems the presence of gallstones increases the risk of carcinomas of the gall bladder.

Management of symptomatic gallstones

Diagnosis of gallstones can readily be confirmed by the use of ultrasound. As gallstones are generated in the gall bladder, cholecystectomy is almost always the treatment of choice for symptomatic disease. If possible this should be carried out using a laparoscopic technique. Removal of the gall bladder, which has been described as the gallstone 'factory', prevents further gallstone formation. (Gall stones may form in the common bile duct after cholecystectomy, but this is rare). As gallstones are so common, an operation is not usually considered unless stones are generating symptoms.

Biliary colic

Pathophysiology of biliary colic

In many people gallstones are present in the gall bladder but cause no clinical features. However, sometimes a stone may pass from the gall bladder where it originated into the cystic duct, or on to the common bile duct (CBD). Stones passing through these ducts cause temporary obstruction, but often there is not enough time for jaundice to develop. The presence of a stone in a bile duct causes vigorous peristaltic muscular contraction of the smooth muscle in the duct walls in an attempt to pass the stone along towards the duodenum. This vigorous muscular activity increases the oxygen demand of the tissue. Also the muscular contraction compresses blood vessels present in the wall of the bile ducts; this reduces blood supply to the smooth muscular walls of the duct. This combination of increased oxygen demand, with reduced delivery, caused by the ischaemia generated by the compressed vessels, means that aerobic metabolism cannot be supported. This results in anaerobic metabolism and the generation and accumulation of lactic acid. Increased concentrations of lactic acid lead to the pain described as biliary colic. As contraction of the gall bladder and bile ducts is normally stimulated by the presence of fatty food in the duodenum, colic often occurs after a meal with a high fat content. As the pain is caused by stone induced spasm, it subsides when the stone is passed into the duodenum.

Clinical features of biliary colic

Pain caused by biliary colic is severe and persistent; an attack lasts from several minutes to several hours. Epigastric pain is a common presentation and pain often develops in the right upper quadrant of the abdomen as would be expected from the anatomical location of the bile ducts. Referred pain may radiate to the right subscapular region and right shoulder. Nausea, vomiting and sweating are frequently associated with this pain. Usually the patient is restless and rolls about in severe pain.

Treatment of biliary colic

Acute episodes of pain should be treated with intravenous opiate analgesia. Patients should not eat for the first 24 hours, to prevent any further stimulation of the gall bladder to contract. Subsequent cholecystectomy (surgical removal of the gall bladder) should be considered. If surgery is delayed the patient should go on to a low fat diet.

Biliary infections

Acute cholecystitis

This is most commonly caused by a gallstone obstructing the cystic duct. As bile cannot leave the gall bladder it becomes progressively concentrated as more water is reabsorbed. This highly concentrated bile is very irritating to the lining of the gall bladder leading to a chemically induced cholecystitis. The inflammation also stimulates the formation of pus and the gall bladder becomes distended.

Distension and inflammation, caused by the stasis of bile, leads to the development of secondary infection in the gall bladder. Infection in turn causes more severe inflammation and associated pain in the right upper quadrant. Therefore acute cholecystitis presents in a similar way to biliary colic but the pain usually develops progressively and is more persistent. In the presence of infection, pain is also associated with tenderness and muscle guarding. As with most serious infections the patient will develop pyrexia which is usually in the range of 38-39°C. Patients will be very unwell with toxaemia and a leucocytosis. Toxaemic refers to a generalised poisoning due to the accumulation of toxins, in this case bacterial toxins. A leucocytosis describes an increase in the numbers of white cells present in the blood in an attempt to combat the infection. If infection is allowed to progress, pus may collect in the gall bladder, a condition referred to as empyema. This causes an intermittent fever with pain and often requires surgical drainage and cholecystectomy.

Treatment of acute cholecystitis usually involves rest, pain control and giving intravenous antibiotics to treat the infection. Patients should be given intravenous fluids and kept nil by mouth. After a few days of this treatment the acute infection should subside. After the acute episode, cholecystectomy should be performed to prevent any recurrence. Another reason for cholecystectomy is that the gall bladder wall will have been stretched due to distension. This will have resulted in a thinning of the wall, leading to a possible disruption in blood supply and drainage. Although uncommon, it is possible that disruption to the blood supply will eventually result in necrosis and subsequent perforation. Perforation of the gall bladder is dangerous as it will allow bile to leak into the peritoneal cavity causing a very severe peritonitis.

Chronic cholecystitis

Chronic cholecystitis may develop after several episodes of obstruction and acute cholecystitis. Repeated episodes of inflammation lead to fibrosis and chronic thickening of the gall bladder wall. The patient usually suffers from recurrent episodes of pain as a consequence of mild cholecystitis. Discomfort is often experienced after eating fatty foods as the thickened gall bladder wall contracts down onto gallstones. Treatment is cholecystectomy which should be curative.

Acute cholangitis

If a gallstone obstructs the common bile duct it will cause biliary colic as described above. If the obstruction is prolonged jaundice will also develop. The levels of jaundice caused by this disorder usually fluctuate, depending on the degree and duration of obstruction. If a gallstone is obstructing the CBD, the duct above the level of obstruction will dilate and the bile will be static. As is common in any form of stasis, infection is likely to develop. Bacteria, such as Escherichia coli, may enter the biliary ducts from the duodenum. Normally, a few bacteria would not cause a problem as they would be washed back into the duodenum in the normal flow of bile. However, an obstruction gives plenty of time for microorganisms to divide and subsequent infection to develop. The presence of bacteria, and the toxins they produce, causes acute inflammation of the bile ducts; a condition referred to as cholangitis. In this bacterial infection, in addition to colic and jaundice, there will be a high fever. Infected bile is serious and potentially fatal. Some bacteria usually enter the blood and may lead to the development of toxaemia. The combination of obstruction and infection of bile will also result in infected bile damming back into the liver leading to liver failure.

Treatment principles in acute cholangitis

These patients should be treated with intravenous antibiotics to kill the bacteria causing the infection. Emergency drainage of the infected bile is a life saving procedure. This is usually done by the endoscopic retrograde approach. An endoscope is passed down the oesophagus, through the stomach, into the duodenum. Here the sphincter of Oddi is opened and the gallstones can be removed using a balloon catheter. This is passed up into the CBD, past the level of the obstruction, and then inflated. As the now inflated balloon is drawn back down the CBD, the stone or stones are also drawn down into the duodenum. Once the stones are removed the infected bile may drain freely into the duodenum relieving the stasis and cholangitis. After the acute episode cholecystectomy is performed to prevent any recurrence of gallstones entering the bile ducts. Prior to any interventions patients are usually given intravenous vitamin K. This is because lack of bile salts in the gut prevents the absorption of this fat soluble vitamin. Lack of vitamin K will prevent normal blood clotting, leading to excessive haemorrhage.

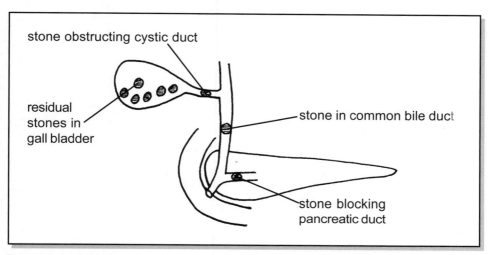

Diagram 20.2
Complications of gallstones, a stone obstructing the neck of the gall bladder or cystic duct will cause acute cholecystitis, while a stone passing through any of the bile ducts is likely to cause biliary colic. Stones may also lodge in the common bile duct leading to cholangitis with biliary colic, jaundice and pyrexia. If a stone lodges in the pancreatic duct this may cause acute pancreatitis. Note the gallstones which remain in the gall bladder cause no or minimal acute problems.

Cancer of the gall bladder

This type of cancer accounts for about 1-2% of all cancers and is more common in women. Most cases present in the 60-80 year old range. The majority of patients have gallstones and these may well be involved in the aetiology. About 90% of gall bladder malignancies are adenocarcinomas and about 10% are squamous carcinomas. Local invasion involves the bile ducts, liver and associated lymph nodes. Clinically the presentation is usually similar to chronic cholecystitis with right upper quadrant pain, nausea and vomiting. Later there is weight loss, obstructive jaundice and a palpable mass. Unfortunately, spread has already occurred by the time the condition generates many clinical features, although if it can be caught early the prognosis is good.

Primary cancer of the bile ducts (cholangiocarcinoma) is still uncommon but is increasing in incidence. It is more common in men and is often associated with inflammatory bowel disease and sclerosing cholangitis.

CHAPTER 21

Disorders of the Pancreas

Acute pancreatitis

An episode of acute pancreatitis may vary in severity from some mild pancreatic oedema to one with severe necrosis and haemorrhage. Mortality in a severe attack may be over 30%.

Background physiology

The pancreas contains two principal types of cell. Most pancreatic cells are exocrine. These produce digestive enzymes which are exported from the gland via ducts, into the duodenum, where they digest food. Secondly the pancreatic islets of Langerhans contain endocrine cells which produce hormones; these are absorbed directly into the blood. The pancreas is therefore an exocrine and an endocrine gland.

In normal physiology the pancreas produces pre-enzymes in an inactive form. For example, the pancreas produces an enzyme called trypsinogen which passes out of the exocrine cells and into the pancreatic ducts. After passing through the pancreas via the main pancreatic duct the trypsinogen enters the duodenum. It is only when trypsinogen is safely in the lumen of the duodenum that another enzyme called enterokinase converts it into the active protein digesting form called trypsin. Production in an inactive form is essential as synthesis of an active protein digesting enzyme within a cell would mean it would start digesting the cell as soon as it was manufactured. The pancreas also produces a fat digesting enzyme called pancreatic lipase and a carbohydrate digesting enzyme called pancreatic amylase.

Aetiology

The most common cause of acute pancreatitis in the UK is gallstones. If gallstones are present, the risk of acute pancreatitis is increased by 25 times, in comparison to the general population. It has been suggested that gall stones may block the ampulla, leading to a backlog of pancreatic juice causing increased pressure within the pancreatic ducts. This backlog in turn affects the pancreatic enzyme producing (acinar) cells. These cells contain granules of digestive pre-enzymes called zymogen granules which fuse with lysosomes prematurely activating the pre-enzymes, converting them into active digestive enzymes. Once activated these enzymes will start to digest the cell and will also escape and activate pre-enzymes in adjacent cells. This leads to a chain reaction of digestive enzyme activation. For example, trypsinogen will be converted to trypsin within the cytosol of the cells.

Other possible mechanisms of enzyme activation include bile entering the pancreatic ducts. This could also be caused by obstruction of the ampulla. In the pancreatic ducts, bile may activate pre-enzymes into their active forms. Reflux of duodenal contents into the pancreatic duct will also prematurely activate pancreatic enzymes. Once protein digesting enzymes have been activated, they start to progressively digest the tissue of the pancreas. Pancreatitis is therefore a process of self or autodigestion.

The second most common cause of pancreatitis is drinking too much alcohol, especially binge drinking. It has been suggested that alcohol causes spasm or oedema of the sphincter of Oddi, leading to a backlog of pancreatic juice as described above. Alcohol also stimulates secretions from the duodenum which in turn triggers the pancreas to secrete more pancreatic juice. This means there is an increased secretion of pancreatic juice at the same time as there is an obstruction of the flow from the pancreatic ducts into the duodenum. This will greatly increase the pressure of pancreatic juice in the pancreatic ducts.

Despite these two well known causes of acute pancreatitis it remains true that a large group of patients present with idiopathic disease, meaning no specific cause can be identified. However, several additional uncommon causes have been identified including trauma, as a side effect of some drugs, some viral infections, congenital disorders and renal failure.

Pathophysiology

Many cases of acute pancreatitis are relatively mild with areas of acute inflammation leading to oedema and congestion. This form of the condition is self-limiting and will recover without active treatment. However, in some cases autodigestion proceeds, with areas of more intense inflammation leading to haemorrhage and necrosis. This serious form is described as acute haemorrhagic necrotising pancreatitis. Haemorrhage may be caused by extensive inflammation or free activated digestive enzymes may digest the walls of blood vessels. Bleeding can be extensive and large areas of the pancreas will be destroyed. In areas of the

Diagram 21.1
A gall stone blocking the ampulla allows bile from the common bile duct to enter the pancreatic ducts, possibly activating pancreatic pre-enzymes. Also a stone blocking the ampulla prevents free drainage of pancreatic secretions leading to an increase in pressure within the pancreatic ducts; this probably triggers activation of intracellular pre-enzymes by an increase in free calcium.

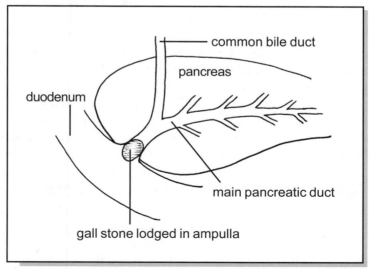

common bile duct

pancreas

duodenum

main pancreatic duct

gall stone lodged in ampulla

pancreas which survive, areas of inflammatory fluid and oedema may be surrounded by fibrous tissue, forming cysts. These are referred to as pancreatic pseudocysts. As enzymes leak out of the damaged pancreas they may spread around the peritoneal cavity leading to peritonitis.

Extensive inflammation will lead to the formation of large volumes of inflammatory fluid. Collection of this fluid within the peritoneal cavity will lead to ascites and abdominal distension; this is an example of fluid third spacing. As inflammatory fluids derive from the blood the accumulation of inflammatory exudates will contribute to hypovolaemia. Any haemorrhage will also lower blood volumes. Both of these mechanisms may therefore contribute to the development of hypovolaemic shock. This in turn will lead to complications of shock such as renal, respiratory and cardiovascular failure. After the acute inflammatory period the necrosed pancreas may become infected leading to sepsis.

Clinical features

The principle symptom of acute pancreatitis is severe upper abdominal pain. Pain from the pancreas is usually fairly well localised in the epigastrium. Usually the pain is sudden in onset and builds up in less than one hour to become constant. Often the pain radiates through to the back. While the abdomen is tender, patients with early stage acute pancreatitis do not usually have the muscle guarding and rebound tenderness associated with conditions which cause early peritonitis. This is because the pancreas is posterior, behind the peritoneal cavity. Usually there will be nausea and vomiting with anorexia. Diarrhoea is also possible. Patients often find the intensity of the pain can be modified by position with less pain being experienced in a supine position (lying on their back). Most patients will develop a fever and tachycardia. Bowel sounds are often reduced as the inflammation spreads to the adjacent areas of the GI tract. The principle diagnostic test used in suspected pancreatitis is increased serum amylase. As this digestive enzyme leaks out of the damaged pancreas, some is absorbed into the blood, where elevated levels may be detected. Ultrasound or CT scanning will demonstrate pancreatic swelling. As with other inflammatory conditions C-reactive protein (CRP) levels in the blood will be increased. Higher levels of CRP indicate more serious disease with a poorer prognosis. Obesity often indicates a poorer prognosis; this may be because lipase will digest readily available fat, which will result in larger areas of inflammation.

Treatment principles in severe acute pancreatitis

As fluid loss may be extensive these patients should be kept under strict fluid balance observation. Intravenous fluids will be required to compensate for the volumes of fluid lost into the abdominal cavity, (this is an example of third spacing of fluids). A central venous pressure line will allow monitoring and aid the process of fluid replacement titration. A urinary catheter should be in situ to monitor hourly urine volumes. Electrolyte replacement should be guided by regular serum biochemistry. Hypocalcaemia is a particular risk. Nasogastric drainage prevents gastric distension and vomiting if paralytic ileus is present.

Pain control may include pethidine. However, morphine based analgesics have a side effect of contracting the sphincter of Oddi so should be used with discretion. Antibiotics are given as infection is likely to complicate the condition. Arterial blood gases and peripheral oxygen saturations should be monitored and oxygen given as required to treat hypoxia. Patients should not be given oral food as this will stimulate the pancreas to produce more enzymes and so make the condition worse. If the patient remains ill for a period of time they may be fed by giving enteral feed, directly into the jejunum via a nasojejunal tube. This provides the patient with nutrition which can be absorbed from the ileum. However, as the pancreas is bypassed it is not stimulated to produce more digestive enzymes. In severe disease this enteral feeding should be started at an early stage as the pancreatitis causes a severely catabolic state and nutritional support is required. Feeding also reduces the risk of endotoxaemia as bacteria from the gut are less likely to enter the blood. Prophylaxis of thromboembolism (DVT and PE) with low dose subcutaneous heparin must be considered.

Surgery has a high mortality in acute pancreatitis as it aids the spread of digestive enzymes and potential infection over a large area. However, after about 7 days it may be necessary to resect necrotic areas as these act as a focus for potentially overwhelming infection. After the patient has recovered from an acute attack the causes of the problem should be removed to prevent recurrence. If the underlying cause was gallstones, cholecystectomy will be advisable. If the cause was alcohol this should never be consumed again.

Chronic pancreatitis

Aetiology

In developing countries, chronic pancreatitis is often associated with malnutrition, particularly a lack of protein. This environmental factor may act on a genetic predisposition. In developed countries, excess alcohol consumption accounts for the majority of cases. Typically there is a history of persistent heavy drinking. Chronic obstruction of the pancreatic duct and cystic fibrosis are other possible causes. As in acute pancreatitis, the underlying cause is premature activation of protein digesting enzymes within the pancreas. In chronic pancreatitis alcohol may inhibit the natural proteins which prevent activation of trypsinogen, as well as causing disease via the mechanisms described below.

Pathophysiology

Alcohol has the effect of stimulating the pancreatic exocrine (acinar) cells to secrete more enzyme proteins. However, alcohol does not stimulate the secretion of correspondingly increased volumes of water. This means the proteins secreted are in less water which makes the secretions viscid. These thick secretions do not flow out of the small pancreatic ducts as normal and start to form protein plugs. These plugs then block the ducts, leading to an increase in pressure and dilation of the obstructed area. Enzymes will then be activated in the secretory acinar cells which then digest and necrose a local area of tissue. There will be chronic inflammation and it is common for damaged areas to fibrose and calcify. Blockage of ducts may also lead to cyst formation. As more and more healthy tissue is lost to these ongoing processes, there is progressive destruction of the exocrine and endocrine tissues of the gland.

Clinical features

Most patients complain of epigastric pain, often radiating through to the back. Pain may occur in episodes or be chronic. The pain may occur either after meals or independently of meals, and usually lasts for several hours. In other

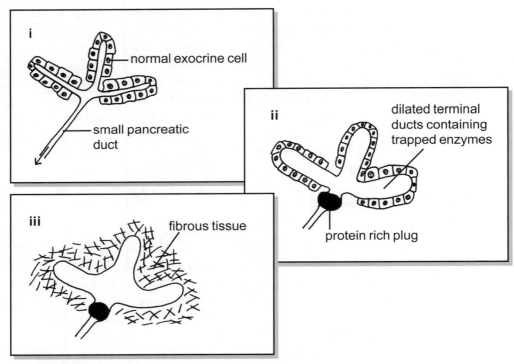

Diagram 21.2
Pathophysiology in chronic pancreatitis;
i   Normal small pancreatic duct; cells surrounding the terminal passages secrete exocrine products into the ducts; arrow shows secretions leaving the small duct.
ii Duct is occluded by a protein rich plug; this leads to dilation and increased pressure behind the plug.
iii Healthy tissue is progressively digested and necrosed to be replaced with fibrous, scar tissue. Ultimately the area may calcify.

patients pain may be an ongoing constant problem for many years. If a patient can stop drinking alcohol the severity of the pain should be reduced in the longer term. Some patients experience reduced pain when leaning forward. The pain is caused by congestion of the pancreatic ducts or by inflammation affecting pancreatic nerves or other sensory nerves close to the pancreas. Diarrhoea is a possible chronic feature.

As a result of progressive damage to the exocrine tissue there are reduced volumes of pancreatic digestive enzymes available for normal digestion of food. This results in incomplete digestive breakdown with associated reduced rates of absorption. Consequences of this include malnutrition, malabsorption and weight loss. Periods of anorexia may compound the problems of malnutrition and weight loss. In more advanced disease fat is not digested as insufficient pancreatic lipase is produced by the failing gland. This means fats are not absorbed giving rise to the bulky, offensive stools seen in steatorrhoea. In some patients destruction of pancreatic islets means there is a loss of the insulin secreting beta cells resulting in diabetes mellitus. Serum amylase levels may be normal most of the time as there is very little functional pancreatic tissue left to produce the enzyme.

Treatment

Pain should be treated using NSAIDs, tramadol and sometimes tricyclics. For severe ongoing pain surgical resection may be considered; sometimes it is possible to improve ductal drainage which may also reduce pain. Giving oral pancreatic enzymes helps the digestion of food, and reduces steatorrhoea. This works by replacing enzymes the pancreas is no longer able to produce. These oral enzymes may also reduce pain, as they result in less stimulation of the pancreas to produce enzymes. Any underlying cause of chronic pancreatitis should be treated and alcohol is totally forbidden. If a patient stops drinking alcohol the progression of the disease should be halted and pain reduced. Diabetes mellitus will probably require insulin injections.

Carcinoma of the pancreas

This is the eleventh most common primary cancer diagnosed in the UK. Incidence increases with age.

Aetiology

Smoking is the most common environmental risk factor for pancreatic carcinoma. This is probably due to the absorption of carcinogens from the lungs into the blood, which then circulates to the pancreas. If a person stops smoking their risk will decline over a 5-10 year period to approximately that of nonsmokers. Obesity, especially central obesity, is a risk factor as is red meat consumption, especially processed red meat such as burgers, meat pies and sausages. A diet rich in fresh fruits and vegetables is protective. Fruits and vegetables rich in folate and lycopenes (such as tomatoes) may be especially good at reducing the risk of developing pancreatic cancer. Approximately 5-10% of patients with pancreatic carcinoma have some genetic predisposition to developing the disease. Patients with long standing chronic pancreatitis are at increased risk, although alcohol alone does not appear to be a factor.

Pathophysiology

Pancreatic cancer is almost always an adenocarcinoma, arising from the pancreatic ducts. The pancreas is described as an organ with a head, body and tail. The majority of tumours are found in the head area. As the common bile duct passes through the head of the pancreas, tumours in this area compress this duct, leading to obstruction and jaundice. Jaundice is often severe with extreme pruritus (itching).

Pain results from invasion of local neurological structures (the coeliac plexus) and is usually constant and boring. Radiation of pain from the upper abdomen to the back is common and the patient may experience limited relief by leaning forward. Tumours affecting the body or tail of the pancreas usually present later with dull pain, anorexia and weight loss. Weight loss, which is likely to be extensive, is caused by malabsorption and steatorrhoea, anorexia and the metabolic effects of the tumour. Many patients develop the severe muscle wasting, weight loss and weakness seen in cachexia. With all pancreatic tumours it may be possible to feel a mass in the epigastrium. A distended gall bladder may also be palpable. Unfortunately pancreatic cancers usually metastasise to involve local structures and regional lymph nodes at an early stage. As the pancreatic veins drain into the splenic vein, which carries blood directly to the liver via the hepatic portal vein, metastasis to the liver is common.

Treatment

Pancreatic cancer has a very poor outlook with a very low 5 year survival rate after diagnosis. Sometimes, if the condition is detected at an early stage it may be possible to surgically resect a localised tumour. Chemotherapy and radiotherapy may be used as part of curative treatment or palliative strategy. Locating a stent in the common bile duct may allow bile to pass from the common bile duct into the duodenum and so relieve obstructive jaundice. Pain should be managed with analgesia and sometimes the coeliac plexus can be injected with pure alcohol to kill the nerves generating the pain.

Insulinomas

These are tumours of the beta cells in the pancreatic islets (of Langerhans), most of which are benign. Increased numbers of beta cells leads to an increase in insulin production and the patient presents with hypoglycaemia.

CHAPTER 22

Genitourinary Disorders

Urinary stones (calculi)

This is a common disorder affecting about 12% of men and 5% of women at some time during their lives. A calculus describes any concretion (a deposit of hard material) which forms in passages which transmit secretions or in cavities associated with secretions. Urinary calculi are often described as 'stones'. 'Lith' or 'litho' are prefixes used to describe calculi. Urolithiasis describes the process of stone formation in the urinary tract. Nephrolithiasis literally means kidney stones.

Aetiology

Several factors may induce and develop stone formation. Reduced urine volumes are a major factor. This will result in more concentrated urine which contains a higher proportion of waste products which in turn increases the likelihood of crystal precipitation. Bacterial infection may also trigger crystal formation. Once the initial precipitation has occurred more salts can crystallise onto the forming stone making it bigger.

Another group of possible causes of urinary calculi are metabolic abnormalities. For example, increased levels of calcium in the blood will lead to increased concentrations in the urine (i.e. hypercalcaemia leads to hypercalciuria) making stone formation more likely. Very acid or alkaline urine and increased concentrations of sodium or calcium in urine are other risk factors.

Overall, men suffer from urinary stones more than women. They are also more prevalent in some geographical areas such as the Middle East. Stone formation in the bladder in adults is usually caused by bladder outflow obstruction. This in turn may be caused by an enlarged prostate, a urethral stricture or a bladder which has an interruption of normal neurological function, e.g. after spinal injury. In children, malnutrition is a common global cause of bladder stones. The treatment for this is to provide children with an adequate balanced diet.

Secondary prevention

Once a person has developed a urinary stone they have a significantly increased risk of developing another one. Recurrence rates are as high as 50% over 5 years. Such people should drink plenty water and aim to pass at least 2.5 litres of urine per day. A useful guide is for patients to monitor the colour of their urine; dark yellow urine is too concentrated. Patients should be advised to drink enough water to pass large volumes of very light coloured urine. People often produce more concentrated urine overnight; this should be avoided by drinking water before going to bed and during the night if they wake up. While this means they may need to get up in the night to pass urine, this is preferable to stone recurrence.

Dehydration should be avoided. This is particularly likely during periods of hot weather, exercise or after alcohol consumption. Patients should also be advised to eat less red meat, refined sugar, dairy products and sodium intake should be limited. Vitamin D supplements should not be taken. They should eat more citrus fruit and oily fish. Any urinary infections should be treated promptly.

Pathophysiology and clinical features

Stones forming in the urinary tract vary in size; some are like small grains of sand, while so called 'staghorn' calculi may almost fill up the renal calyces. Smaller stones under 4 mm in diameter will normally be passed naturally but larger stones may well require some form of intervention to remove them. Urinary stones are usually composed of a protein matrix or framework. This framework supports crystallised material, most commonly calcium salts such as calcium oxalate or phosphate. Other stones are composed primarily of magnesium ammonium phosphate (stuvite) and are associated with infection. Less commonly stones are composed of uric acid or cystine.

Urinary stones may be single or multiple. Most stones probably form in the upper urinary tract and pass down to the bladder; however some stones also form in the bladder. Stones in the kidney may cause pressure and subsequent localised necrosis of renal tissue. Calculi in the kidneys or ureters may obstruct the flow of urine leading to hydronephrosis with subsequent renal impairment. In obstructive hydronephrosis there is a reduced outflow of urine which leads to distension of the renal pelvis with urine. If obstructive hydronephrosis is not treated it will cause renal atrophy and eventual failure.

Pain is a common presentation. Some pain is generated when calculi move around within the calyces; this is sometimes referred to as calyceal colic. Ureteric colic occurs when a stone is passing down the ureter which may lead to spasm of the ureter with obstruction. Ureteric colic is one of the worst of all pains and must therefore constitute a medical emergency. The patient suddenly becomes aware of loin pain, with radiation to the flank, groin and often into the testes or labium. The intensity of the pain increases over a few minutes and then remains constant and severe. Some patients vomit and there is usually pallor and sweating. Pain often passes off after about 2 hours but may be present for much longer. After an acute episode of pain there is often lingering dull pain in the loin or back. The presence of the stone passing down a ureter leads to haematuria. Urine should always be tested for the presence of blood as this helps to confirm the diagnosis.

Another presentation of calculi is urinary tract infection. A ureteric stone may lead to an obstruction, damming back a volume of stagnant urine. This is another case of stasis leading to possible infection. Bladder stones may cause cystitis and stones in the kidney may lead to acute pyelonephritis. There is also the risk of a bladder infection ascending to cause pyelonephritis.

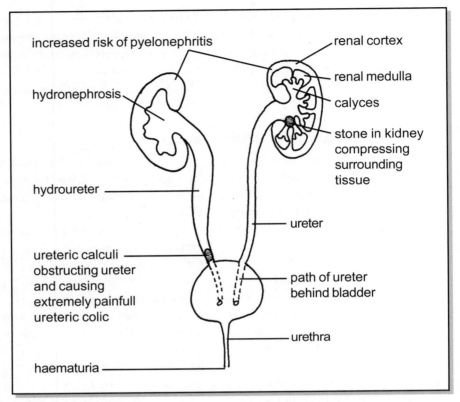

Diagram 22.1
Pathophysiology and possible complications of urinary calculi.

Management

Renal colic should be managed with adequate doses of morphine. Intravenous morphine works rapidly and provides some relief; 10 mg may be titrated as an initial adult dose. NSAIDs such as diclofenac may be helpful. It also seems logical to give the patient a high fluid intake. This is sometimes called hydrotherapy and may involve giving intravenous fluids and possibly a diuretic. People who favour this approach argue that the increased flow of urine down the ureters helps to flush the calculi into the bladder. Once a calculus has entered the bladder any ureteric colic will subside.

Some stones in the kidneys, renal pelvis or ureters can be broken down by using shock wave lithotripsy. In this treatment, targeted shock waves are externally generated, passed through a water medium and into the patient to fragment stones within the urinary tract. Once stones are fragmented, the pieces are small enough to be passed naturally.

Stones in the kidney or renal pelvis can be removed using percutaneous (through the skin) nephrolithotomy. This involves passing an instrument directly into the urinary tract through the upper abdominal wall or lower chest, then removing the stone. Calculi in the lower ureter can be removed by passing a catheter with a stone removal device into the ureter, via the urethra and bladder. Bladder stones can be physically broken up using an interventional cystoscopic technique. Open surgery is only indicated in a small minority of cases, usually for much larger stones.

Benign prostatic hyperplasia (BPH)

Hyperplasia refers to an increase in the number of cells present. Benign means that the condition is not malignant. Benign prostatic hyperplasia is also sometimes referred to as nodular hyperplasia of the prostate. This condition is very common in older men and some prostatic enlargement is part of the normal ageing process.

Aetiology

BPH is caused by an imbalance between cellular proliferation and programmed cell death. There is some stimulation of prostatic tissue by testosterone; however this male hormone has a much more active metabolite called dihydrotestosterone. If there is an increase in dihydrotestosterone this will stimulate an increased cellular proliferation. This hormonal influence is consistent with the observation that BPH never develops in eunuchs, as long as castration occurred before puberty. In addition to this hormonal over-stimulation of cell division there is a reduction in programmed cell death via the process of apoptosis. The combination of increased stimulation of cell division with reduced rates of cell death results in an increase in the total number of cells present in the gland. As cells take up space the gland enlarges and becomes bulky. Apoptosis rates may be reduced due to a deficiency of a factor which normally stimulates cell death, called transforming growth factor beta. Changes in the size and consistency of the prostate gland can be detected in men from the 40s onward, although this does not usually become clinically significant until a man is in his 60s. The condition is common in men of African and European extraction but less common in Asia.

Pathophysiology

Hyperplasia involves the connective, smooth muscle and glandular tissues of the prostate gland. Early hyperplasia begins in the submucosa close to the urethra and expands outwards. This inner area of prostatic tissue is also referred to as the transitional zone. Anatomically the urethra passes through the prostate, this means that the hyperplasia results in periurethral swelling with progressive compression of the prostatic urethra. Compression can result in a highly narrowed, slit like passage through the prostatic urethra. As a result of this urethral narrowing there is bladder outflow obstruction making it progressively more difficult to pass urine. This means the bladder needs to generate higher pressures to overcome the increased outflow resistance.

Increased outflow resistance therefore results in higher pressures within the bladder. This in turn means the workload of the muscle in the bladder wall (the detrusor muscle) is increased. When the workload of a muscle is increased, the individual cells respond by increasing in size, an example of hypertrophy. As the distribution of smooth muscle fibres over the wall of the bladder is irregular, some areas of bladder wall hypertrophy more than others resulting in trabeculation. This results in areas between bundles of muscle hypertrophy where the bladder wall is relatively weak. The increased pressure within the bladder will push a weaker area outwards to form a blind ended pouch called a diverticulum. These blind ended spaces cause stasis of urine, leading to increased risk of infection, stone formation and malignancy.

Progressive inability to empty the bladder, as a result of outflow obstruction, leads to chronic retention of urine. After passing some urine, there is a residual volume retained in the bladder which may lead to dribbling, referred to as overflow. If the condition is not treated, residual volumes of urine increase over time, eventually resulting in failure of the valves which prevent reflux from the bladder back into the ureter (the vesicoureteric valve) with subsequent hydroureter and hydronephrosis. BPH also results in the prostatic tissue being gradually compressed and there is interference with normal uretheral sphincter function.

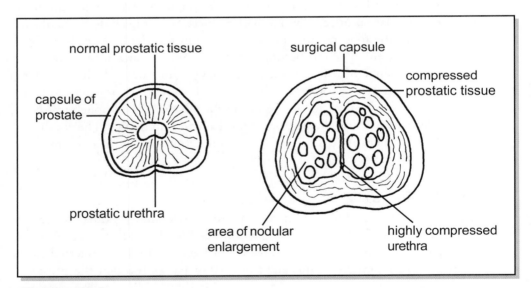

Diagram 22.2
Cross section of a normal prostate gland and urethra in comparison to a gland showing BPH. In the enlarged gland a periurethral area of nodular enlargement is obvious, this has compressed the urethra and normal prostatic tissue. Internal enlargement also causes compression of peripheral prostatic tissues leading to fibrosis and the formation of a so called 'surgical capsule'.

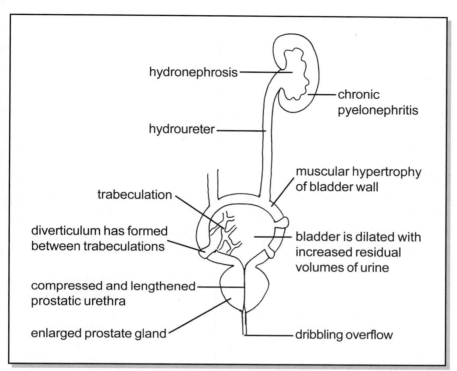

hydronephrosis

chronic pyelonephritis

hydroureter

muscular hypertrophy of bladder wall

trabeculation

diverticulum has formed between trabeculations

bladder is dilated with increased residual volumes of urine

compressed and lengthened prostatic urethra

enlarged prostate gland

dribbling overflow

Diagram 22.3
Benign prostatic enlargement and associated complication.

Clinical features

Patients feel the desire to pass urine often. This is called frequency but only small volumes of urine are passed at any one time. There is also urgency which describes the feeling of immediate need to pass urine. Despite the urgent need it often takes time before a flow of urine can be initiated, referred to as hesitancy. Even when urination has begun, the flow is weak and the patient often strains to expel the urine. High residual pressures in the bladder may lead to dribbling incontinence. Often the patient needs to get up several times during the night to urinate, a feature termed nocturia. Collectively, the features generated by an enlarged prostate gland are termed lower urinary tract symptoms (LUTS). In addition to detrusor hypertrophy and diverticulum formation, bladder stones and urinary infections are possible complications. An enlarged prostate can be palpated by a per rectum digital examination through the anterior surface of the rectum.

Over time, as the bladder wall stretches, large volumes of urine can be painlessly retained. The dilated bladder can be palpated and percussed in the pelvis. Volumetric ultrasound scanning is also useful for estimation of the retained volume of urine. Typically when the retained volume reaches 1 litre the urine will reflux back into the ureters and kidneys leading to hydroureter and hydronephrosis. If left untreated these complications will lead to features of renal failure and uraemia. Eventually, an untreated patient will die from renal failure.

Blood may be tested for levels of prostate specific antigen (PSA). Serum levels of PSA increase with increasing mass of the prostate gland; this means PSA levels can be used as a crude proxy for the degree of gland enlargement. Prostate cancer and acute bacterial prostatitis will also lead to increased levels of PSA.

Management

Some medical treatments are available for management of moderate BPH, for example 5 alpha reductase inhibitors act by inhibiting the enzyme which converts testosterone into dihydrotestosterone. The preferred surgical option is transurethral resection of the prostate (TURP). In this procedure the inner layers of the gland are 'shaved' off using a resectoscope and a cutting diathermy loop. In some cases of advanced disease open surgical prostatectomy is indicated. Episodes of acute retention may occur, possibly precipitated by urinary infection, alcohol or constipation. These may need to be managed with temporary urinary catheterisation.

Carcinoma of the prostate

This is the single most common malignancy diagnosed in men in the UK and US having overtaken bronchogenic malignancy as the most common cancer. In the UK prostatic cancer accounts for 21% of all malignant neoplasms diagnosed in men. The mean age of presentation is 70 years and post mortem studies suggest that the majority of men aged over 80 have malignant prostatic changes.

Aetiology

The precise cause is unknown, but genetic, hormonal and dietary factors are all potentially influential. Incidence of prostate cancer is higher in men with relatives who have developed the disease, indicating a possible genetic factor. As about 10% of cases probably have a genetic basis, first order relatives of patients should probably be screened for the disorder. Men with a family history of the disease also tend to develop the condition at an earlier age. Several specific genes have been identified which are strongly associated with prostate cancer development. Some reports have suggested a shared familial risk for prostate and breast cancer. Hormonal factors are also relevant in the development of the condition. Eunuchs do not develop adenocarcinoma of the prostate, probably because testosterone is needed to stimulate mitosis in the prostatic glandular tissue.

Interestingly, carcinoma of the prostate is rare in China and Japan and while this may be partly genetic it has been suggested it is because there is less fat in the diet. Japanese men living in the United States, eating a higher fat diet, suffer from more prostate cancer than their relatives living in Japan. Overall, the condition is less common in vegetarians and eating soy seems to be protective. Vitamin E and selenium may be protective as these are both antioxidants. It is also probable that vitamin D and skin exposure to sunlight are protective. Epidemiological studies strongly indicate that tomatoes are protective, probably because they contain an antioxidant called lycopene.

Pathophysiology

The vast majority of cases are adenocarcinomas. Carcinoma means a malignant neoplasm derived from epithelial tissue, and adeno relates to glandular tissue. Most commonly carcinoma arises in the peripheral tissues of the gland. From here the cancer can spread out of the prostatic capsule leading to early metastasis to the pelvic lymph nodes and then to distant sites. There may also be direct invasion into the bladder. As the tumour grows, the urethra may be constricted generating lower urinary tract features.

Clinical features

Most commonly patients present with features of LUTS which are indistinguishable from those of benign prostatic hyperplasia. These features include urinary retention, decreased urine stream, urinary frequency, urgency and possible haematuria. Less commonly patients present with evidence of metastatic disease including obstruction of the ureters, bone pain, pathological fracture, weight loss or anaemia.

Screening and management

If serum PSA levels are raised this may arouse suspicions and a biopsy may be taken to diagnose the cause. On rectal examination, a malignant prostate gland feels hard and irregular. Treatment options include radiotherapy and radical

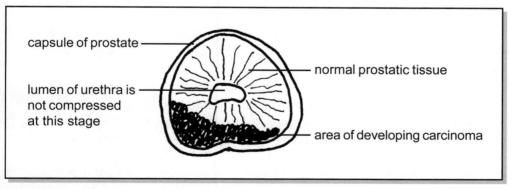

Diagram 22.4
Unlike the pathology in BPH which starts immediately around the urethra, carcinoma of the prostate usually arises from peripheral tissues. This means early urinary symptoms are usually absent in the initial stages of the disease.

prostatectomy. Like breast cancer, prostate cancer is sensitive to hormonal influences. Reducing the levels of male androgen hormones will slow progression of the disease by reducing rates of cell division in prostate derived cells. This can be done surgically by bilateral orchidectomy, or more likely by giving drugs which reduce androgen levels or activity.

Prostatitis

Inflammation of the prostate gland may be acute or chronic. Acute prostatitis is usually associated with other urinary infections and is caused by reflux of infected urine into the prostate gland. There are febrile symptoms with perineal pain. (The perineum is the area between the anus and the base of the penis.) There may also be other urinary features such as dysuria, bladder irritability, obstruction, abscess formation and haematuria. Haematospermia (blood in the seminal fluid) is another possible feature. Infection is caused by the growth of bacteria within the gland and antibiotics may need to be given for several weeks.

In the chronic form of prostatitis, infection may come from the urethra and is often difficult to eradicate. Patients complain of aching in the perineum, low back pain, low grade fever, possible burning during ejaculation and urinary features. Long courses of antibiotics may be indicated, sometimes they need to be taken long term to suppress the condition.

Carcinoma of the bladder

The bladder is the most common site for urinary tract tumours. The condition usually presents in older people and is more common in men. Smoking is a causative factor. Cancer causing chemicals are absorbed into the body from inhaled smoke, through the lungs. As carcinogens, these chemicals are treated as waste products, so are excreted by the kidneys. As a result, carcinogens accumulate in the bladder with the urine. This gives a time when the bladder lining is exposed to these chemicals and malignant changes may develop. Other possible factors are carcinogens from the dye and chemical industries and analgesic abuse. The most common cause world wide is chronic cystitis caused by schistosomiasis.

The pathology is transitional cell carcinoma, arising from the pear shaped epithelial transitional cells comprising the lining of the bladder. The most common presentation is painless haematuria with blood well mixed in the urine. It should be assumed that painless, visible haematuria is from a tumour until proved otherwise. Retention of urine and UTI are other possible presentations. Bladder tumours are diagnosed by cystoscopy. Treatment depends on the stage the disease process has reached and the degree of spread. Local resection or diathermy may be possible in early disease. It is also possible to infuse intravesical chemotherapy directly into the bladder. Later options include more radical surgery, radiotherapy and systemic chemotherapy.

Testicular cancer

Fortunately these tumours are relatively rare; however they are important to know about as they affect young men. Testicular cancer is the most common malignancy in men in the 15-35 years age group. Unfortunately this is the age group who often feel embarrassed, and may delay asking for medical help. There is no clear cause of testicular cancer but a history of undescended testis in childhood is a recognised risk factor. Pathologically a seminoma arises from the seminiferous tubules and is usually a fairly low grade malignancy. A teratoma arises from primitive germ cells and may be more aggressive. Tumours arising from Leydig cells are rare.

Most patients present with a painless lump or swelling in one of the testis. Others present with a testicular ache. Testicular self examination is best carried out when they are warm, e.g. after a hot bath when the testes are well descended. The earlier the condition is detected and treated the better. Any lump discovered in the testes should be considered malignant until proved otherwise and ultrasound scanning usually provides an accurate diagnosis. Without treatment the disease will metastasise to areas such as the lungs, liver and retroperitoneal area. The primary treatment is orchidectomy and most forms of the disease respond very well to chemotherapy giving rise to a reasonably good prognosis in most cases.

Cervical Cancer

Aetiological factors

The risk of developing cervical cancer increases with an early age of first sexual intercourse. The more sexual partners a woman has, and the more partners any one of her sexual partners has had, the greater the risk. From this it can be seen that incidence of the disease could be reduced if young women postpone beginning sexual activity and choose a partner who has had few, if any previous partners himself. The explanation for the sexually transmitted nature of cervical cancer is that 95% of cases are caused by human papilloma virus (HPV) infection, a virus which is passed on during sex. Evidence for this viral aetiology is that HPV viral DNA is found in more than 90% of cervical squamous malignant tissue which is examined.

However, not all women infected with HPV develop cervical cancer, so other factors must be involved in disease development and progression. These factors probably reduce the effectiveness of local immunity, allowing the viral damage to accumulate. These factors include multiparity (having many babies), poor nutritional status and vitamin deficiencies, smoking, oral contraceptive use and HIV infection. There are also many different types of HPV (77 have been identified so far) with varying degrees of pathogenisity (disease causing potential). HPV types 16 and 18 are the most common forms seen in cervical cancers.

The incidence of cervical cancer has been falling in most developed countries as a result of effective screening programmes. However, it remains a leading malignancy in women of less developed countries.

Pathophysiology

Cervical cancer is a squamous cell carcinoma in most cases. Most commonly, malignant changes arise in the cervical os. The cervical os is the opening of the cervix into the vagina. In this area, there is a boundary between the stratified squamous cells of the vagina and the columnar cells of the cervix, known as the squamocolumnar junction. The columnar cells in the area of the squamocolumnar junction form a region called the transformation zone. It is the cells in this area which can change into malignant squamous cells. This process of cellular transformation is referred to as metaplasia and results in a dysplasia with a distinct change from normal to abnormal cells.

Cytologists grade dysplasia in cervical cells using the CIN classification. CIN stands for cervical intraepithelial neoplasia. CIN-1 is mild dysplasia, CIN-2 moderate and CIN-3 describes severe dysplasia and carcinoma in situ. It was believed that the sequence of abnormal cell development progressed through mild, moderate and severe dysplasia before finally becoming malignant. However, most current thinking suggests that CIN-1, CIN-II and CIN-III lesions arise as such.

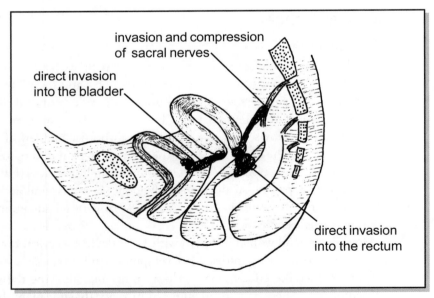

Diagram 22.5
Direct invasion of adjacent tissues in cervical cancer can lead to the formation of fistulae between the vagina, bowel or bladder. Posterior direct spread can compress and invade the sacral nerve roots. Chronic secondary infection may also be present.

HPV infection without CIN changes and CIN-I are grouped together as low grade squamous intraepithelial lesions (SILs) while CIN-II and CIN-III are classified as high grade SILs. It is more likely that high grade SILs will develop into an aggressive tumour which will invade and metastasise. However CIN-I, low grade SIL, still has some potential to become malignant.

Less commonly, cervical cancer may also arise from the glandular tissue associated with the columnar epithelium of the endocervix; this is an example of an adenocarcinoma.

Clinical features

Early disease is asymptomatic, after this bleeding is usually one of the first features. This may be post coital (coitus means sexual intercourse) or there may be blood spots or light bleeding between periods. Post menopausal or intermenstrual bleeding should always be investigated and explained as this may arise from a malignancy. Irregular shaped tumours increase the probability of infection becoming established. This leads to the development of an infective vaginal discharge, which is often very smelly. Chronic infection is a common problem in cervical cancer and may generate signs of chronic pelvic inflammation.

As the disease develops there will be pain during sex. Pain at other times usually indicates spread of the disease to the pelvic cavity. Local invasion often involves the bladder or rectum resulting in fistula formation. A fistula is an abnormal communication between two body cavities. If there is a fistula between the rectum and vagina or bladder and vagina, faeces or urine may come out of the vagina. Direct spread backwards involves the sacral nerve plexus leading to severe sciatic pain. Systemic metastatic spread is via the lymphatics with distant spread commonly affecting the liver, lungs and bones.

Screening

The incidence of cervical cancer has fallen greatly in western countries as a result of cytological screening. Cells smeared from the cervix can be examined and classified using the CIN classification. Progress from normal to malignant cells normally takes several years meaning the developing disorder can be detected and treated before the first malignant cells appear. Screening protocols vary but as a general principle sexually active women should be screened every 3 years.

Management

If detected and treated at an early, preferably pre-malignant stage, the outlook for this disorder is very good. Examination and early treatment is often aided with the use of colposcopy. A colposcope is an instrument which allows clear binocular inspection of the cervix with magnification allowing for visualization of possible erosions, ulcer or increase in cervical size. Early local treatment may involve cryosurgery, diathermy or CO_2 laser ablation. Resection of a cone of tissue from the cervix may also be curative although long term follow up is necessary. In more advanced disease, hysterectomy may be appropriate. Radiotherapy is the other main option.

Diagram 22.6
Cervical smears are taken from the os in the region of the transformation zone, just past the squamocolumnar junction.

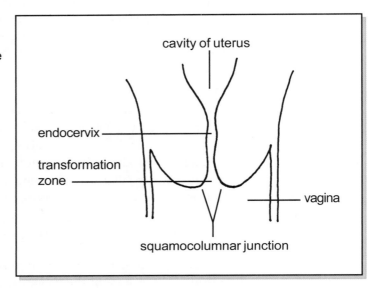

Diagram 22.7
Histology of the squamocolumnar junction. Cells of the transformation zone are shaded in this diagram and are the ones which are at risk of developing CIN and malignant changes. A cervical smear must harvest some of these cells for examination. In postmenopausal women the transformation zone is deeper in the endocervix. (Cells are not drawn to scale.)

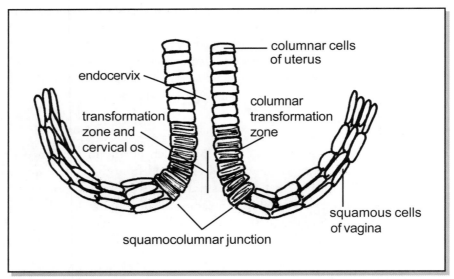

Urinary tract infections (UTIs)

UTIs are infections in any part of the urinary tract. Clearly infection will lead to inflammation. Cystitis refers to inflammation of the bladder while pyelonephritis is inflammation of the kidney. UTI is common in women but relatively uncommon in men. In children UTI has special significance so will be considered separately.

Urinary tract infection in adults

Aetiology

Most UTIs are caused by coliform bacteria from the patient's bowel, such as Escherichia coli or Streptococcus faecalis, gaining access into the urinary tract. While infection may spread to the urinary tract via the blood, lymphatics or a fistula, the most common route is for bacteria to enter then ascend through the lumen of the urethra. In women, the urethra is much shorter than in men and the urethral orifice (opening) is close to areas which may be heavily colonised with bacteria.

Bacteria migrate from the anus to colonise the area around the lower vagina and urethra. Bacteria may migrate up the short female urethra into the bladder to cause cystitis. Sexual intercourse greatly assists the passage of bacteria up the urethra making cystitis more likely. This explains why more infections are reported when young women become sexually active. Once in the bladder, bacteria may multiply to cause infection.

Urine in the bladder is normally sterile. This sterility is maintained by the one way flow of urine from the bladder out of the urethra. If the odd bacteria does manage to enter the bladder, it is usually washed out in the flow of urine. Large volumes of urine will flush bacteria out of the bladder and urethra efficiently. This is why low urine volumes and infrequent emptying of the bladder predispose to infection while passing large and regular volumes of urine helps to prevent and treat cystitis.

Other factors may predispose to UTI including any anatomical abnormality of the tract such as a tumour or scarring from previous infections which provide bacteria with a site to colonise. An enlarged prostate will lead to stasis of urine which means that any bacteria which do enter the bladder have plenty of time to reproduce. Urinary stones are another possible site of chronic infection which may multiply and spread causing occasional acute exacerbations. Glucosuria, in poorly managed diabetes mellitus is another risk factor as the sugar provides a ready food supply for bacteria. Catheters and other instruments passed into the bladder will traumatise the urethra and so predispose to infection. UTIs are common in pregnancy. There is a risk that infection may ascend to the kidneys, leading to pyelonephritis, which may stimulate premature delivery. All pregnant women should be screened for bacteria in urine at their first prenatal visit and given antibiotics if indicated.

Diagram 22.8
Bacteria may migrate from the anus, forward to the area around the vagina and urethral orifice. From here they may ascend the urethra, (possibly assisted by sexual intercourse) into the bladder, (A to B to C on the diagram). Growth of bacteria in the bladder causes cystitis. This is why nurses have traditionally been advised to wipe female bottoms (when the need arises) from the front, backwards.

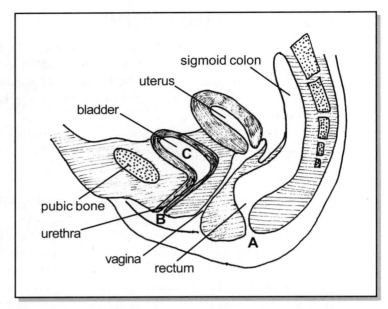

Clinical features in UTI

In cystitis there is frequency and urgency, often a desperate need to pass urine is experienced, but little or no urine comes out. These features are probably produced by irritation of the lower bladder and sphincter. Passing urine is painful (dysuria), often with a burning sensation which is largely due to urethral inflammation. There may be some pain over the bladder in the suprapubic area. The internal lining of the urinary tract is referred to as the urothelial surface. This is a constant surface from the bladder up to the renal pelvis. This allows for the possible spread of infection from the bladder to the upper urinary tract. If infection ascends, the kidneys may become involved resulting in serious infection. In acute pyelonephritis there is fever and the patient feels very unwell with significant malaise. Loin pain usually develops as the kidneys become inflamed. In any urinary infection there may be frank blood and pus in the urine.

Diagnosis

Detection of pus cells or nitrite in urine is a good indication of bacterial infection. If UTI is suspected a mid-stream sample of urine should be obtained and sent for culture. A mid-stream sample prevents collecting bacteria from the urethra in the early flow. Traditionally a UTI has been diagnosed when there are over 100,000 organisms found per 1 ml of urine. However, infections much less serious than this can be clinically significant. A 'low count bacteriuria' is considered to be at least 1000 organisms per ml. Further urological tests may be indicated if an underlying cause of the infection is suspected. These may include ultrasound, intravenous pyelogram, intravenous isotope studies and cystoscopy.

Treatment of UTI

Antibiotics may be commenced on clinical grounds with a positive dip stick test for leucocyte esterase and nitrite. The antibacterial agent can later be modified in the light of sensitivity testing. Commonly used preparations include amoxicillin, oral cephalosporin and trimethoprim. For more serious infections intravenous antibiotics may be indicated.

UTIs may be partly prevented by ensuring an adequate to high fluid intake. This should include plenty of water as tea, coffee and alcohol all have a diuretic effect. The bladder should be fully emptied when urine is passed. If women empty the bladder after sex, then any bacteria which have been propelled up the urethra should be flushed out. Clearly if any underlying cause of a UTI is identified, this should be corrected if possible.

UTIs in children

Young children may develop potentially serious urinary tract infections as a result of congenital abnormalities such as vesicoureteric reflux, obstruction or bladder dysfunction. If these UTIs are not identified, and treated, they may lead to chronic pyelonephritis. Such chronic renal infection will lead to scarring and permanent renal damage. This can give rise to chronic renal failure and hypertension. It is therefore essential that such infections are identified and treated as this will prevent irreversible renal damage. Many adults who have to be admitted for long term renal dialysis have suffered from chronic pyelonephritis which had its origins in childhood. Without dialysis or transplant end stage renal failure will of course result in death.

Presentation

This problem is relatively common as 2% of boys and 8% of girls develop UTIs in childhood. While not all children who develop a UTI will need long term treatment they should all be referred to a specialist for investigations. Neonates usually have a non-specific presentation with irritability, poor feeding and vomiting. Other children may develop general features of infection as bacteria spread around the body. This may present as sepsis or even meningitis. Older babies and toddlers often present with vomiting, diarrhoea, irritability and fever. In school age children the clinical features are more similar to those presenting in adults with dysuria, frequency and possible suprapubic and loin pain.

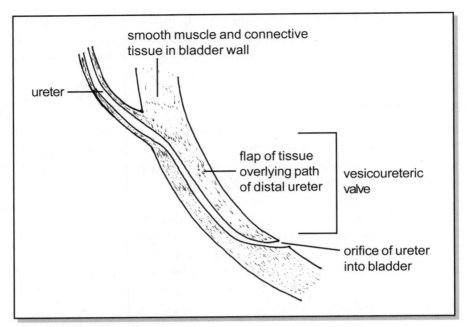

Diagram 22.9i
In normal anatomy the ureters follow a long course through the bladder wall at a shallow angle. This forms a flap to close off the orifice of the ureter.

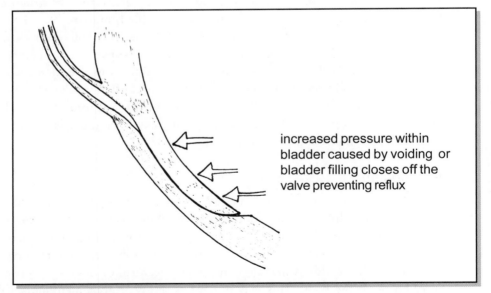

Diagram 22.9ii
When the pressure in the bladder is increased to facilitate voiding, the ureter is 'pinched off' forming a seal or valve to prevent reflux. Also as the bladder fills with urine the increasing pressure within the bladder leads to firmer closure of the vesicoureteric valve.

Diagram 22.9iii
In some congenital abnormalities the ureter passes through the bladder wall at a steeper angle, nearer 90°. This means there is no bladder wall to form a flap, the valve is therefore lost and urine, with any bacteria it may contain, is free to reflux into the ureter.

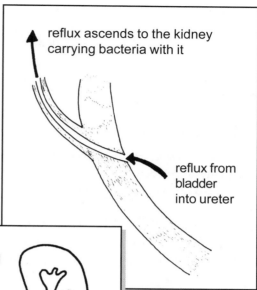

reflux ascends to the kidney carrying bacteria with it

reflux from bladder into ureter

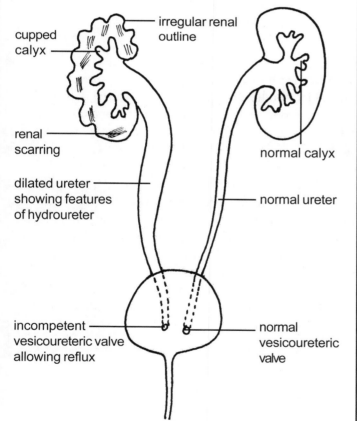

cupped calyx

irregular renal outline

renal scarring

dilated ureter showing features of hydroureter

normal calyx

normal ureter

incompetent vesicoureteric valve allowing reflux

normal vesicoureteric valve

Diagram 22.10
The left kidney is normal, but the right shows features of damage caused by chronic pyelonephritis. There is renal scarring with permanent renal damage.

Whenever UTI is remotely suspected in any child, a specimen of urine should be collected for culture and sensitivity. This should be mid-stream if possible. You will need to be imaginative or have fast reflexes to get a good sample from babies. Sometimes it may be necessary to obtain a suprapubic sample of urine by aspiration. This involves passing a needle directly into the bladder through skin when the bladder is full.

Pathophysiology

The main cause of chronic pyelonephritis in children is vesicoureteric reflux. Potentially infected urine from the bladder passes backwards, up the ureter to infect the kidneys. Reflux occurs when the child passes urine as this process increases the pressure within the bladder. Normally this would close off the vesicoureteric valve and be synchronised with a relaxation of the urethral sphincter. In reflux the increase in pressure within the bladder still causes urine to be voided, but also propels some to reflux into the ureter.

Management

In young children intravenous antibiotics should be given to prevent the dissemination of infection. Older children can normally be treated with oral antibiotics such as trimethoprim, second generation cephalosporin or amoxicillin with clavulinic acid. Renal scarring is most likely to occur before the age of 5 years, when the kidneys seem to be most sensitive. When infection is caused by vesicoureteric reflux, the child should be given prophylactic antibiotics. For example, one dose of trimethoprim or nitrofurantoin should be given every night. This will probably need to be continued for several years. Over time, as the bladder develops, the reflux disappears as vesicoureteric valve function develops. Antibiotics therefore prevent infections, pyelonephritis, renal damage, renal failure and hypertension. Most children do very well on prophylactic antibiotics and should not need surgical reimplantation of the ureters.

Reflux normally ceases at puberty as a result of growth of the bladder base. However, damage already done to the kidneys tends to progress with ongoing fibrosis, even though there is no ongoing infection.

CHAPTER 23

Renal Disorders

Acute Renal Failure (ARF)

In renal failure there is a reduction in glomerular filtration rate (GFR) resulting in a failure of the kidneys to perform their usual excretory function. Glomerular filtrate is normally generated by the process of ultrafiltration that occurs between the glomerular capillaries and Bowman's space, at the start of the nephron. As a result of a depressed GFR, the kidneys are no longer able to excrete waste products, or maintain homeostasis of water, electrolytes and acid-base balance. Interruption of renal homeostasis can therefore lead to chemical disturbances which are life threatening. This is why ARF is a medical emergency. There may also be a reduction in other renal functions including activation of vitamin D, release of renin and production of erythropoietin.

Acute renal failure will result in increased levels of urea in the blood (uraemia) as the kidneys are no longer able to excrete this nitrogen containing waste product. Sometimes this increase in nitrogen containing waste products in the blood is referred to as azotaemia. Inability to excrete potassium will cause an acute hyperkalaemia. In ARF there is usually an oliguria, which is production of an abnormally low urine volume. In some cases there may be anuria, which means a total absence of urine production. However, in a minority of patients with ARF urine volumes may be normal, but the kidneys are unable to concentrate excretory substances into the urine which is produced. Again this results in the accumulation of urea, potassium and other waste products in the blood.

Clinically, it is essential to distinguish between urine production and voiding. For example, a patient may be producing normal urine volumes but may not pass any for several hours due to a urinary obstruction or simply choosing not to urinate. In this case the urine produced by the kidneys will accumulate in the bladder. If we suspect that urine is being produced but not voided it is usually possible to palpate and percuss a full bladder. Ultrasound scanning will also immediately detect the presence of urine retained in the bladder. Unless a lower urinary tract obstruction is suspected, patients with ARF should not normally be catheterised. While it is interesting for us to be able to accurately chart hourly urine volumes, the patient is at increased risk of developing a catheter related urinary tract infection.

Most types of acute renal failure are reversible if they are detected and the patient is correctly managed. Aetiology of ARF is usually described as prerenal, intrinsic renal or postrenal.

Acute prerenal failure

This is when renal failure occurs as a result of reduced blood flow through the kidneys resulting in renal hypoperfusion. This may occur secondary to a period of systemic hypotension caused by any of the clinical forms of shock. Some drugs may also reduce renal blood supply.

Oliguria

The process of ultrafiltration between the capillaries of the glomerulus and Bowman's space requires adequate hydrostatic blood pressure. If blood pressure in the glomerulus drops, there will be corresponding reductions in production of glomerular filtrate. As the volume of glomerular filtrate is reduced, urine volumes will suffer a corresponding fall.

Renal hypoperfusion

After blood has passed through a glomerulus it leaves via the efferent arteriole. Despite carrying blood away from capillaries, this vessel is still referred to as an arteriole, rather than a venule. This is because the efferent arteriole goes on to perfuse the network of capillaries which surround the renal tubules, i.e. the proximal and distal convoluted tubules and loop of Henle. In normal physiology this second capillary network selectively reabsorbs required components from

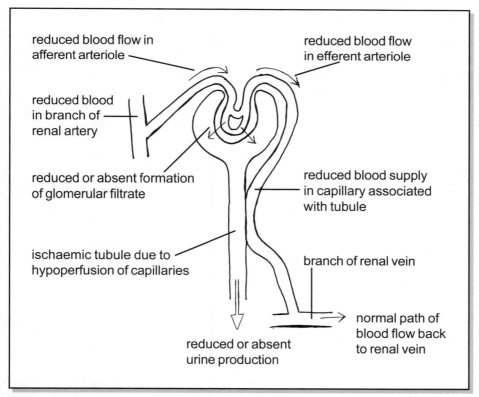

Diagram 23.1
In prerenal failure there is a reduced blood flow through the kidney. This results in reduced hydrostatic pressure in the glomerulus with reduced production of filtrate. Reduced blood flow through the tubule capillaries results in ischaemia and ultimately necrosis.

the nephron tubules. Some materials are also secreted from the capillaries into the tubules via the process of tubular secretion.

In addition to these reabsorption and secretory functions, the capillaries around a nephron provide nutrients and oxygen to the renal tubules. This means if there is a reduced blood flow through the capillaries, the nephron tubules will become ischaemic. Renal tubules are particularly prone to ischaemia as they have a high metabolic rate with a consequently high oxygen requirement. Over time tubular ischaemia will result in acute tubular necrosis which is a common cause of intrinsic renal failure.

Acute intrinsic renal failure

This is also referred to as intrarenal failure and results from damage to structures within the kidney. Causes may be renal ischaemic, inflammatory, nephrotoxic or obstructive. Pre-renal ischaemia can cause intrarenal damage via the mechanism of acute tubular necrosis.

Acute tubular necrosis (ATN)

Reduced perfusion and oxygenation of the nephrons leads to the death of some of the cells lining the tubules. Necrotic cells slough off the internal surfaces of the renal tubules and these dead cells may cause tubular obstruction. This obstruction means the flow of filtrate through many nephrons is blocked which will reduce urine output. In addition the blockage of the nephron will lead to back pressure into the area of Bowman's space which will reduce glomerular filtration rates further.

If the underlying cause of the renal hypoperfusion can be rapidly corrected, then ATN will not have time to develop. Also if the disorder causing the ATN can be corrected fairly quickly, the cells lining the nephron will regenerate leading to a full recovery. Clinical recovery normally takes 1-2 weeks. If the cause of the ATN is not reversed the condition will continue to deteriorate, potentially leading to renal cortical necrosis and irreversible renal failure. This is one reason why it is essential to reverse shock as soon as possible.

Other intrinsic causes of ARF

Inflammatory causes include acute glomerulonephritis and pyelonephritis which damage the glomeruli. Severe systemic infections may also contribute to acute renal failure as toxins released from bacteria sensitise renal tubules to ischaemic effects.

Various drugs and toxins can damage the kidneys and are referred to as nephrotoxins. Some drugs may directly damage the renal tubules such as aminoglycoside antibiotics, including gentamicin, streptomycin and neomycin. Nephrotoxicity is dose and duration of exposure related and is more likely to occur if there is previous renal impairment. Blood levels of potentially nephrotoxic drugs may need to be monitored during treatment to ensure toxic levels are not reached. Lead, mercury and some industrial organic solvents are also nephrotoxic. Tubular necrosis caused by renal toxins may also lead to ATN with tubule epithelial cells sloughing off into the nephrons where they fill up the lumen leading to obstruction.

If there is a sudden increase in haemolysis (the break-up of red blood cells) there will be a release of free haemoglobin with a resultant haemoglobinaemia. This may occur as a result of a haemolytic crisis or a blood transfusion mismatch. Haemoglobin is filtered into the glomerular filtrate resulting in a haemoglobinuria. However, the relatively large haemoglobin molecules tend to clog up the nephrons resulting in tubular obstruction and a form of acute tubular necrosis.

A similar mechanism operates in rhabdomyolysis caused by muscle injury. In cardiac and skeletal muscle there is an oxygen storing compound called myoglobin (this is why muscle tissue and red meat are red). If muscles are damaged, such as during a crush injury, then muscle cells will be disrupted and

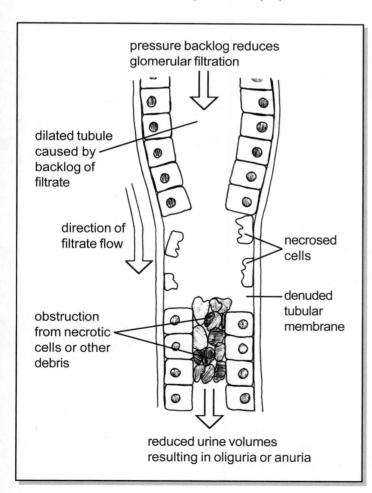

pressure backlog reduces
glomerular filtration

dilated tubule
caused by
backlog of
filtrate

direction of
filtrate flow

necrosed
cells

denuded
tubular
membrane

obstruction
from necrotic
cells or other
debris

reduced urine volumes
resulting in oliguria or anuria

Diagram 23.2
Acute tubular necrosis describes death of some cells which compose the nephrons. ATN can be caused by ischaemia, nephrotoxins, severe systemic infections or tubular obstruction. Necrosed (dead) cells slough away from the epithelium and may block the tubule. Obstruction causes backlog of the filtrate within the upper tubule, this increases the pressure in the area of Bowman's capsule. Increased pressure in the Bowman's capsule reduces filtration rates. Obstruction may also be caused by haemoglobin or myoglobin. As the tubules are obstructed, little or no urine will be produced.

split open. This will allow myoglobin molecules to escape into the tissue fluids and plasma. As myoglobin is also filtered into glomerular filtrate this too may lead to an intratubular obstruction and ATN. Both myoglobin and haemoglobin discolour urine giving a dark red, brown or even black colour.

Acute postrenal failure

This is renal failure which develops as a result of urinary obstruction. If there is obstruction of urine flow this will lead to the development of hydronephrosis and eventual renal failure. Obstructions may be located in the ureters, bladder or urethra. Most commonly the cause is urethral obstruction, secondary to prostatic enlargement. Normally the condition can be managed by ensuring adequate bladder drainage via a urethral or suprapubic catheter. This will allow plenty of time to stabilise the patient prior to surgical correction of the underlying cause. Renal stones or tumours may also lead to post renal obstruction.

Diagram 23.3
Acute renal failure may be prerenal as a result of reduced renal blood flow, intrinsic caused by damage to structures within the kidney or postrenal caused by obstruction of urine flow from the kidneys.

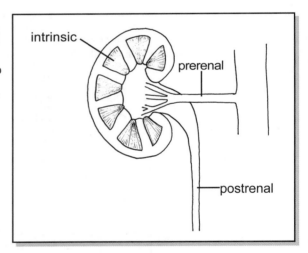

Evolution of acute renal failure

Onset

The onset or initiating phase lasts from the development of the underlying cause to the time when tubular damage occurs. After this there is an oliguric phase.

Oliguria

During this time urine volumes are low. Fluid retention in the body gives rise to systemic oedema with a raised jugular venous pressure. Pulmonary oedema with basal crackles may develop in the lungs. If the acute renal failure persists, levels of urea in the blood will rise. Urea adversely affects the CNS resulting in anorexia, nausea, hiccoughs, drowsiness, coma and eventually death. Serum potassium levels will increase resulting in hyperkalaemia. This may cause ECG changes and muscular weakness. If potassium levels continue to rise cardiac arrest is a possibility.

Recovery phase

Sometimes urine volumes start to gradually increase. There may also be a diuretic phase in which large volumes of dilute urine are generated very abruptly. Diuresis occurs because glomerular filtration recovers and the tubules are cleared of obstruction. However, the ability of the tubules to reabsorb and concentrate filtrate takes more time. The diuretic phase normally only lasts for a few days but intravenous fluid replacement may be needed. Blood levels of sodium, chloride and potassium need to be carefully monitored and supplements may be indicated. Urine volumes start to return to normal levels as tubular reabsorption mechanisms recover.

Management of acute renal failure

The underlying cause should be identified and corrected. Following this, the aim in acute renal failure is to keep the patient alive until spontaneous recovery of renal function develops.

Fluid retention

As the kidneys are not producing urine, the body has no mechanism for removing excess water. This means that fluid intake must be restricted. Patient input and output volumes should be accurately recorded. Insensible water may be lost in sweat, as moisture in exhaled air, as a component of faeces and some water simply transpires from the skin surface into the air. Fluid losses from any urine produced, vomiting or other forms of loss should be calculated, and to this figure 500 mls should be added per day for insensible loss. The patient's fluid intake over the next 24 hours should then be limited to this volume to prevent overload developing. If the weather is very hot, or the patient has a fever, the 500 ml allowance for insensible loss will need to be increased. Accurate daily weights should be recorded as changes from day to day are mostly due to fluid volumes in the body.

Pulmonary oedema

Oxygen saturations should be closely monitored as pulmonary oedema may develop as a result of fluid retention. Pulmonary oedema should be treated with high concentrations of oxygen with the patient in a sitting position. Intravenous diuretics such as furosemide should help to remove the unwanted excess tissue fluid. If high doses of intravenous diuretics fail to stimulate a diuresis more invasive methods such as haemofiltration, peritoneal dialysis or haemodialysis will be indicated.

Electrolyte balance

As the kidneys are not able to excrete sodium and potassium effectively the intake of these elements must be minimised and their blood levels monitored. Retention of sodium will increase osmotic retention of water. However, the main risk is the danger posed by hyperkalaemia (increased blood potassium levels). Developing hyperkalaemia may not cause any clinical features until the patient goes into cardiac arrest. Asystole is a risk because high levels of potassium in the plasma and tissue fluids alter the electrical function of the myocardial cells, eventually preventing muscular contraction. In addition to blood analysis, regular ECG recordings can also indicate the presence of a hyperkalaemia of 7.0 mmol/L or higher. This is in contrast to normal serum potassium levels of 3.5-5 mmol/L so represents a substantial percentage increase. In hyperkalaemia the QRS complexes broaden and the T waves develop a spiked appearance.

Hyperkalaemia is a medical emergency and ion exchange resins can be given orally or rectally. Giving intravenous glucose together with insulin will increase the shift of potassium from the plasma into the cells. Other patients will need dialysis which is an effective intervention. Acidosis may also develop as the kidneys are not able to excrete hydrogen ions. The likelihood of this can be reduced by effective nasogastric drainage to reduce absorption of acid from the stomach.

Diet

As discussed, sodium and potassium will need to be severely restricted in most patients. Traditionally, patients have been managed on a low protein diet. If more proteins are eaten than the body immediately requires, they are broken down to produce energy. When proteins are metabolised in this way, waste nitrogen is generated. This waste nitrogen is converted to urea in the liver. However, as the kidneys are not able to excrete this nitrogen containing waste in the urine, it accumulates in the blood leading to accelerated development of uraemia. It is probably best to give about 40g of protein per day. This level of ingestion will help prevent body proteins being broken down by catabolism but will not be enough to exacerbate uraemia. If patients are to be dialysed they may be given additional protein.

Patients should eat plenty of carbohydrate and fat. These will provide adequate fuels for energy and prevent the body breaking down stored proteins in muscle. If the body does start to utilise stored proteins for energy production, waste nitrogen will be released into the circulation. Patients who do not feel like eating may be given carbohydrates and fats via a nasogastric tube. Parenteral feeding may be used as a last resort.

Dialysis and haemofiltration

Options include peritoneal dialysis, haemodialysis and haemofiltration. These treatments may become necessary for a period of time if significant complications of acute renal failure develop. Indications for these treatments include hyperkalaemia, other significant chemical disturbances, severe acidosis, pulmonary oedema and uraemia.

Drugs

It is the kidneys which excrete a lot of drugs and their metabolites from the body. Therefore in renal failure this function will be inhibited. One effect of this is that drugs may accumulate in the body and reach toxic levels if repeated doses are given.

Chronic Renal Failure (CRF)

In this disorder there is irreversible destruction of renal tissues, usually following a progressive course resulting in loss of renal function.

Aetiology

The most common aetiologies vary in different parts of the world. For example, in much of Africa the most common cause is glomerulonephritis secondary to malaria. The most common cause in most western countries is diabetic nephropathy, followed by hypertension and chronic glomerulonephritis. Chronic pyelonephritis, hydronephrosis, tuberculosis, schistosomiasis and various vascular diseases are other possible causes.

Some causes of chronic renal failure are genetic, the most common example being adult polycystic kidney disease, a condition transmitted by an autosomal dominant gene. About 50% of persons with polycystic disease eventually develop end stage renal failure. The condition usually becomes symptomatic in the 35 to 55 age range. Around a third of patients with polycystic kidney disease also develop cysts in the liver. In a few patients there are also cysts in the spleen and pancreas. Some congenital abnormalities of renal structure can also lead to failure.

Evolution of chronic renal failure

Reduction in the number of functional nephrons results in a reduced level of renal function. This in turn means that there is less glomerular filtrate produced. Progression of chronic renal disease usually follows four stages; diminished renal reserve, renal insufficiency, renal failure and end stage renal disease.

Diminished renal reserve

Human design incorporates a significant reserve of renal function. Young healthy people are able to produce much more glomerular filtrate than is needed to remove waste products from the blood and maintain homeostasis. If one kidney is lost or fails to develop, the individual can usually live a full normal life. Diminished renal reserve is normally diagnosed when glomerular filtration rate

Diagram 23.4
In polycystic disease the kidneys are grossly enlarged and the normal tissue is ultimately, almost completely replaced by cysts of varying size. The outline of the kidney is irregular due to the presence of the cysts, which are filled with a straw coloured fluid.

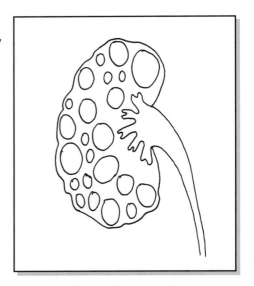

(GFR) falls to 50% of the normal rate. In this situation blood urea and creatinine (a waste product of protein metabolism) levels remain normal and there are no clinical features.

Renal insufficiency

This is normally diagnosed when GFR lies between 20% to 50% of normal. During this stage urine volumes may be normal but the ability to concentrate urine is progressively reduced. This means the urine which is produced is not carrying a sufficient load of waste products therefore blood urea and creatinine will start to rise. Hypertension and anaemia may also develop at this time.

Renal failure

This develops when GFR is less than 20% of normal. This will result in the development of hyperkalaemia, fluid retention with oedema, uraemia and metabolic acidosis.

End stage renal disease

This is diagnosed when GFR falls to below 5% of normal. There is atrophy and fibrosis of the kidney tissue. Patients will die without regular dialysis or renal transplantation.

Clinical features in chronic renal failure (CRF)

Clinical features in renal disease are often difficult to attribute to specific pathophysiological changes. However, affects on the central nervous system such as malaise, nausea, vomiting, anorexia, loss of energy and insomnia may be attributable to uraemia. Itching (pruritus) is a common complaint and may be caused by uraemia and retention of other metabolic waste products. Dialysis usually helps with pruritus, but for some patients it is an ongoing problem with no clear cause or treatment.

Salt and water retention may cause systemic and pulmonary oedema. Anaemia presents in the majority of patients with CRF due to reduced production of erythropoietin and the adverse effects uraemia has on red bone marrow function. Many patients complain of 'restless legs' syndrome where the patient needs to keep changing the position of their legs.

Bone disease called renal osteodystrophy complicates renal failure. Vitamin D increases calcium absorption from the gut and helps to control calcium deposition in bones. However, the form of vitamin D in the diet, or synthesised in the skin on exposure to sunlight, is not very metabolically active. In order to be physiologically useful this form of vitamin D must be converted into a much more active form. It is converted into active vitamin D by an enzyme called 1 alpha-hydroxylase which is produced by the kidneys. With progressive renal damage this essential converting enzyme is not produced in adequate amounts meaning less vitamin D is activated. Lack of the active form of vitamin D (called dihydroxycholecalciferol) means calcium metabolism cannot be properly controlled resulting in abnormal bone structure. Patients may be treated with an active form of vitamin D called calcitriol, along with calcium supplements.

Numerous other features and complications may present in CRF. These include gastrointestinal complications, gout due to urate retention, endocrine effects and cardiovascular disease which is a major factor in reduced life expectancy.

Management in chronic renal failure

As in all conditions any underlying pathology should be identified and corrected as far as possible.

Blood pressure control

Blood pressure control is important as hypertension develops in about 80% of patients with CRF. Reduction of high blood pressure is also an important factor in slowing the progress of diabetic nephropathy. BP should be reduced to 130/80 or lower if the patient does not become clinically hypotensive. Diuretics may be needed to help remove excess sodium and water from the body, although in end stage renal disease these will have little effect. ACE inhibitors are a mainstay of blood pressure control in renal disease, and other antihypertensives may also be indicated.

Cardiovascular disease

Atherosclerosis and cardiovascular disease are common in patients with CRF. This is partly due to the hypertension which is common. Also, high blood levels of cholesterol are seen in almost all patients with proteinuria. Statins should probably be given to lower serum cholesterol levels.

Glycaemic control

This must be tightly controlled in diabetic patients. If the blood sugar levels and blood pressure can be kept low, progress of diabetic nephropathy will be retarded.

Fluid and electrolyte control

As the kidneys lose the ability to concentrate urine they may still be able to excrete all of the required metabolic waste products by increasing urine volumes. This means they will produce larger volumes of more dilute urine. These patients need to drink enough water to maintain a urine output of 3 litres per day.

Some patients lose excess amounts of salt in their urine (so called salt wasting disease) and therefore must eat enough to compensate for the loss because sodium depletion will lead to fluid depletion and consequent reduced renal perfusion and function. Hyperkalaemia is a constant threat and in later disease but most patients respond well to dietary potassium restriction. It is important that patients realise how important it is not to allow their potassium to rise because of the risk of cardiac arrest. Sodium may also need to be restricted in later disease, if there is evidence of accumulation. Calcium and phosphate levels also need to be monitored and controlled.

Diet

Restrictions in protein are usually needed but if patients are restricted for a long time they become malnourished. Where renal replacement therapy is available protein restriction should be moderate with about 60g per day allowed. This is allowed because dialysis will remove excess nitrogen which can be generated as a result of eating proteins. Adequate amounts of energy giving foods should be eaten to prevent protein breakdown. Dehydration and fluid overload both need to be avoided.

Infections

Immune mechanisms are impaired in CRF leaving the patient vulnerable to infections. Infections must be recognised and treated promptly as they can be life threatening.

Renal replacement therapy

Renal function can be replaced by the process of dialysis. In end stage renal failure dialysis is life sustaining. The two forms of dialysis are haemodialysis and peritoneal dialysis.

The basic principle behind haemodialysis is that blood is temporarily taken out of the patient and separated from dialysate (dialysis fluid) by a semi-permeable membrane. Diffusion then takes place through the semi-permeable membrane. This means if the levels of urea in the blood are high but low in the dialysate, there will be a diffusion gradient from the blood to the dialysing fluid. This means urea will diffuse from the blood into the fluid. As a result the blood which is returned to the patient contains less urea than it did. The same is true for potassium, creatinine, hydrogen ions and numerous other waste products. These are all removed from the blood and will be discarded in the used dialysate. Venous access may be gained via a surgically created arteriovenous fistula or by a tunnelled line into a central vein. It is essential not to use veins in dialysis and pre-dialysis patients for casual venepuncture or cannulation purposes as this results in unnecessary damage.

In peritoneal dialysis a catheter is placed in the peritoneal cavity and dialysate is run in. This converts the potential peritoneal space into an actual space. The peritoneal space lies between the visceral and parietal peritoneal membranes which cover a large number of small blood vessels. This means there are large volumes of blood close to the dialysing fluid. It is the capillaries and the peritoneal membranes which act as the semi-permeable membrane. As in haemodialysis, unwanted components in the blood such as urea, creatinine, phosphate and potassium diffuse down their gradients into the dialysate. After a period of time the dialysate is allowed to drain, carrying the waste products with it.

Renal transplantation

A donated kidney can essentially fulfil all of the functions of a natural one. While good anaesthetic and surgical techniques are essential the main factor is how good a match can be found in terms of tissue typing. Clearly the donor must have the same blood group as the recipient. However, tissues have many other biochemical features which need to be as closely matched as possible. The closer the match the less the recipient's immune system will recognise the new kidney as foreign tissue and so less immunological rejection will occur. After transplantation it is essential that the recipient takes immunosuppressive therapy. This will be needed as long as the new kidney remains in the recipient. The risk of immunological rejection is highest in the first 3 months after a transplant. The only cases where rejection is not a factor is when the donor and recipient have identical tissue types. This only occurs in monozygotic twins, when two individuals have identical genes determining these tissue factors.

Glomerulonephritic (nephritic) syndrome

This syndrome is caused by a group of disease processes which can damage the glomeruli; they are often referred to as the glomerulonephritides. The glomeruli are damaged by a systemic disease process and because both kidneys contain the same types of tissue the disease is bilateral.

Pathophysiology

In all forms of glomerulonephritis there is glomerular inflammation which is usually caused by immunological mechanisms. However, there are 2 possible groups of pathophysiological immunological mechanisms which may give rise to glomerular inflammation. These are immune complex causes and anti-GBM (glomerular basement membrane) antibody-mediated causes.

Immune complex mediated glomerular inflammation

Physiologically, antibodies (i.e. immunoglobulins) are synthesised by the B lymphocytes as a result of the presence of infectious antigens such as bacteria or viruses. These antibodies then bind onto antigens, which means antibodies may agglutinate (bind together) several antigens prior to phagocytosis. The combination of some antigens with the antibodies which agglutinate them is referred to as an immune complex.

It was believed that immune complexes formed in the circulatory system and then migrated into a glomerulus. It now seems more likely that only the antibodies migrate into the glomerulus where they attach to glomerular antigens or to bacterial or viral antigens which had previously migrated in to infect a glomerulus. This is described as in situ immune complex formation. It is the combination of the antibodies with the antigens which triggers a destructive inflammatory response. The presence of immune complexes in the glomerulus attracts white blood cells and activates the complement cascade (which is an immune mechanism) resulting in inflammatory injury.

Diagram 23.5
This is a simple example of an immune complex, 2 antigens have been agglutinated by an antibody molecule. In practice many antigens may be agglutinated by groups of antibodies giving rise to a relatively large complex.

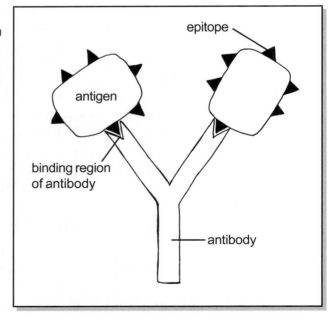

Anti-GBM (glomerular basement membrane) antibody-mediated causes

These disorders are mediated by an autoimmune attack on the collagen which is an important structural component of the glomerular basement membrane. Autoantibodies bind to and damage the GBM. This form of glomerulonephritis may also be associated with damage to collagen in the basement membrane of the alveoli, leading to pulmonary haemorrhage. The majority of patients with anti-GBM nephritis also have glomerular crescents (which are discussed below). Clinically anti-GBM glomerulonephritis presents with rapidly progressing nephritic features and renal failure.

General clinical presentations in nephritic disease

The clinical features which may present in glomerulonephritic disorders are proteinuria, haematuria, oliguria, uraemia, sodium retention, oedema and hypertension. However, these features may present, resolve or become chronic in a variety of ways. In some nephritic conditions, such as acute glomerulonephritis, manifestations may develop rapidly and present as an acute syndrome. This will lead to acute renal insufficiency which will usually resolve after a period of time. Some presentations of chronic glomerulonephritis are continuous or intermittent over many years eventually resulting in irreversible renal failure. In other conditions, such as Goodpasture's syndrome, there is a rapidly progressive crescentic proliferative glomerulonephritis causing renal insufficiency. As this description suggests these disorders rapidly deteriorate leading to chronic renal failure.

Glomerulonephritis

The forms of glomerulonephritis which will be discussed here are proliferative, crescentic, acute post-streptococcal, membranous, IgA and Goodpasture's syndrome.

Clinical features in glomerulonephritis

Inflammatory changes in the glomeruli cause injury of the glomerular capillaries. Capillary damage leads to an increase in permeability, causing them to become leaky which results in a loss of blood and protein into the glomerular filtrate. This explains the presence of a variable degree of proteinuria and haematuria in glomerulonephritic syndromes. In addition to a ward-based urinalysis for protein, a definitive diagnosis of significant proteinuria should be made by measuring the amount of protein lost over 24 hours. Inflammatory damage and associated proliferative changes may also impair blood flow through the glomerular capillaries resulting in a decreased glomerular filtration rate. This will lead to oliguria and reduced renal clearance of nitrogen containing waste products such as urea and creatinine. As these wastes are not excreted in the urine they will accumulate in the blood. Salt and water are also retained leading to fluid overload, oedema and hypertension.

Proliferative glomerulonephritis

Proliferative changes develop in many immune complex related nephritic syndromes. In proliferative glomerulonephritis there is an increase in the number (i.e. a proliferation) of cells in the glomerulus resulting in a diffuse glomerular

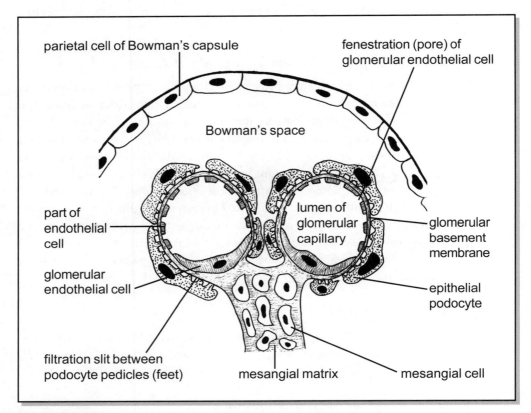

parietal cell of Bowman's capsule

fenestration (pore) of glomerular endothelial cell

Bowman's space

part of endothelial cell

lumen of glomerular capillary

glomerular basement membrane

glomerular endothelial cell

epithelial podocyte

filtration slit between podocyte pedicles (feet)

mesangial matrix

mesangial cell

Diagram 23.6

Normal structure of the glomerulus in health. Each of the one million glomeruli in each kidney is composed of a ball of capillaries. Ultrafiltration takes place from the lumen of the glomerular capillary into Bowman's space. From here the glomerular filtrate passes on into the nephron. The walls of the glomerular capillaries are composed of endothelial cells that contain pores (or fenestrations). Mesangial cells are located between the glomerular capillaries. Under the glomerular endothelial cells is the glomerular basement membrane (GBM), this forms a structural base for the glomerular capillary endothelial cells and also acts as a dialysing membrane. Glomerular capillaries are surrounded by podocytes; these specialised cells have numerous pedicels which are foot like extensions of cytoplasm which wrap around the capillaries forming filtration slits. A thin membrane called the slit membrane extends across each filtration slit.

enlargement. There is also an increase in the number of capillary endothelial cells and mesangial cells. The acute phase begins 1 to 2 weeks after an initial infection and in most patients this resolves after several weeks. Usually the cellular changes completely resolve after several months. Proliferative changes in glomerulonephritis may be diffuse or focal. In diffuse proliferation all of the glomeruli are affected in a similar way. In focal disease some of the glomeruli show evidence of proliferative changes while others are normal.

Crescentic proliferative glomerulonephritis

Crescentic means that crescents form in Bowman's space within the capsule. When the walls of a glomerular capillary are severely damaged, plasma components including clotting factors and inflammatory mediators enter

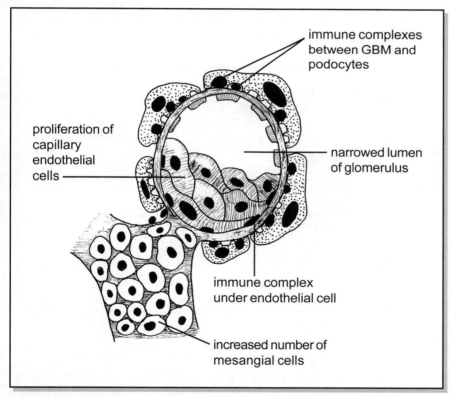

immune complexes between GBM and podocytes

proliferation of capillary endothelial cells

narrowed lumen of glomerulus

immune complex under endothelial cell

increased number of mesangial cells

Diagram 23.7
In proliferative glomerulonephritis there is an increase in the number of endothelial and mesangial cells present. An increase in the number of mesangial cells will cause thickening of the stalk. Increased numbers of endothelial cells obstruct the lumen of the glomerular capillaries. Immune complexes accumulate under the endothelial cells and are associated with the cellular proliferation and increased capillary permeability which causes the loss of protein and blood into the glomerular filtrate.

Bowman's space. This results in fibrin formation and an accumulation of macrophages. These changes trigger a proliferation of parietal epithelial cells (which form the wall of Bowman's capsule) into Bowman's space. As Bowman's capsule surrounds the glomerulus the cellular proliferation forms a crescent shape around the glomerulus giving rise to the crescentic description. Crescents are therefore associated with severe glomerular damage and this means the glomerulonephritis will rapidly progress to complete renal failure. This crescentic form of the disease is most commonly caused by the presence of immune complex, but a few are caused by anti-GBM autoimmune antibodies.

Acute post-streptococcal glomerulonephritis

This form of acute nephritic syndrome is most common in childhood and typically follows about 10 days after a streptococcal infection, often of the throat, tonsils or ears. This is why it is often referred to as post-streptococcal glomerulonephritis. The time delay between the initial streptococcal infection

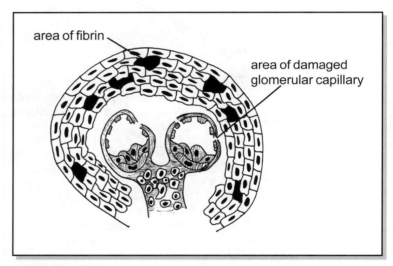

area of fibrin

area of damaged glomerular capillary

Diagram 23.8
Damage to the glomerular capillaries allows leakage of plasma contents and inflammatory mediators into Bowman's space where this material comes into contact with the parietal cells of Bowman's capsule. This leads to a proliferation of parietal cells which adopt the shape of a crescent around the glomerulus. Within the crescent there are deposits of fibrin. This derives from fibrinogen which has leaked from the damaged glomerular capillaries. Crescentic glomerulonephritis is severe and rapidly progressive. Note there is also a proliferation of mesangial and glomerular endothelial cells within the lumen of the glomerular capillary. (Podocytes are not illustrated and in reality the glomerulus is a complex cluster of capillaries.)

and the onset of renal features represents the time taken for the formation of antibodies, their deposition in the glomerular capillaries, and the development of the associated inflammatory damage. As immune complexes develop in the walls of the glomeruli they trigger an inflammatory response resulting in a diffuse proliferative glomerulonephritis.

Clinical features and prognosis

As would be expected the clinical features are proteinuria, frank or hidden haematuria, oliguria, systemic and pulmonary oedema, uraemia and hypertension. As long as the patient is well managed during the acute phase of the illness the prognosis in children is excellent. However, after apparent full recovery a small number of adult patients go on to develop hypertension or renal impairment. These people should have their creatinine checked every few years and annual blood pressure checks.

Treatment principles

As this is essentially a form of acute renal failure the management in acute glomerulonephritis is aimed at preventing complications while awaiting the spontaneous remission that usually occurs. Ongoing immune complex formation may be prevented by eliminating any possible bacterial antigens by giving a course of penicillin. Regular blood pressure readings should be taken and any hypertension managed.

Outbreaks of post-streptococcal glomerulonephritis may occur in individuals who live closely together. This occurs when a haemolytic streptococcus of a nephritogenic type spreads from one person to another. (Nephritogenic refers to a form of bacteria which has the potential to cause glomerulonephritis.) If spread to contacts is a possibility, individuals at risk should be given 500mg of prophylactic phenoxymethyl penicillin daily.

Membranous glomerulonephritis

Membranous glomerulonephritis is a common cause of nephrotic syndrome in adults. In most patients the initial antigen which triggers antibody formation is unknown. However, in the tropics Plasmodium malariae is a frequent cause. There is an accumulation of immune complexes between the visceral epithelial cells (i.e. the podocytes which surround the glomerular capillaries) and the GBM. These are probably formed in situ rather than being derived from circulating complexes. Antibodies cross the GBM and bind onto the podocytes which they pathologically recognise as antigens. The presence of immune complexes causes a thickening of the adjacent GBM which eventually engulfs the complexes. As the inflammatory pathology progresses the glomerular capillary lumens are narrowed with eventual sclerosis resulting in chronic glomerular disease. (In sclerosis there is an increase in the amount of collagen present, this is essentially scar tissue.) Despite the GBM thickening the membrane also becomes more permeable to protein, which results in the proteinuria of nephrotic syndrome. Protein loss in turn leads on to hypoproteinaemia and oedema.

Over a 20 year period about 25% of patients make a spontaneous recovery, 25% develop renal failure and 50% have persistent proteinuria but maintain, or only suffer partial loss, of renal function. It seems likely that patients with more severe protein loss or progressive impairment of renal function will benefit from steroid and immunosuppressant therapy.

IgA nephropathy

This is a focal proliferative glomerulonephritis, formally referred to as Berger disease. The nephropathy is caused by the accumulation of IgA based immune complexes in the mesangial cells and in more severe cases there is also IgA deposition in the capillary walls. The condition usually follows upper respiratory or gastrointestinal infection, but other infections may also be implicated. Most patients fall into the 16-35 years of age range. Haematuria is most often microscopic but there may be episodes of frank blood loss in the urine. Some patients only suffer from very mild features while a minority develop a rapidly progressive glomerulonephritis. If acute renal failure does develop it normally resolves spontaneously. Most patients have a good prognosis but about 20% will develop renal failure after 20 years.

Goodpasture's syndrome

This disorder presents with a severe form of anti-GBM antibody mediated glomerulonephritis which is often crescentic. This means the disorder is severe and will progress on to chronic renal failure. In addition to the renal involvement there is recurrent haemoptysis, a feature more likely to occur in smokers. Coughing up of blood occurs because of lung haemorrhages. Lung haemorrhages occur because the autoantibody responsible for the disease attacks a form of collagen which is found in the GBM and in the alveolar capillary basement membrane. This illustrates a cross reactivity of the autoimmune response.

Focal segmental glomerulosclerosis (FSGS)

In this group of disorders there are focal lesions as only some of the glomeruli have sclerotic changes while others appear normal. Segmental means that only parts, or segments, of the glomeruli are affected; other segments of an individual glomerulus appear normal. FSGS may have several different causes. Many cases are primary and idiopathic, with no obvious aetiology. Secondary disease may complicate several conditions including obesity, reduced renal mass, cyanotic congenital heart disease and sickle cell disease. Pathologically there is segmental solidification of the glomerular tufts. These solid areas are caused by the deposition of lipids, collagen and other protein based material. Most patients have a persistent proteinuria with a progressive decline in renal function. About 50% of patients with FSGS go on to develop end stage renal failure within 10 years.

Minimal-change glomerular lesion

Minimal change disease (MCD) is the most common single cause of the proteinuria of nephrotic syndrome in children. MCD is not a form of glomerulonephritis as it is not an inflammatory condition.

Aetiology

The pathological changes seen in MCD are probably autoimmune and may be caused by disordered T lymphocytes. It has been suggested that these T cells release a cytokine which increases glomerular permeability; this allows protein to pass through the glomerular membrane.

Pathophysiology

Minimal-change refers to the nature of the histopathology seen in the glomeruli which is limited to loss of the foot processes of the podocytes. Increased glomerular permeability leads to significant loss of albumin and lipoproteins into the glomerular filtrate. This leads to a hypoalbuminaemia. The liver attempts to compensate for the reduced blood levels of proteins and lipoproteins by synthesising more lipoproteins resulting in a hyperlipidaemia.

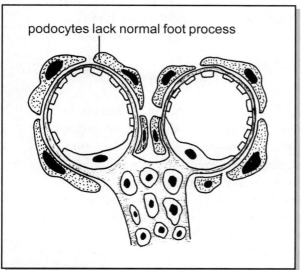

podocytes lack normal foot process

Diagram 23.9
In minimal-change disease there is loss of the foot processes from the epithelial podocytes. Apart from this change the microscopic appearance of the glomeruli is normal.

Treatment principles

As long as any complications are well managed these patients do well in the long term. Infections such as peritonitis are possible as a result of reduced levels of antibodies in the blood. These are lost as they are composed of proteins and some escape into the glomerular filtrate with albumin as a result of the increased permeability of the glomerular membrane. Infective complications should be managed with antibiotics. Another possible complication is hypovolaemic shock as a result of excessive oedema formation. Hypertension is a complication in a minority of individuals. Thromboembolic complications may also occur including peripheral arterial occlusions and DVT.

The likely autoimmune basis of MCD is supported by the effects of corticosteroid therapy. The majority of children enter complete remission after 2 months of treatment but with adults it usually takes longer. While some patients may have intermittent relapses over a 10 year period, minimal change disease does not progress onto chronic renal failure.

Nephrotic syndrome

The characteristic feature of nephrotic syndrome is the loss of protein in the urine. There will be heavy proteinuria resulting in a protein loss of more than 3.5g over 24 hours. Normal urine should contain no detectable protein.

Aetiology

All forms of glomerulonephritis may lead to nephrotic syndrome. In children living in developed countries the most common cause is minimal-change glomerular disease, while in many tropical areas infections such as malaria account for most cases. Other possible causes of nephrotic syndrome include diabetic glomerular disease, systemic vascular inflammatory conditions such as systemic lupus erythematosus (SLE), uncommon drug reactions and some allergic reactions.

Pathophysiology

In normal physiology large molecules such as protein should not pass from the glomerular capillaries into the glomerular filtrate; there should be ultrafiltration on the grounds of molecular size with only smaller molecules passing through. In nephrotic syndrome glomerular capillaries are excessively permeable allowing large protein molecules to pass from the blood into the filtrate. The pathology is usually located in the basement membrane of the glomerular capillaries.

As more protein is lost in the urine there is a proportional reduction in plasma protein concentration resulting in hypoproteinaemia. Albumin is the principle plasma protein which generates plasma osmotic pressure. When levels of albumin are reduced there is a hypoalbuminaemia with a corresponding reduction in plasma osmotic pressure. Reduced plasma osmolarity reduces the volume of tissue fluid which can be reabsorbed at the venous end of the capillaries. This leaves more fluid in the tissue spaces resulting in oedema. In addition, retention of sodium contributes to oedema.

As antibodies are made of protein these too can be lost from the plasma resulting in hypogammaglobulinaemia. This can lead to reduced immune function predisposing to infections such as pneumococcal pneumonia.

Some factors which inhibit normal blood clotting are lost into the urine. The liver may also over produce factors which promote blood coagulation. Both of these effects predispose to an increased risk of venous thromboembolism with deep venous thrombosis and possible pulmonary embolism.

Another effect of hypoproteinaemia is that the liver is stimulated to synthesise more proteins in an attempted compensation. Some of the proteins which are synthesised are low density lipoproteins resulting in hypercholesterolaemia with an increased risk of the development of atherosclerosis.

Investigations

Diagnosis is confirmed by examination of 24 hour urine protein levels which will be above 3.5g in adults. In children protein levels may be proportionately lower depending on urine volume. Blood will be tested for serum albumin concentrations which are likely to be less than 30g per litre of blood as opposed to a normal range of 35-50g/L. Serum cholesterol concentrations are very likely to be raised. Sodium retention leads to hypernatraemia. The overall level of renal function is estimated by measuring serum urea and creatinine and urinary creatinine clearance.

Management principles

Adequate amounts of protein should be eaten, but high protein diets have not been found to confer additional benefit. The levels of sodium in the diet should be reduced and diuretics such as bendroflumethiazide given. Sodium restriction will reduce the total amount of sodium in the body and so reduce water retention. Use of diuretics will reduce the volume of water in the circulatory system and so increase the osmolarity of the blood which will lead to reabsorption of more tissue fluid and so reduce oedema. With diuretic use the patient must be carefully monitored for possible hypotensive effects. Cholesterol lowering drugs such as statins and anticoagulant therapy should be considered. Intravenous infusions of albumin will temporarily increase the osmotic potential of the plasma and so reduce oedema. Clearly the underlying causative condition should be identified and corrected. In children high doses of corticosteroids may be used to treat minimal change glomerulonephritis. Malaria should be treated if present.

Malignant renal tumours

Primary tumours affecting the kidneys account for about 3% of newly diagnosed cancers in the UK. Metastatic and benign tumours may also develop in the kidneys.

Aetiology

Men are affected more commonly than women with the peak age of presentation being about 55 years. The overall incidence, in the UK and globally, has increased over the past 20 years. Obesity is a risk factor for renal carcinoma probably because it leads to endocrine changes, particularly for women. Smoking is also a risk factor as chemical carcinogens are systemically absorbed from tobacco smoke and subsequently concentrated in the kidney prior to excretion in the urine. Exposure to some occupational chemicals also increases risk. While most cases are sporadic, about 5% have a recognised autosomal dominant genetic base.

Pathophysiology

The majority (about 80%) of malignant neoplasms affecting the kidney are renal cell carcinomas (RCC). Malignant cells arise most commonly from the proximal tubular epithelial cells. Typically a large irregular neoplasm develops in a kidney but multiple and even bilateral tumours may also occur. As the tumour invades branches of the local veins there may be blood borne metastatic spread to the other kidney, lungs, bone, lymph nodes or liver.

Clinical features

The most common presenting sign is haematuria. The other two classical features are pain in the loin and a palpable mass in the flank. Pain may develop and become severe. Some patients complain of anorexia, weight loss, pyrexia or malaise. Anaemia is another possible feature explained by reduced secretion of erythropoietin. Unfortunately it is not uncommon for patients to present with features of metastatic disease. RCC may cause several paraneoplastic effects as a result of ectopic hormone production. For example, hypertension develops in some patients as a result of increased release of renin which then activates the angiotensin mechanism. A minority of patients secrete increased volumes of erythropoietin and so develop polycythaemia. Release of an ectopic parathormone-like chemical will lead to hyperparathyroidism.

Treatment and prognosis

Nephrectomy is the treatment of choice. As long as the other kidney is healthy, overall renal function will remain adequate. The most important factor influencing prognosis is tumour stage. If nephrectomy can be performed before the tumour has invaded through the renal capsule and before metastasis has occurred the outlook is fairly good (75% five year survival). Later stages of the disease are associated with a poorer prognosis. Drug treatments may include medroxyprogesterone to control metastatic disease and some patients enter remission with immunotherapy using interleukin-2 and alpha-interferon.

CHAPTER 24

Alteration in Body Temperature

Pyrexia

Pyrexia refers to an increase in body temperature resulting in a fever. A person with a fever is said to be febrile. When the body temperature is not raised the person is described as being apyrexial (the prefix 'a' or 'an' always means without). It is the hypothalamus which regulates body temperature by comparing the temperature of the blood circulating through the structure with a set point, usually between 36.5-37°C. When blood temperature drops, the hypothalamus initiates mechanisms to increase body temperature; conversely when blood temperature rises above the set point, heat loss mechanisms are initiated. In a fever the set point is increased to a new higher setting.

Cause of fevers

Fevers are most commonly caused by infection but also occur after tissue damage which may be caused by trauma, surgery or disease processes. For example, pyrexia is not uncommon after a myocardial infarction when part of the myocardium is damaged by an occlusion of the coronary arterial blood supply. Neoplasm is another possible cause and fever may be an early sign of a developing cancer.

Infection is caused by the presence of microorganisms, such as bacteria or viruses, in a tissue. As the presence of bacteria or viruses causes a febrile response these infectious agents are often referred to as exogenous pyrogens. Exogenous means the cause is from outside the body, the infection comes from the environment. 'Pyro' literally means fire or heat, 'gen' refers to genesis which means beginning, so a pyrogen is something which 'begins heat'.

Leucocytes (white blood cells) are able to detect the presence of infectious agents in a tissue. Upon detecting infection these white cells, especially the macrophages, respond by producing cytokines. Cytokines are hormones produced by individual cells which have the potential to affect other cells or tissues in the body. Two of the cytokines produced by macrophages in response to the presence of infection are interleukins (ILs) and tumour necrosis factor (TNF). It is the presence of these cytokines in the blood that increase the set point of the hypothalamus in order to generate a fever. Because these pyrogenic cytokines are released from the body's own cells they are referred to as endogenous pyrogens.

Damaged tissue cells can release cytokines directly. In addition damaged tissues can activate macrophages to release cytokines. These pyrogenic cytokines from damaged tissue and activated macrophages are also able to increase the set point of the hypothalamus. Cancer cells can release pyrogenic cytokines which explains why fever can sometimes occur in patients with cancer, even in the absence of infection.

Fever increases immune function

By being able to recognise these cytokines the hypothalamus becomes aware of the presence of infection or damaged tissue. This allows for the initiation of a fever as part of the systemic response to infection. It has been suggested that pathogenic microorganisms are less viable at febrile temperatures. While there is some truth in this for some organisms, the main reason fever is generated is to increase the efficiency of the immune system.

It has been demonstrated that neutrophils exhibit greater motility and bacterial killing activity as the temperature rises from 36 up to 40°C. Some studies indicate that macrophages function more efficiently at about 39°C. As neutrophils and macrophages are the most active phagocytic cells it follows that this process of white cells 'eating' bacteria and viruses works most efficiently at these increased temperatures. At temperatures around 39°C other activities of the immune system such as release of interferons, release of cytokines, activation of complement and the activity of lymphocytes have all been shown to be enhanced. Pyrexial temperatures also increase the likelihood that virally infected cells will self destruct, therefore killing the viral particles they contain.

If the immune system is working more efficiently as a result of a fever, then the infection will be combated more aggressively and quickly. This will in turn limit the course of the infection, promoting rapid recovery. As infection is efficiently combated by the immune system in febrile patients, tissue damage as a result of the infection is less likely to occur. In addition to these benefits of fever there will also be an increase in the metabolic rate of the body which will allow tissues to regenerate more rapidly.

Damaged tissue is often caused by wounds, which are at risk of becoming infected. The ability of the hypothalamus to recognise endogenous pyrogens means that the body temperature can be increased above normal. As an increase in body temperature will increase the working efficiency of the immune system, any infection can be combated more aggressively at an early stage, hopefully before it becomes established.

Stages of a fever

When the set point of the hypothalamus is increased by the presence of pyrogens, mechanisms are initiated to warm up the whole body. The aim of this response is to warm up the body to reach the new set point. Initiation of heat gain mechanisms will lead to peripheral vasoconstriction, shivering, chattering of teeth, contraction of hair erector muscles and release of epinephrine (adrenaline) from the adrenal medulla. The individual will also experience a feeling of coldness. They will feel cold to the touch as a result of peripheral vasoconstriction, despite the fact that their temperature is rising above normal. Because the person feels cold they will huddle up and pull over bed covers to try and warm up. As a result of these physiological mechanisms and behaviours body temperature will start to rise towards the new, pyrogen induced, set point. This first stage of a fever is called the chills or rigor stage.

After some time the new set point will be reached, the person is now pyrexial. At this point the person has no chills; they do not feel warm or cold. This is because, at this stage, the body is not trying to gain or lose heat. As long as stimulation from the pyrogens persists, the body temperature will be regulated at this higher level. During this stage the patient does not usually feel particularly warm to the touch, as they are not peripherally vasodilated.

When the immune system has overcome the infection, or damaged tissue has been phagocytosed, levels of pyrogens in the blood will drop. This will allow the hypothalamus to return the temperature set point to normal. In this situation the body temperature is still raised but the hypothalamus has returned the set point to normal. In order to reduce body temperature, cooling mechanisms are instigated. These will include vasodilation and possible sweating. During this stage the patient will experience a feeling of warmth and will also feel warm to the touch. The point at which the patient starts to feel warm and vasodilates is referred to as the flush or crisis. Before the era of antibiotics the crisis point was keenly awaited. When a patient had passed the crisis it was likely they were going to recover from an infection rather than die.

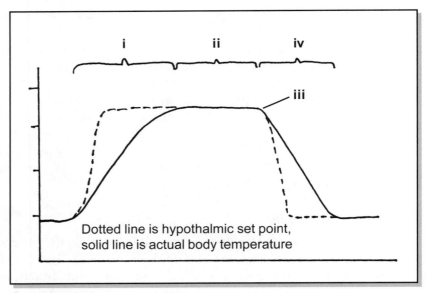

Dotted line is hypothalmic set point, solid line is actual body temperature

Diagram 24.1
The stages of a fever, temperature set point of the hypothalamus plotted against time.
- **i.** rigor or chills phase - heat gain mechanisms in operation, patient feels cold.
- **ii.** pyrexial stage - body temperature is homeostatically maintained at the new higher set level, patient does not feel hot or cold.
- **iii.** crisis - the point at which body temperature starts to fall, the patient feels warm, and so starts to cool down.
- **iv.** cooling - the process of body temperature lowering, the patient feels warm until core temperature returns to normal.

Clinical features of fever

Obviously, in fever there is an increase in recorded temperature, however the degree to which individuals are aware of the stages of a fever described above varies. Some patients are surprised to learn they are pyrexial and have not been aware of a rigor stage. In addition to the temperature, there are other features seen in fever. For every 1°C increase in body temperature the metabolic rate increases by 13%. This will clearly increase the oxygen demand of the tissues, probably resulting in an increased respiratory rate. Typically for every 1°C increase in temperature the pulse rate rises by about 12 beats per minute. This response will circulate oxygen and nutrients at a faster rate to supply the increased demands of tissue metabolism. Fevers are often associated with symptoms of fatigue and malaise (generally feeling unwell). Feeling unwell is also important as it promotes rest, which aids recovery. Exercise in the presence of infection is potentially harmful to the heart, so should be avoided.

Fever management in adults

As pyrexia is part of a physiological response to an infection or injury, it would seem inappropriate to automatically reduce temperature with the use of antipyretic drugs such as aspirin or paracetamol. Some people still treat all pyrexias while others only treat fevers when they reach a particular high level. What now seems clear is that we have been too ready to give antipyuretics in the past. Use of antipyuretics also makes it difficult to follow the evolution of an infection.

After considering the effects of fever on the function of the immune system it would seem that a pyrexial state promotes patient recovery. However, if it is concluded the pyrexia is doing more harm than good then it would seem best to treat the fever. Adverse effects of pyrexia include using up the body's energy reserves more rapidly due to the raised metabolic rate. This can mean that the body's reserves of fats and proteins are used as an energy source leading to depletion, although feeding can replace such losses. If patients have compromised cardiac or pulmonary function an excessive strain may be placed on these systems. Also pyrexial patients will lose more body fluids, partly as a consequence of increased respiratory rate. However, this complication can usually be compensated for by increasing fluid intake. Reducing fever also makes patients feel better in the short term.

Fever management in children

Babies under two months of age have a limited ability to generate fever. This means a baby may have a significant infection but not demonstrate a typical febrile response. Children under the age of 2 years are not able to effectively regulate their body temperatures. As a result a child's temperature may rise rapidly without being detected.

A child with a high fever is at risk from brain damage because the individual neurones which compose the central nervous system are largely made up of proteins. Protein molecules are long chains of amino acids folded to form three dimensional structures. These structures are maintained by the formation of cross bonds between different lengths of an amino acid chain. It is the molecular shape formed by protein molecules which allows them to perform a particular physiological function the individual molecule is designed to fulfil. Increases in temperature will break some of the cross bonds between different lengths of a protein, this will mean the molecule will no longer be held in the correct shape. In essence the protein will unfold; this is referred to as denaturing of the molecule. If this happens extensively within a neurone, the cell will no longer be able to carry out the essential physiology necessary for life and will die. Brain and spinal cord tissues contain very few stem cells, this means that if part of the brain or spinal cord is damaged it has virtually no powers of regeneration. This is why CNS damage is essentially irreversible.

As a consequence it is necessary to monitor a febrile child's temperature closely. Paracetamol or ibuprofen (never both together) should be considered if the child appears distressed or is unwell. These antipyretic drugs are usually very effective in reducing temperature back down towards normal. Pyrexial children should be kept in light clothing and nursed in a cool area. The environment should not be cold as this will simply cause peripheral vasoconstriction, retaining unwanted heat in the body. This is why tepid sponging is no longer recommended. Fluids should usually be encouraged to maintain hydration. Of course the cause of any infection causing the fever should be identified and treated accordingly.

Some children are genetically predisposed to febrile convulsions. These are fits that occur when the child has a fever. The peak age for these episodes is 5 months to 5 years, but older and younger children may still have these febrile fits. Typically, febrile convulsions occur early in the course of a febrile illness. Most febrile convulsions occur when the child has a temperature of over 39°C. Typically the convulsion only lasts for a few minutes and needs no specific treatment other than antipyuretics. Prolonged febrile convulsions (those lasting 15 minutes or longer) are rare but must be treated more actively, as there is the possibility of resulting brain damage. Diazepam is the drug of choice given either by slow intravenous injection or preferably per rectum.

Early detection of infection

In addition to recording temperatures in patients who have a recognised infection, close observations should be maintained in those who are at increased risk. When an infection is detected in the early stages, treatment may be given in order to prevent the condition becoming established. If someone is immunocompromised for whatever reason, they are particularly prone to intercurrent infections. This high risk group includes patients on immunosuppressant therapy following tissue graft surgery (i.e. recipients of organs or tissue from a donor) and patients on steroids or chemotherapy. Diseases such as leukaemia and AIDS predispose to infection and asplenic (without a spleen) patients are also vulnerable.

Heat illness

Heat illness is a general term used to describe the effect of excessive heat on the body. This has nothing to do with the pyrexia associated with fevers. In heat illness the temperature set point in the hypothalamus is normal but the individual still suffers from the effects of excessive heat. There are three forms of heat illness; heat cramps, heat stroke and heat exhaustion.

Heat cramps

These cramps occur in skeletal muscles and can be moderately painful. When there is a lack of salt in the extracellular fluids, which bathe the muscle cells, cramps develop. Historically, these cramps were suffered by people who stoked steam boilers. Stoking was hard physical work in hot conditions which resulted in excessive sweating and therefore loss of salt and water from the body. After a period of this work, the stoker would become thirsty and drink water. This would have the effect of diluting the extracellular fluids, essentially reducing the concentrations of salt. When the concentration of salt was sufficiently depleted the individual would suffer cramp. This is why the traditional term for heat cramps is 'stoker's cramps'. Miners also suffered the same symptoms and compensated by putting salt in their beer. (Despite this tradition, we should recommend against drinking alcohol in hot conditions as it is a diuretic.)

Heat cramps still occur, even in young fit people, often after a days strenuous activity in hot conditions. Adding some salt to drinking water or food can prevent the problem. Long distance runners for example, often take special drinks containing carbohydrates for energy with salt to prevent cramps. From this it can be seen that 'heat cramps' are caused by the effects of being hot and sweating over a period of time, rather than being caused by the heat directly.

Heat stroke

Heat stroke occurs when the body is unable to prevent a rise in body temperature. When core temperature rises to a hyperthermia of 40°C or higher this may be described as heat stroke.

Aetiology

Basically heat stroke will develop whenever heat gained by the body exceeds heat lost to the environment. Heat stroke often occurs in areas of high ambient humidity. (Ambient means in the surrounding environment). When humidity is high, sweat will not evaporate as efficiently as in conditions of low humidity.

If humidity reaches 100%, evaporation of sweat will be essentially zero. This means in high humidity, body temperature will start to rise if air temperature exceeds about 33-34°C. Body temperature will also rise if a person is immersed in water of 34°C or higher. Conversely, when atmospheric humidity is low, people can tolerate air temperatures significantly above body temperature as sweat is free to evaporate, cooling the body. Tolerance of hot conditions is therefore good as long as people have access to plenty of water and salt, to replace losses incurred by sweating.

Exercise causes catabolic processes in skeletal muscles. Catabolism describes any biochemical reaction where large molecules are broken down into smaller ones. Fatty acids and sugars are oxidised in the mitochondria of the cells to produce energy. Most of the energy produced ends up as heat. As blood circulates through skeletal muscles this heat is distributed around the body raising core temperature. (In addition to the generation of energy, water and carbon dioxide are produced as waste products.) As exercise generates heat, the more exercise carried out the more heat will be produced. This will clearly contribute to a developing heat stroke.

Overdressing is another possible cause of heat stroke. This often occurs in military training where it is necessary to wear a lot of kit, often carrying weights while exercising in warm environments. Clothes will prevent the circulation of cooling air and inhibit the ability of sweat to evaporate.

Increase in core temperature will also increase the temperature of the hypothalamus. In many cases of heat stroke this will inhibit the ability of the hypothalamus to stimulate sweating. If this occurs and sweating is no longer stimulated an upward vicious spiral may rapidly result in death.

If the body has been too hot for a period of time prickly heat may develop. In this condition there is inflammation of sweat glands resulting in a blockage of the ducts which prevents sweat reaching the surface of the body. Numerous small pimples develop on the surface of the skin. If prickly heat is widespread, sweat secretion will be inhibited, preventing heat loss by sweat evaporation. Prickly heat may therefore contribute to the development of heat stroke.

Clinical features

An increase in the temperature of the brain above 41°C will lead to features such as dizziness, headache, nausea, vomiting and disorientation. Confusion caused by the hyperthermia may prevent the individual taking logical remedial action to cool themselves down. Eventually there will be loss of consciousness and irreversible brain damage.

Muscle cell membranes are prone to heat injury which can allow myoglobin to escape into the tissue fluids and blood, possibly leading to rhabdomyolysis. Heat can also adversely affect the blood clotting mechanisms leading to disseminated intravascular coagulation with vascular thrombosis and haemorrhage. The liver and kidneys are also vulnerable. There have been cases of people who have survived a period of heat stroke only to die in subsequent days from organ failure.

Management

Treatment is aimed at reducing the temperature back down to normal as rapidly as possible. Some people have suggested placing the patient in cold water to achieve this. However a bath of cold water may well not be available. Even when people are placed in cold water, a peripheral vasoconstriction is caused which will reduce heat loss to the environment. For these reasons most thinking in this area would advise removal from the heat source if possible, followed by rest and tepid sponging in a well ventilated area. When tepid water is used the vasoconstriction associated with cold water is avoided. Direct fanning may also lead to vasoconstriction; this is why the person should be in an area of moving air currents rather than subject to a direct air stream. Plenty of water should be drunk but alcohol should be avoided as it is a diuretic and so contributes to dehydration. Temperature should be monitored until it has returned to normal. Even after effective treatment, the patient may feel weak and unwell for a day or two after the event.

Heat exhaustion

Aetiology

Heat exhaustion occurs when there is a loss of salt and fluids from the body. This may develop over a long or short period of time depending on the balance between loss and replacement. In hot environments active people may lose over 5 litres of sweat per day and as much as 20 grams of salt.

Clinical features

When fluid and salt are lost from the body, blood volume is initially maintained as water moves osmotically from the tissue and intracellular fluid compartments, to replenish the intravascular volume. (Intravascular means within the blood circulatory system.) However, as the condition worsens a hypovolaemia will develop eventually leading to hypotension. Poor blood supply to the muscles will lead to a generalised fatigue. Reduced perfusion of the brain will cause giddiness, syncope and eventually delirium. As dehydration progresses, sweating will be inhibited, leading to an increase in core temperature with the possible development of heat stroke. Dehydration will also lead to reduced urine volumes (oliguria) and eventually there may be a complete cessation of urine production (anuria) resulting in acute renal failure.

Management

These patients should be cared for in a cool shady place. They should drink about 5 litres of water and be given 25 grams of salt in the first 24 hours. More serious cases may require parenteral fluid replacement. If venous access is not attainable, an intraosseous infusion directly into a bone (usually the tibia) may be necessary. Particular attention should be paid to sodium and potassium levels in the plasma as these are vital electrolytes.

Ideally the condition would have been prevented by taking in adequate volumes of fluids and electrolytes before heat stroke developed. A useful guide in hot conditions is that people should drink enough to ensure they are passing regular volumes of fairly light coloured urine.

Acclimatization to heat

When someone moves to a hot environment, or spends a lot of time in the heat, several physiological adaptations occur. There is an increase in the maximal rate of sweating and an increase in plasma volume to allow for this. Increased plasma volume also allows blood pressure to be maintained in the presence of widespread vasodilation. Heat increases levels of aldosterone released from the adrenal cortex. This hormone increases the reabsorption of salt from the glomerular filtrate, resulting in reduced salt losses in urine. Aldosterone will also reduce the concentration of salt in sweat, resulting in sweat becoming more hypotonic (less osmotic than plasma). Basic tropical acclimatisation takes about 10 days but will progress for some months. A person who is acclimatised to heat will be less likely to suffer from heat cramps, stroke or exhaustion.

Hypothermia

Causes of hypothermia

Hypothermia is usually defined as core body temperature below 35°C. Low core temperatures usually occur accidentally. Whenever heat loss exceeds heat gain the body temperature will fall. If a person falls into cold water, heat will rapidly be conducted out of the body into the water. In very cold water death may occur within a few minutes due to rapid cooling. Cold environments, especially if accompanied by wind, can cool the body down; the combination of cold and wind is referred to as wind chill. Wetness is another major risk factor. When someone is wet the latent heat of vaporisation will be extracted from the body to evaporate surface water. This will lead to rapid cooling. Anything causing immobility in cold conditions, such as a fall, may also lead to hypothermia. Other causes of immobility may include an acute illness such as a myocardial infarction or cerebrovascular accident.

Assessment

An accurate core temperature must be determined which could be recorded rectally. In addition to the degree of hypothermia it is important to try and find out how long the patient has been hypothermic for. Rapid onset hypothermia is often defined as developing in less than 12 hours. Insidious onset cases develop over more than 12 hours.

Clinical features

In hypothermia none of the body cells will be working efficiently. This is because the intracellular enzymes, which catalyse all of the biochemistry in a cell, function optimally at normal body temperature. Any cooling will therefore reduce enzymic activity and so retard cell biochemistry and physiology.

Low grade hypothermia, 36 – 35°C

When people start to cool down the skin appears pale because of peripheral vasoconstriction, there will be shivering and piloerection (contraction of hair erector muscles in the dermis) will cause goose pimples.

Mild hypothermia, 35 – 32°C

Below 35°C mental function starts to decline, there will be increasing confusion and decreasing levels of consciousness. Progressive decreased motor function will also present.

Other features of mild hypothermia may be explained by hypothalamic mediated, attempted sympathetic compensation. As cold blood is detected by the hypothalamus, neurones respond by stimulating activity in the sympathetic nervous system. The autonomic nervous system is physiologically divided into sympathetic and parasympathetic branches; the sympathetic is often associated with the 'fight or flight' response. Sympathetic activity is designed to improve the chances of individual survival in difficult and stressful situations. In hypothermia, sympathetic responses attempt to conserve and generate heat. Shivering is maximal at about 35-32°C and the person feels intensely cold as a result of profound peripheral vasoconstriction. As more blood is retained in the core of the body, lower volumes are needed overall and a cold induced diuresis will develop. Tachycardia and increased blood pressure may also present.

Moderate hypothermia 32 – 28°C

As the brain cools, there is a risk of convulsions and a progressive reduction in the level of consciousness. Muscular rigidity will develop. Eventually the hypothalamus itself will no longer be able to function normally and loses the ability to generate sympathetic compensations. Reduced function of the hypothalamus can be explained by the cold reducing the activity of essential intracellular enzymes. This is why there is little or no shivering when core temperature falls below 32°C. Loss of sympathetic tone will also allow peripheral blood vessels to dilate. This will allow relatively warm blood to circulate near the dermal temperature receptors resulting in the hypothermic person beginning to feel warm. Once these sympathetic compensatory mechanisms fail, the rate of temperature reduction will accelerate and the patient is in immediate danger.

Cold oedema develops as the capillaries are no longer able to retain the fluid component of the plasma, eventually resulting in hypovolaemia. In combination with bradycardia and vasodilation this will lead to hypotension. Reduced renal function will complicate hypotension leading to renal failure. Sinoatrial and atrioventricular node depression may cause cardiac dysrhythmias. It is important to realise that hypothermia of 32°C or less is frequently fatal as it may cause ventricular fibrillation.

Severe / profound hypothermia, less than 28°C

If core temperature drops to these levels this will cause coma. Pulse and respirations may not be detectable and the condition mimics death. As the temperature drops further there will be spontaneous cardiac dysrhythmias and death may occur from ventricular fibrillation. If the patient is still alive by the time their temperature drops to 24°C, respirations will cease and below this the heart will stop spontaneously.

Management of hypothermia

There are essentially two ways a hypothermic patient may be warmed up. Firstly; passive rewarming is when the patient is kept warm and the body temperature returns to normal as a result of the person's own metabolic processes. Secondly; active rewarming uses sources of external heat. Active methods are sometimes divided into external and internal rewarming. Active external involves gaining heat by such methods as huddling with warm people or using warm baths or air. Active internal involves the use of inhalation of warmed air, warmed IV fluids and gastric or peritoneal lavage. In all of these methods the trunk should be warmed before the peripheries.

Principles in rewarming management

As a general principle, in patients where hypothermia is of rapid onset, rapid rewarming is indicated. This is because the body temperature may continue to fall, even after the person has been rescued. Rapid rewarming in these cases may prevent cardiac complications. Conversely, when the onset has been prolonged, the patient needs to be rewarmed slowly. Most authorities recommend rewarming should be no faster than 1°C per hour. If temperature rises more rapidly, after prolonged hypothermia, death may result because the cold heart cannot increase output to match increased systemic oxygen demand.

Ideally the patient is cared for in a warm environment if this is available. Further heat loss should be prevented. They should be kept dry and given layers of clothing. As a lot of heat can be lost from the head, some form of hat or head covering should be used. Warm food and drink may be given but these should not be too hot as vasodilation may be induced. Any cause of sudden vasodilation may lead to the phenomenon known as 'after drop'. This occurs when the core temperature falls as a result of cold blood returning from near the body surface and extremities. Warming the torso of the body before the limbs helps to prevent after drop. Mass return of cold blood to the heart may cause ventricular fibrillation so must be avoided. Hypothermic people must be handled very gently as sudden or vigorous movements may precipitate life threatening cardiac dysrhythmias.

If a hypothermic patient needs to be rescued they should be kept flat. This was discovered when people died being hoisted out of cold water by helicopters. As a cold heart is irritable it has a lowered threshold for ventricular fibrillation. If a patient is rescued upright there will be pooling of blood in the lower half of the body resulting in a drop in venous return, which will lead to a proportional reduction in cardiac output. Cardiac output is dependent on venous return; if blood is not being returned to the heart it cannot be pumped out. This drop in cardiac output will result in a reduced perfusion and oxygenation of the myocardium.

During any form of rewarming it is essential to monitor the temperature, cardiac activity, fluid balance and biochemistry, correcting any abnormalities. Oxygen should be given if available; this will improve oxygenation of hypoperfused areas and will reduce the irritability of excitable tissues (i.e. nerve and muscle.) Cases of later post rewarming death may occur in the elderly as oedematous fluid is reabsorbed into the blood leading to fluid overload.

As hypothermic patients may appear to be dead, death should not be diagnosed in the presence of a low body temperature. If a hypothermic patient is warmed and is found to be dead, then it is safe to diagnose death. Other patients, who may appear to be dead, will recover when warmed. This is why 'no one is dead until they are warm and dead'.

Induced hypothermia

In the future we may well see more therapeutically induced hypothermia. For example, after head injuries, hypothermia will reduce the metabolic activity of the brain which will reduce the production of potentially toxic waste products which may cause secondary brain injury. In countries where cardiopulmonary bypass facilities are not available induced hypothermia is used during heart surgery. Induced hypothermia may also improve prognosis in the follow up management of out of hospital cardiac arrest.

Temperature observations after surgery or trauma

Temperature should be monitored in all postoperative patients. Lowered body temperature may occur after surgery as a result of exposure to cool air during surgery, as an effect of the anaesthetic or due to the period of immobility. Traumatised patients are also at risk of hypothermia from cold environments, immobility or infusions of cool intravenous fluids. Whatever the cause hypothermia will reduce the ability of the blood to clot.

Conversely, an increase in temperature may occur as a consequence of tissue damage suffered during surgery or trauma; this is why low grade pyrexia in the days after surgery or injury may be normal. However, pyrexia in later days could indicate the development of an infection. This may be associated with the operation or injury site or be related to other interventions such as intravenous therapy. In fact any invasive procedures carry some infection risk, as external devices are in contact with the blood or body fluids. Continued observation of temperature may also discover pyrexia caused by the development of complications. For example, patients with reduced mobility have an increased risk of hypostatic pneumonia. This is an infection affecting all lobes of the lungs and pyrexia may be an early indicator of this complication. Urinary tract infection or DVT may also complicate surgery. Pyrexia is also a complication of blood transfusions, indicating a possible mismatch.

Health and the weather

In warmer weather there are more pollen and fungal spores and these lead to an increased prevalence of hay fever and asthma. Hot weather also causes an increase in thromboembolic disease. This may be because sweating reduces the proportion of water in the blood, leading to increased viscosity. In the United Kingdom there is an increase in mortality and morbidity every winter of approximately 20-30% compared to summer. Mortality describes the death rate and morbidity the number of people suffering from a disease. After a spell of cold weather there is a delayed effect on morbidity and mortality. For example, incidence of myocardial infarction increases after 3 days; this may be explained partly by an increase in blood pressure caused by cold induced vasoconstriction. Cold also seems to increase fibrinogen plasma levels, arguably making thrombus formation more likely. Thrombosis describes a pathological blood clot in a vessel. Fibrinogen is the precursor of fibrin which is long sticky strands of protein. Because fibrin is sticky it adheres to and collects blood cells to form a clot. These factors, caused by exposure to cold, may also explain the increase in strokes which occurs 5 days after a cold spell.

When someone becomes chilled and shivery they increase the probability of developing a respiratory infection. As cold air causes vasoconstriction of the blood vessels in the nose, there will be a reduced blood supply. This in turn will reduce the circulation of white blood cells to the area. It has therefore been suggested that the deficiency of these defence cells may allow any infections in the air to become established, leading to infection. Another factor leading to an increased incidence of respiratory infections in winter is crowding in poorly ventilated spaces. During cold weather this can clearly lead to contagion and is a factor in the development of flu epidemics. Another effect of cold weather is an increase in injuries from falls on icy and slippery surfaces. The elderly are at particular risk from such falls which can lead to broken bones and other injuries.

In the UK, the proportion of people admitted into hospital during winter time who are hypothermic may be 2% of all admissions. Much of the explanation for this is that the British do not adapt dress and lifestyle sufficiently when the ambient temperature is low. In other cold countries, people tend to account for the cold more effectively. This may explain why the winter increase in mortality in many colder countries is actually less than in the UK.

CHAPTER 25

Wounds and Healing

Introduction

Wound healing occurs whenever there is injury to the tissues of the body. An injury describes an area of loss of continuity in any body tissue, this may occur as a result of trauma, infection or a pathological process. The mode of wound healing depends on the powers of regeneration a particular tissue possesses. The following are some examples at specific sites.

Liver

Liver is able to regenerate very well. For example, acute hepatic injury caused by viral hepatitis or toxin exposure, can regenerate completely restoring full form and function. However, chronic insults such as ongoing exposure to alcohol or hepatitis C virus, may result in the formation of collagen based scars and the development of cirrhosis. This latter process is associated with loss of functional liver tissue, so may progress to liver failure. This gives hope for heavy drinkers; liver function may be restored, sometimes after many years of abuse, as long as the person stops drinking before cirrhosis is established.

Kidneys

In the kidneys, epithelial tissues lining renal tubules may regenerate but whole nephrons do not. This means that mild damage to the kidneys will heal completely but more extensive injuries will result in scar formation. The glomeruli are the balls of capillaries within a Bowman's capsule and do not regenerate after injury. However, if one kidney is removed, the glomeruli in the other kidney enlarge to compensate.

Lungs

Damage to the alveoli may occur as a result of infection, inhalation of irritants or shock. As long as the basement membranes of the alveoli remain intact there can be complete healing. However, more severe damage can lead to areas of pulmonary fibrosis. The epithelial lining of the respiratory tract may regenerate effectively after injury, provided that the underlying structures and extracellular matrix framework is preserved. In the trachea and bronchial passages, there is restoration of epithelium from adjacent cells after injury.

Muscle

Skeletal and cardiac muscle cells do not have the potential for significant mitosis in adults. This means that damaged muscle cells are not effectively replaced. In skeletal muscles, if there is a relatively small area of injury, other muscle cells can enlarge to restore overall muscle strength. Damage to the myocardium which results in necrosis is permanent, as cardiac muscle cells do not divide. Healing is by the formation of granulation tissue and fibrosis (i.e. fibrous scar tissue). This means affected areas of myocardium become non-contractile. This is why early thrombolysis is so important after coronary thrombosis, to prevent necrosis developing.

Nervous system

Most neurons do not divide and are not capable of mitosis after injury. Any functional recovery which occurs after death of CNS neurones is primarily as a result of reorganisation of surviving nerve cells to re-establish neural connections. In the peripheral nervous system axons may slowly regrow, but even this does not occur in most of the CNS. Damage to the CNS results in the formation of gliosis, this is a permanent scarring of the nervous system. Gliosis occurs as a result of proliferation of glial cells, which are the supportive and structural non-neuronal cells of the nervous system. Once gliosis is established, there is no ongoing recovery of neurones; this explains why transverse spinal cord injuries cause permanent paralysis, and why dementia is irreversible.

Common types of wound

Contusion

A contusion is more commonly called a bruise. It is usually caused by a blunt blow, the overlying skin is unbroken, but tissues and blood vessels below are damaged. The discolouration is caused by bleeding from small vessels into the tissues. Red blood cells trapped in the tissue spaces become deoxygenated and

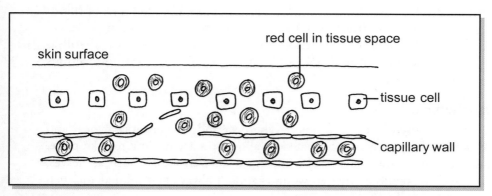

Diagram 25.1
A contusion or bruise represents the presence of blood cells in the tissue spaces. This causes a characteristic discolouration of the area. Initially a bruise is 'black and blue' due to the presence of reduced haemoglobin in the tissues. Over time macrophages phagocytose the red cells in the tissues and the haemoglobin is converted to bilirubin. This is why the discolouration changes from blue to yellow as the bruise fades.

dark coloured. Bruising can also develop after deeper tissues, such as bones are damaged, and may only become apparent after a period of time as blood tracks towards the body surface.

If blood collects in a discrete pool within the tissues this is described as a haematoma. As the blood in a haematoma is well consolidated it may cause pressure effects on surrounding tissues, these may include pain and nerve compression. There is a risk a haematoma may become infected and some need to be surgically evacuated.

Abrasion

An abrasion is a scrape or graze. Typically, there is a superficial surface wound involving the epidermis and part of the dermis. As dermal nociceptors are exposed in the damaged dermis, these wounds are often very painful. Some abrasions can however, be deeper wounds involving tissues below the level of the skin. Abrasions are most commonly caused by friction injuries, falling off bikes is a common cause. These wounds need to be well cleaned to remove dirt and grit which may be sticking to the wound surface.

Avulsion

This term describes a wound where there is tissue loss, preventing the closure of the wound edges. An avulsion may be caused by gouging or tearing of tissue.

Laceration

Laceration describes a wound made by a blunt object, and has often involved considerable force. The wound edges are usually split or torn with ragged edges as the skin has been burst rather than cut. After significant trauma there may be lacerations involving internal organs. Lacerations of the liver, kidneys, or spleen may be associated with serious haemorrhage requiring urgent surgical intervention. This is why traumatised patients should be managed as still as possible, as movement may dislodge blood clots and result in more serious internal haemorrhage.

Incised wound

This is a cut caused by a sharp object. These wounds usually appear neat and the edges can be readily approximated to allow primary healing to take place. In incised wounds the cut may also involve deeper structures such as nerves, blood vessels or tendons. Incised wounds should always be explored for such deeper injuries and treated as required.

Puncture wounds

These may well present as misleadingly small wounds and are also described as penetrating wounds. They are made by pointed or sharp objects. As the edges of the wound may be closed above areas of bacterial contamination, infection is a potential hazard. Also puncture wounds may penetrate down into body cavities or other significant structures such as blood vessels. If the base of a wound cannot be seen it should be surgically explored as a matter of urgency.

Strains

Strains are injuries to muscles, fascia or tendons caused by stretching forces. Patients complain of pain and stiffness and there may be some associated swelling. It is usually important to exclude other injuries such as fractures. Strain injuries usually resolve with rest followed by progressive mobilisation.

Sprains

A sprain describes an injury to the fibrous tissues surrounding a joint. Fibrous ligaments around the joint are injured, usually as a result of excessive movement of the joint. A mild sprain may involve tearing a few of the fibres in a ligament, in more serious cases there will be associated haematoma formation. In severe cases there may be complete tearing and disruption of a ligament. Patients usually present with local heat, pain, swelling, disability and possible discolouration over the area. Ankles are commonly sprained; if the ankle is turned inwards there will be injury to the lateral ligaments. Sprains usually take longer to recover than strains as ligaments have a poor blood supply.

Priorities in wound management

Systemic stabilisation

In any person with a wound, priority is always given to their systemic condition, only after this has been assessed and stabilised as required, is the wound considered in detail. After trauma, the first priority is always airway with cervical spinal protection followed by breathing and ventilation, then comes circulation with haemorrhage control. These priorities must all first be assessed and managed as required.

Haemostasis

Haemostasis means the arrest of haemorrhage and is clearly essential. Haemostasis is normally achieved by the application of firm direct pressure over the wound. This pressure will close off local blood vessels and give the blood time to clot. The principles of haemostasis are discussed in more detail in Chapter 8.

However, with some wounds, bleeding should be encouraged. This is true when the wound is likely to be contaminated and when blood loss will not be too severe. For example, in case of accidental needle stick injury you should encourage bleeding as much as possible by squeezing the wound and running it under warm water. Warm water will bring about a localised vasodilation, which will increase the volume of bleeding. The outward flow of blood may wash out potential disease causing agents, such as bacteria and viruses. The same is true for other potentially dirty wounds such as animal or human bites.

Wound assessment

After bleeding has been stopped the wound should be anaesthetised if required. The wound should be explored to carry out an accurate assessment. Whenever a practitioner is confronted with a wound, they must identify which form of healing is indicated for the particular wound under consideration. This will usually involve healing by either primary or secondary intention.

Healing by primary intention

A wound will heal by primary intention if the edges of the wound can be approximated together. Some form of wound closure is normally employed to keep the wound edges closed. Common ways of achieving closure and stability of the wound edges include adhesive strips, sutures or super glue.

Advantages of healing by primary intention

Approximation and stabilisation will allow the edges of a wound to heal directly into each other. In primary healing the process is fairly rapid, normally wound edges will be closed with sufficient tensile strength to remove the sutures after 7-10 days. However, it takes much longer than this to restore full strength to the wound, even after 2 weeks the wound only has 20% of full strength. If the edges of a wound are closed, the surface area of the wound is reduced. This means that there will be a minimal amount of scar tissue formed, giving good cosmetic and functional results. As the wound is closed, there is less opportunity for secondary colonisation or infection to enter the wound from outside sources of microbiological contamination.

Potential problems with primary intention

Because the wound edges are closed, there is the possibility that foreign material or bacteria may be enclosed within the wound. This will allow any bacteria present to multiply and lead to wound infection with possible abscess formation. Also the presence of foreign material can lead to future complications such as pain and damage to tissues. If foreign material can be removed before closure, this particular complication may be prevented; this is one reason why wound exploration is so vital. If the wound is likely to be contaminated with bacteria from the implement which made the wound, then again it is unwise to close the wound, unless the practitioner feels they are able to adequately wash away the contamination with irrigation or other wound cleaning procedures. When primary healing is not possible, or is not advisable, healing by secondary intention will be used.

Healing by secondary intention

In this form of healing the wound is left open and allowed to heal by granulation. It is appropriate to use secondary healing when there is tissue loss and a wound cannot be closed because the edges will not approximate. In addition, if a

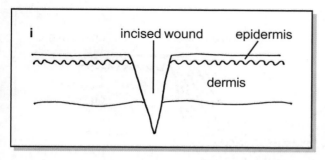

Diagram 25.2

i. Cross section of a wound. This is an incised wound; a sharp object has cut through the epidermis, dermis and some underlying tissue. When the skin is cut the edges 'fall apart' or 'pull open', this is because intact skin is under a degree of tension.

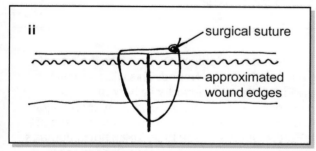

ii. The edges of this wound have been pulled together as close to their original position as possible, after this approximation a suture has been inserted to hold the wound edges together to promote primary healing.

wound is contaminated secondary healing may be chosen to prevent infective complications. All chronic wounds, such as ulcers, will be colonised with bacteria and so should not be closed.

It is particularly dangerous to close a wound if there are anaerobic organisms present. If a wound is closed, the amount of oxygen the wound is exposed to is reduced; this lack of oxygen promotes the growth of anaerobic bacteria, such as Clostridium strains, which may lead to tissue necrosis and gangrene. Prior to the advent of antibiotics, gangrene was the most common indication for limb amputation. Tetanus is caused by Clostridium tetani, a gram positive bacillus which is also anaerobic.

Disadvantages associated with secondary intention

Because the wound is left open to heal by granulation the time taken can be much longer than for primary healing. As secondary healing may be a protracted process, more nursing time will be required before the patient can be fully independent again.

A large wound may take several months to heal. Because the wound is larger, more scar tissue will form resulting in poorer cosmetic and functional than in primary healing. In secondary healing there is a risk that a wound may become infected from outside sources of contamination. All chronic wounds are colonised with various forms of bacteria but this does not adversely affect the healing process unless it develops into infection. Bacteria from a colonised or infected wound may however be transferred to another wound, or the wound of another patient, if we are not careful in preventing cross infection. Some wounds may be managed open for a time to allow for cleaning or removal of devitalised tissue. After this time of cleaning such wounds may be subsequently closed, this is a delayed primary closure (or DPC).

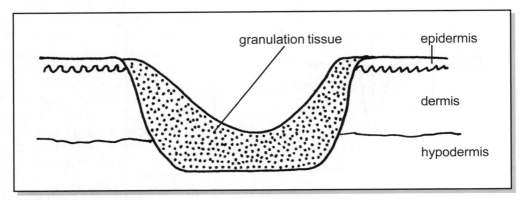

granulation tissue   epidermis

dermis

hypodermis

Diagram 25.3
Cross section of a wound healing by secondary intention, this involves the formation of granulation tissue which is progressively filling the wound. This will promote the processes of tissue healing with residual granulation eventually becoming scar tissue. An important part of management is the preservation of healthy granulation tissue; this will involve the use of non adhesive dressings and the maintenance of a moist wound healing environment. Particular care needs to be taken not to damage this important but delicate tissue during procedures such as dressing changes.

Delayed primary closure

This means a wound is allowed to heal by primary intention, but only after being managed open for a period of time after the initial injury. First the wound is treated to ensure it is clean enough to permit healing by primary intention. This may involve using agents to clean the wound and the removal of any devitalised tissue, which would necrose if left. After this, the wound is closed to facilitate primary healing. Skin grafting is an example of a delayed primary closure. The donated skin is placed over the recipient area and heals in direct contact with the underlying tissue, so the healing is primary in nature.

Wound healing by regeneration and/or repair

Healing of wounds occurs by two physiological processes called regeneration and repair. In regeneration the wound heals as the lost tissue is replaced by cells from adjacent healthy tissue. Mitosis occurs in these adjacent cells to replace the cells lost as a result of the injury. This means the tissue is restored, more or less as it was, by the process of cellular and tissue regeneration. This is the ideal form of healing giving good cosmetic and functional results.

Repair is an efficient method of closing and 'patching' damaged tissues. The damaged specialised tissue is replaced with collagen. Collagen is a tough protein with high tensile strength; it is the main component of fibrous scar tissue. In repair, the original tissue is replaced with fibrous tissue, so the functional and cosmetic results are poor. Most wounds heal by a combination of regeneration and repair.

Stages in wound healing

It is traditional to describe wound healing in terms of stages; however in practise there is overlap. These stages and the physiology involved apply to wounds healing by primary and secondary intention.

Inflammatory phase

This is the first stage and is essential if the wound is to progress on to further stages of healing. Damaged blood vessels undergo a reflex vasoconstriction, this is to reduce blood loss and allow the blood time to clot. As a result of haemorrhage the wound fills up with clotted blood. Shortly after the vasoconstrictive phase, release of inflammatory mediators from damaged tissue and mast cells causes an inflammatory vasodilation.

Vasodilation leads to increased local blood flow, a reaction termed a hyperaemia. This increases the flow of nutrients to the injured area as these will be needed as raw materials in the process of repairing damaged cells and producing new ones by mitosis. The increased flow of red blood cells increases the delivery of oxygen, to keep the damaged area well oxygenated. This is vital as wound healing is a very energy demanding process. Anabolic reactions are needed to build and repair cells, and like any building work, large amounts of energy are required. All energy production is dependent on the oxygenation of food based fuels, so if a wound is hypoxic, energy production and hence healing will be impeded. This explains why a good blood supply and effective tissue oxygenation is vital in the process of wound healing.

Inflammatory vasodilation has the effect of increasing the physical size of the gaps between adjacent capillary endothelial cells. This promotes increased capillary permeability resulting in them becoming 'leaky'. Increased capillary permeability allows larger molecules, such as fibrinogen, to escape into the tissue spaces. In the wound and tissue spaces, fibrinogen is converted into long sticky strands of the clotting protein fibrin. Networks of fibrin strands form a physical barrier to compartmentalise the injured area and may play a vital role in preventing the spread of infection to healthy tissues. The framework generated by fibrin also acts as a provisional matrix through which healing can start. Also fibrin and other proteins, within the first 4 hours, provide the initial mechanical stabilisation of a wound.

Destructive phase

White blood cells are also able to migrate from the blood into the tissue spaces; they can squeeze through the enlarged gaps between the capillary endothelial cells. Neutrophils arrive via the blood and migrate into the tissue spaces of the wound within the first 24 hours. Neutrophils phagocytose any foreign organisms which may have been introduced clearly reducing the risk of infection. Neutrophils also phagocytose debris in the wound such as dead tissue cells.

The trauma will have killed local tissue cells and if these are not removed from the wound they will become a ready food supply for bacteria. Monocytes also migrate into the wound after about 24 hours. Once in the tissues, these monocytes also phagocytose bacteria and dead tissue, this causes them to grow and they become large cells called macrophages. ('Macro' means big and 'phage' relates to eating, so these cells are literally 'big eaters'.)

Neutrophils and macrophages are able to move independently through the tissue spaces using a process called amoeboid movement. They are chemically attracted to bacteria and dead tissue, so their phagocytic activity is well targeted. This means bacteria and dead tissue are destroyed in a physiological process of debridement. To debride a wound in surgery means to clean by removing foreign, infected or devitalized material.

In addition to phagocytosis, macrophages also coordinate much of the healing process by release of growth factors. These locally acting chemicals stimulate the regrowth of epithelium, new capillaries and the migration of fibroblasts. At least 20 different growth factors are involved in normal wound healing. In the absence of macrophages, there are no growth factors to stimulate mitosis in adjacent healthy tissues. This means that regeneration of damaged tissues cannot occur.

Proliferation phase

This phase of wound healing starts about 2 to 3 days after the initial injury. By this time the phagocytic cells should have cleaned out the wound and disposed of any dead tissue. It is now necessary for fibroblasts to migrate into the wound. A 'blast' cell produces and secretes a product, so fibroblasts produce the extracellular material needed for fibrous tissue formation. Fibroblasts are attracted into the wound by growth factors released from macrophages and by chemicals released from damaged matrix. (Matrix is the ground substance of a tissue; it fills up the spaces between the cells and other extracellular components. It is composed of a variable mixture of carbohydrate and protein molecules called glycoproteins.) Like phagocytes, fibroblasts are able to actively migrate through tissues, but more slowly.

Fibroblasts are essential for wound healing; they synthesise and secrete collagen and ground substance. Fibroblasts also secrete further growth factors which stimulate and regulate the regeneration of new blood vessels, a process called angiogenesis. 'Angio' relates to blood vessel and 'genesis' means beginning, this process is also sometimes called angioneogenesis, literally the beginning of new blood vessels.

Once in the wound cavity, the fibroblasts secrete collagen strands, these form a three dimensional 'scaffolding' through which repair can occur. As soon as 1-2 days after the injury, granulation tissue begins to form. Granulation tissue is a combination of fibroblasts, collagen, new capillary loops, new matrix and macrophages. Later it also contains numerous plasma cells. These are derived

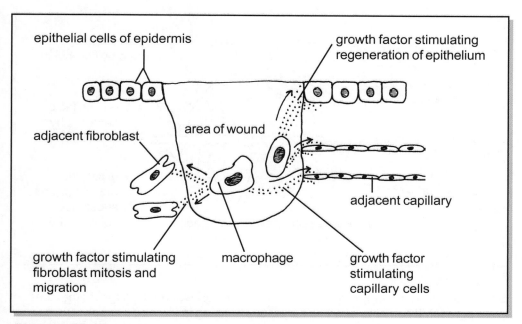

Diagram 25.4
In the tissues or in a wound, monocytes become large cells called macrophages. As well as ingesting and digesting bacteria and dead tissue in the process of phagocytosis, they coordinate much of the regenerative process, by synthesising and releasing growth factors. These growth factor chemicals diffuse through the tissue fluids and stimulate mitosis and migration of adjacent healthy cells. This cellular stimulation is responsible for the processes of fibroblast migration, angioneogenesis and re-epithelialization.

from B lymphocytes and secrete antibodies. The combination of antibodies and phagocytic cells makes granulation tissue very resistant to infection. Because circulating blood can be seen through the translucent new tissue, granulation tissue is bright red in colour. Granulation tissue is fragile and bleeds readily because of the new thin walled blood vessels it contains.

Re-epithelialization is also part of the proliferation phase. This refers to the re-growth of epithelial tissue. Viable epidermal cells divide by mitosis and start to migrate over the surface of the granulation tissue. Epithelialization occurs in wounds that heal by primary as well as by secondary intention. In primary intention the epithelial migration begins within a few hours, and if no complications occur, should have effectively sealed off the underlying wound within about 48 hours. This should be the case with sutured surgical wounds, and explains why surgical patients are usually allowed to shower 2 days after surgery.

Re-epithelialization may develop from the wound edges. Anatomically, epidermis dips down into the hair follicles, into the dermis and even hypodermis. This means there are reserves of epidermal cells in these deeper structures. As a

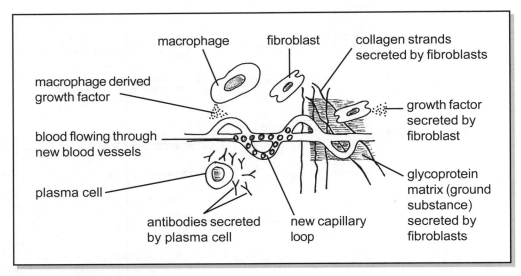

Diagram 25.5
Granulation tissue is only produced when required for wound healing, at other times it is not present. It contains new capillary loops bringing in the blood supply. Collagen strands, ground substance and some growth factors are secreted by fibroblasts. Macrophages phagocytose bacteria and dead tissue and secrete most of the growth factors. Plasma cells derived from B lymphocytes secrete immunoglobulins (i.e. antibodies).

result, the epidermis may regenerate from these preserved deep elements. This means that even when the full thickness of the epidermis is lost, full regeneration is still possible.

In wounds healing by primary intention re-epithelialization takes place over the granulation tissue but below the scab on top of the wound, the scab is mostly the residue from the initial blood clot. This scab is very useful as it helps to keep bacteria out of the wound until it can be sealed by the new epithelium. It also prevents the new epithelium and granulation tissue from drying out. This is essential as these new cells and tissues can dry out and so dehydrate. This would kill the new cells so prevent re-epithelialization.

Larger wounds healing by secondary intention also need to have a moist environment to preserve the granulation tissue and promote cellular migration. This is best achieved by using some form of dressing to keep in the natural tissue fluids. As well as keeping the wound moist, these physiological fluids also contain essential growth factors released by macrophages and fibroblasts.

Remodelling phase

This is also referred to as the maturational phase. It typically begins about 3 weeks after the injury and may go on for a year or more, depending on the size of the wound. Collagen fibres progressively align themselves with the tensile forces passing through the wound, this gives progressively increasing strength.

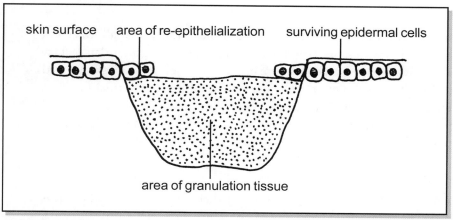

Diagram 25.6
The process of re-epithelialization in a wound healing by secondary intention.
In these wounds, re-epithelialization is seen as pink tissue around the wound
edges. (Re-epithelialization may also develop from preserved 'islands' of
epithelium within a wound.)

Eventually the strength of the wound is about 75% that of uninjured tissue.
Especially in wounds which have healed by secondary intention there is
contraction of the scar tissue. This is a useful feature of remodelling as it means
scars become smaller. However, contractures may develop over joints, especially
after burns and may inhibit movement. Such contractures may need to be
surgically divided. Wound contraction occurs because specialised fibroblasts,
called myofibroblasts, join up and contract in a similar way to smooth muscle.
Scar vascularity also reduces with time. Young scars have a pink/red appearance,
due to blood flowing through the tissue. As vascularity decreases the scar fades
and will eventually become a similar colour to the surrounding skin. So we can
reassure patients that scars will shrink and fade.

Hypertrophic and keloid scars

You may have come across cases of healing wounds where the proliferation of
scar tissue continues, resulting in the formation of a hypertrophic or keloid
scar. Hypertrophic scars do not proliferate beyond the limits of the original
wound, do not increase in size and often regress after 2-3 months. Keloid scars
however, normally extend beyond the original wound area and may continue
to grow for years. Both of these abnormalities are benign.

Factors which may delay wound healing

Local and systemic factors may influence the rate of wound healing. Local factors
describe the conditions in the immediate wound environment while systemic
factors refer to 'whole body' influences on the local wounded area.

Infection

It is a common observation that infected wounds heal slowly, if at all. Infection means that bacteria are present in the wound and are generating an inflammatory host response. Living bacteria secrete waste products of their metabolism referred to as exotoxins. These substances are toxic, and so inhibit the normal function of local cells and tissues e.g. they may interfere with protein synthesis. Infected wounds need to be well cleaned and often systemic antibiotics are needed. Any foreign bodies in a wound are also likely to be associated with infection.

Poor hygiene

Patients with poor personal hygiene may infect their wounds from other areas of their body or from outside sources of contamination. This can also be a problem in people who interfere with wound dressings.

Local blood supply

Good blood supply to a wound is one of the main factors promoting healing. Wounds on areas of the body with copious blood supplies, such as the face or scalp, tend to heal quickly. Conversely areas of the body with a poorer blood supply, such as the back or feet, heal more slowly. Blood supplies leucocytes, nutrients, oxygen, removes waste products, and keeps the wound warm; all factors which promote healing. Wound ischaemia may occur as a result of the initial trauma, if blood vessels are damaged or compressed by swelling. Pre-existing vascular insufficiency is a significant adverse factor in healing. Ischaemia results in very poor rates of healing or no healing at all. For example, foot or leg wounds in patients with peripheral vascular disease are notoriously difficult to heal. Venous deficiency is an adverse factor in wound healing, as seen in venous leg ulceration. Systemic conditions affecting the cardiovascular system may also reduce local wound perfusion; these may include heart failure or shock. Immobility will also reduce the circulation of the blood and so reduce wound perfusion.

Oedema

The presence of oedema, for whatever reason, adversely affects wound healing. All cells of the body receive nutrients and oxygen from the capillary blood, via tissue fluid, by the process of diffusion. If there is an increased volume of tissue fluid, as is the case in oedema, then there will be an increase in the distance from the capillaries to the tissue cells. This increased distance means nutrients and oxygen have further to travel to reach the cells, so supplies are reduced. The result is that cells become relatively embarrassed and their ability to function is reduced. If cell function is reduced wound healing will be correspondingly adversely affected.

Inhibited wound oxygenation

This may occur secondary to wound ischaemia. Lack of oxygen in the wound is a consequence of a poor blood supply, as it is the blood which transports oxygen to the area. Any systemic cause of hypoxia will also reduce wound oxygenation and healing rates. This means if you are able to improve any underlying causes of wound hypoxia, such as respiratory infection or anaemia, wound healing will be promoted.

Smoking

Smoking may adversely affect wound healing. Nicotine causes vasoconstriction, therefore reduces blood supply to the skin and periphery. This reduces the perfusion of wounds. Smoke also contains carbon monoxide which increases the proportion of carboxyhaemoglobin in the blood. Another problem is that smokers lose more vitamin C than non-smokers. Smoke causes the breakdown and increased excretion of vitamin C from the body, resulting in a chronic shortage. As vitamin C is essential for collagen formation wound healing will be correspondingly inhibited.

Cooling of the wound

Cooling leads to localised vasoconstriction which reduces wound perfusion. As wound healing is dependent on a good blood flow to supply nutrients and oxygen, the process will be inhibited. Removal of metabolic and respiratory waste products will also be correspondingly inhibited. Wound cooling will inhibit the biochemical processes in local cells as this chemistry is dependent on the action of intracellular enzymes. Enzymes are made of proteins and only function within a narrow temperature range. Wound cooling should therefore be prevented as far as possible and should be a consideration in wound redressing procedures. In hypothermia when the whole body is cool, peripheral vasoconstriction will result in wound bed cooling. Also when the body is hypothermic, all metabolic processes will be retarded.

Insufficient diet or malnutrition

For a wound to heal it needs to be supplied with the nutritional building blocks required for the regeneration of tissues. To optimise wound healing the patient should eat an adequate balanced diet including adequate proteins, carbohydrates, fats, vitamins, minerals, fibre and water. Balanced means the dietary components should be eaten in the profile required by the body. Adequate means the components must be eaten in sufficient quantities. Malnutrition delays healing.

Proteins

Proteins in the diet are broken down into component amino acids during digestion. Amino acids then circulate in the blood and are taken up by tissues where they are needed. Human proteins contain 20 different forms of amino acids. A single protein may contain hundreds or thousands of amino acid units. For a wound to heal new cells and tissues must be constructed, amino acids are required as building block components for the new proteins. Without amino acids from the diet, wounds fail to heal properly and may even break down. Lack of protein specifically inhibits angiogenesis, collagen and matrix synthesis and fibroblast proliferation. Severe lack of protein will also lead to hypoproteinaemia and consequent oedema.

Carbohydrates

Carbohydrates are energy giving foods. Wound healing is a very energy demanding process so carbohydrates are important to fuel metabolic processes in the cells and tissues involved. Patients with extensive wounds, e.g. large burns, will need an increased intake of energy giving foods. When adequate carbohydrates are available the body does not need to break down amino acids for energy production.

Fats

Fats are composed of sub-units called fatty acids in much the same way proteins are composed of amino acids. Some components of cells and tissues e.g. cell membranes, are composed of fatty acids, so a supply of these is required for tissue regeneration. In addition to supplying essential fatty acid building blocks, fats also act as a source of energy for cell metabolism in a similar way to carbohydrates.

Vitamins

Vitamins are micronutrients which are vital in the diet. Vitamins A, D, E and K are fat soluble and so may be stored in the body. Vitamins B_1-B_{11} and C are water soluble so cannot be stored. Vitamin C (ascorbic acid) is particularly important for wound healing as it is essential for protein and collagen formation. When a person is very deficient in vitamin C, old wounds may fall apart as collagen in scar tissue is not adequately maintained. Vitamin A is important for regenerative processes such as re-epithelialization, collagen synthesis and angiogenesis. Vitamin A also helps to reverse the anti-inflammatory effects of corticosteroid drugs and so may promote wound healing in such patients. Vitamin B is needed to facilitate the action of several enzymes needed for normal tissue regeneration. Adequate vitamin K is needed for blood clotting and the prevention of haematoma formation.

Minerals

Minerals are inorganic nutrients required in small quantities for health. One essential mineral required for wound healing is zinc, this is probably essential for re-epithelialization.

Psychological Stress

Stress has adverse effects on the immune system; this may make wound infection more likely. During periods of anxiety, people release the hormone adrenaline from the adrenal medulla. Epinephrine (adrenaline) is a very powerful vasconstricting agent. Peripheral vasoconstriction will reduce perfusion of the wound, with a corresponding reduction in local blood supply. Steroid hormones, such as hydrocortisone, are released during periods of stress from the adrenal cortex; these hormones inhibit the inflammatory response. As in other conditions, the way you approach and communicate with your patient has the potential to significantly reduce their anxiety levels. If the patient believes you are trying your best to help them and have the ability to do so, they will feel psychologically better and should therefore heal more rapidly.

Delayed inflammatory response

The inflammatory response may be delayed for local or systemic reasons. If the area is cold, there will not be significant inflammation as the vasoconstricting reaction to cold will act against the vasodilatory effect of the inflammatory process. A reduced inflammatory response is also seen in patients who are receiving corticosteroids as these drugs are very anti-inflammatory. Corticosteroids work by decreasing capillary permeability and inhibiting fibroblast activity and the phagocytic capacity of leucocytes. As discussed above, inflammation is the first essential stage in the physiology of wound healing so any factor which reduces this response will delay wound healing.

Age effects

Children and young adults usually heal well. It is important to remember that children with wounds need adequate nutrients for wound healing, in addition to the normal requirements of growth and development. Wound healing in the elderly may be slow due to a reduced number of fibroblasts in their tissues and consequent reduced rates of collagen formation. Re-epithelialization and wound contraction are also slower in older people. The elderly are more likely to have underlying disease processes which may adversely affect wound healing such as diabetes mellitus, heart disease and peripheral ischaemia. They are more likely to have reduced mobility, with increased risk of pressure sore formation.

Poorly managed or unrecognised diabetes mellitus

It is a common observation that people with diabetes mellitus often have poor wound healing. Adverse effects on wound healing are related to poor glycaemic control. Higher blood sugar levels inhibit wound healing. Reasons for this include high levels of glucose in the tissue fluids and basement membrane thickening in arterioles, capillaries and venules.

CHAPTER 26

Fractures

Introduction

A fracture describes any loss of continuity in the substance of a bone; this may range from a hair line crack to massive disruption of a bone.

Open and closed fractures

In a closed fracture the skin overlying the break is intact, if there are any injuries to the skin these are superficial and not related to the fracture. In an open (formally called compound) fracture there is a wound connecting the broken ends of the bone with the outside air. In some cases the broken end of bone may protrude through the skin. However, broken ends of bone may penetrate the skin from inside and not be externally visible. This is why even small wounds around a fracture site must be treated with extreme suspicion as they may indicate that a fracture is open. Outside trauma may also cause a wound which is continuous with a fracture. If there is any communication between the broken bone and the surface there is the potential for infection to enter the bone. This may lead to osteomyelitis which can be very difficult to eliminate.

Causes; traumatic, pathological and stress fractures

Direct and indirect trauma can cause fractures. Whenever the force applied to a bone exceeds its strength a fracture will result. Pathological fractures occur as a result of some abnormality in a bone which leads to weakness. Osteoporosis is the most common cause of pathological fractures. Other causes include metabolic disturbances, bone cysts, tumours and infection. In some bones with pathology present, relatively mild trauma may lead to a fracture. Stress fractures, sometimes termed march or fatigue fractures, develop as a result of repeated mild trauma to a bone. Repeated stress induces microfractures which eventually unite to cause a true fracture through the bone cortex. Common causes include long distance walking or running.

Descriptions of fractures

Hairline fractures are caused by minimal trauma or repeated stress, there is no displacement of the bone ends. Greenstick fractures occur in children as their bones are not as brittle as adults. A fracture line is caused part way through the bone on the opposite side to the causal traumatic forces. Simple fractures are uncomplicated and closed and are described by the orientation of the fracture line seen. In a simple transverse fracture the break runs at a right angle to the shaft of the bone or has an angle of less than 30°. If the angle is more than 30° the fracture is described as oblique. A simple spiral fracture spirals around the shaft of a bone. In contrast to simple, a complicated fracture is one which involves important soft tissue damage such as injury or compromise of blood vessels, nerves or internal organs.

Comminuted fractures are also described as multifragmentary and are usually caused by high energy trauma, such as a road traffic accident (RTA) or high falls.

Comminution describes a fracture with more than two fragments; in severe cases there may be multiple small pieces of bone. These fractures are often associated with significant soft tissue injuries, can be difficult to reduce and heal slowly. Crush fractures occur as a result of compression forces; these may involve the vertebral bodies or heels. Avulsion means to 'tear away' so a breach in the continuity of the bone is caused by tearing. Avulsion fractures are therefore caused by tractional forces such as those generated by sudden muscular contractions when a tendon or ligament may tear off a fragment of bone. Impacted fractures occur when one bone fragment is driven into another. If the skull is struck by a blunt object, such as a hammer, a piece of bone may be forced down into the brain tissue; this is termed a depressed fracture. An unstable fracture is one which is displaced or has the potential to be displaced. Displacement is when the bone ends have shifted relative to one another. This is important as soft tissues may be damaged or the fracture may become open. For example, a displaced vertebral fracture may cut the spinal cord resulting in complete loss of motor and sensory function below the level of the lesion.

Clinical features of fractures

Fractures are very painful. The periosteum and endosteum, lining the outside of a bone and the medullary cavity respectively, are well supplied with nociceptors. When a bone is broken these tissues are disturbed, often resulting in extreme (often called exquisite) pain. This pain is worse with movement and when any stress is applied to a limb. Direct pressure over a fracture line causes extreme pain. Fractures cause loss of function, so a person will not be able to use a fractured limb. This is partly due to the pain as well as the mechanical deficit caused by the fracture. Crepitus describes the sound of two broken ends of bone grating together, for example when a patient is being moved. While this will confirm the presence of a fracture it should not be elicited as it damages the bone ends and soft tissues. Any abnormal movement in a limb should be noted, for example a leg may flex abnormally if there is a fracture in a long bone, but again this feature should be observed not elicited. Numerous limb deformities may be seen if a bone is displaced as a result of a fracture. A limb may lie in an abnormal position or there may be shortening. Displaced fractures may also be seen as displacements of the skin if they are applying pressure from underneath. In some open fractures a bone end may protrude through the skin and be obvious. Swelling from inflammation and haematoma will develop around a fracture site and after some time bruising usually develops.

Dislocation injuries

Trauma involving joints may lead to disruption of the normal anatomy of the articular surfaces. Dislocation describes the complete loss of congruity of the joint surfaces, with one bone end being greatly displaced from the other bony component of the joint. A subluxation is a partial loss of contact between the

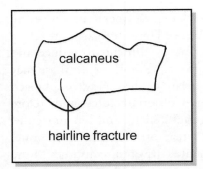

Diagram 26.1
Hairline fracture.

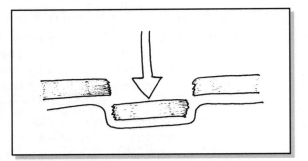

Diagram 26.2
In a depressed fracture a bone fragment penetrates inward into underlying tissues.

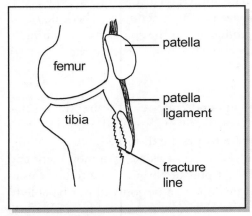

Diagram 26.3
Avulsion fracture, in this case of the tibia.

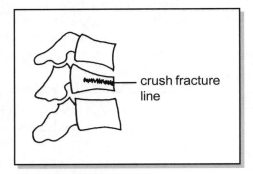

Diagram 26.4
Crush or compression fracture.

joint surfaces. The articular surfaces will be partly displaced, but there will not be gross displacement of the bones involved. As the bone ends displace there is stretching and injury to the joint capsule causing a lot of pain. Common sites of dislocation injuries include the shoulder, fingers, wrists, elbows, hips and knees. Dislocations and subluxations are normally manipulated back into position under anaesthesia or sedation. Dislocations may interrupt the normal blood supply to the bone ends or to other tissues, so should be reduced as soon as possible.

Healing in bones

Given time bone healing is a very effective process; once healing is complete the bone is as strong as before the fracture. Healing in bones is a continuous ongoinig process from acute inflammation, through repair to remodelling. Despite this the following descriptive stages are useful; these are haematoma formation, cellular proliferation, callus formation, ossification and remodelling.

Diagram 26.5
Simple transverse fracture.

Diagram 26.6
Simple oblique fracture.

Diagram 26.7
Simple spiral fracture.

Diagram 26.8
Greenstick fracture.

Diagram 26.9
In an impacted fracture the two bone ends have been forced together.

Diagram 26.10
Multifragmentary or comminuted fracture.

Diagram 26.11
Fracture showing displacement.

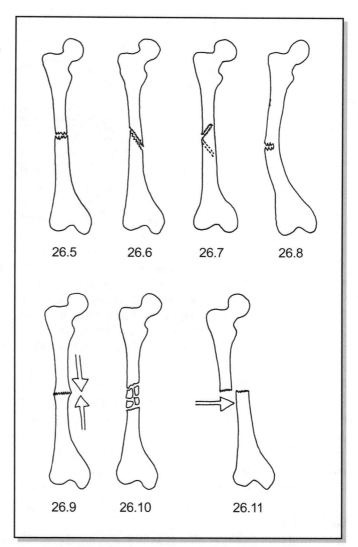

26.5 26.6 26.7 26.8

26.9 26.10 26.11

Haematoma formation

As bones are highly vascular, fractures will tear blood vessels present in the bone. This results in local haematoma formation. It is likely that signal molecules derive from the haematoma which stimulate some of the cellular activities needed for subsequent bone healing. The fracture ends are jagged and will damage surrounding tissues if they are not well immobilised. Fibrinogen in the haematoma is converted into strands of fibrin which act as a provisional framework for future cellular migration and healing. About 7 days after the initial injury most of the haematoma is organised with new blood vessels and early collagen based fibrosis. Over time the blood clot is dissolved and replaced with granulation tissue.

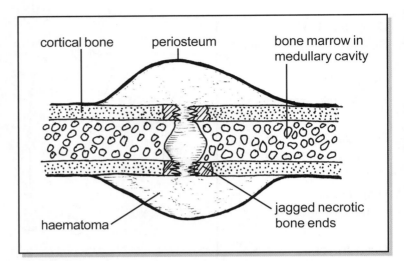

Diagram 26.12
Cortical bone ends are necrotic as the trauma has disrupted blood vessels within the bone and perforating vessels from the periosteum, this results in avascular areas. Bone edges at the fracture site are jagged as a result of the initial trauma. The haematoma is essential to initiate the process of bone healing.

Cellular proliferation

Fractures in bone activate local osteoblasts in the periosteum, endosteum and bone medullary cavity. Osteoblasts are the bone forming cells; they synthesise and secrete collagen which forms the principle structural framework of bone. The combination of new proliferated cells and the extracellular material they secrete forms soft callus. Cellular proliferation will also restore any damaged areas of periosteum.

Callus formation

Within about 2 weeks the osteoblasts, and the collagen they secrete, form bridging or soft callus which is composed mostly of fibrous tissue with some cartilage (sometimes called fibrocartilaginous callus). This substance is relatively soft and flexible and grows outwards from the broken edges of bone forming a bridge connecting the broken ends of the bones together. After 3 to 4 weeks mineral salts are deposited onto the soft fibrocartilaginous callus to form a hard, but immature, callus which is often referred to as woven bone.

Ossification

At this stage of consolidation the fracture has been firmly fixed and the callus is progressively replaced with mature bone. This mature bone is referred to as lamellar bone as it contains concentric lamellae which are well organised rings of calcified collagen. In other words the normal histology of the bone is restored.

The fracture site now appears united on X-rays and feels firm and immovable. At this stage plaster casts or other fixation devices may be removed. Excess callus is reabsorbed by the action of osteoclasts.

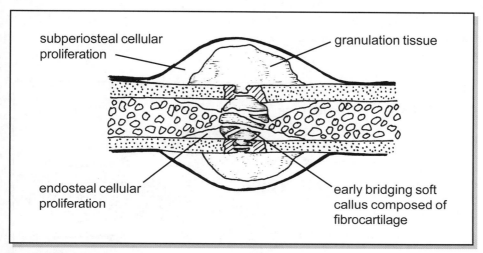

Diagram 26.13
The haematoma has now been organised into granulation tissue. Cellular proliferation has lead to soft callus formation. Areas of cellular proliferation have developed into fibrocartilaginous callous. This new tissue is evident within the medullary cavity, under the periosteum and forming bridges between the broken ends of the bone.

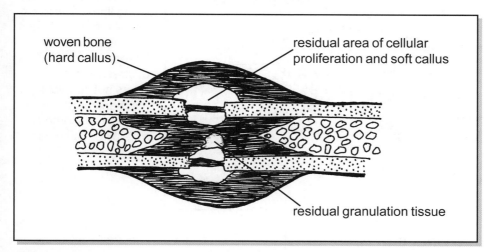

Diagram 26.14
Mineralisation of the soft callus leads to the formation of hard callus, which is woven bone. Jagged and necrotic edges of the original cortex have been removed by the action of osteoclasts. Some soft callus and haematoma remain in the fracture site.

Remodelling

Reabsorption of excess callus from the medullary cavity and from around the fracture site continues. Remodelling is directed by the lines of mechanical stress which run through a bone, mostly generated by weight bearing. The result of this process is the restoration of the normal anatomy of the bone cortex and medullary cavity. This process may go on for several years after the fracture has clinically healed.

Diagram 26.15
Mature lamellar bone progressively replaces the immature woven bone resulting in solid fixation of the bone ends. The union is now solid and strong.

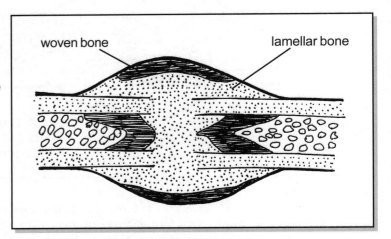

woven bone   lamellar bone

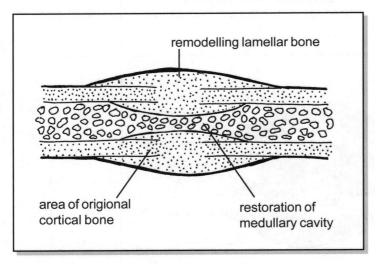

remodelling lamellar bone

area of origional cortical bone

restoration of medullary cavity

Diagram 26.16
New bone is organised along lines of stress and mechanical forces. Osteoblast activity increases along lines of stress, while in areas not subject to mechanical stress, bone is reabsorbed as a result of osteoclast activity.

Factors affecting bone healing

Blood supply and bone blood flow is the most important requirement for fracture healing. Blood supply is required to provide oxygen for metabolic processes and essential nutrients required for reconstruction. Good nutrition is needed for bone healing with essential nutrients including vitamins A, C and

D. If there is extensive associated soft tissue injury around a fracture this will delay bone healing, partly because there may be disruption of the blood supply. Generally, thicker bones such as the femur or tibia take longer to heal than thinner bones such as the ribs or clavicle. In children bone healing is quicker than in adults; however old adults do not heal significantly more slowly than young adults. Other factors include the site of the fracture and the overall health of the patient.

Nicotine from smoking slows the process of bone healing, reduces the strength of callus and increases the probability of non-union. Significant use of NSAIDs also delays bone healing. Non-union is when a fracture does not heal. Causes include interposition of soft tissue at the fracture site as this prevents bridging of the gap between the bone ends. If the gap between two bone ends is too large non-union may also result. Other causes of non-union include infection, excessive motion of the bone ends and a poor blood supply.

Treatment principles

Reduction

Reduction describes the process of restoration of a normal alignment of broken bones with the establishment of apposition of bone ends. If this is not carried out the bone ends may heal in the wrong position; this is termed malunion. Traction may be necessary to restore normal length of a limb and promote bone alignment. This process of stretching will prevent the broken ends of the bone causing further damage to the bone ends or to soft tissues, explaining why it often reduces pain. Traction may also improve blood supply to a limb by re-stretching kinked blood vessels. Closed reduction involves the manipulation of a fracture, normally using a combination of traction and manual pressure. Anaesthesia is needed for this process as it is likely to cause severe pain. Once the fracture has been reduced it is normally held in place using a plaster cast. Pins may be inserted into a bone and connected using an external fixation device. Open reduction involves a surgical procedure to pin a fracture using metal plates which are screwed into the bone ends. Alternatively intramedullary nails may be used.

Immobilisation

In order to heal the fracture ends must be immobilised, as mentioned this is maintained by plaster casts, internal or external fixation. In the first aid situation splints may reduce bleeding, further bone or soft tissue injury, pain and nerve or blood vessel compression. Good levels of immobilisation reduce the amount of excess callus formed and improve the rate of bone healing. If a fracture is not immobilised this may result in the formation of a pseudoarthrosis; this is when a joint forms where there should not be one. Fibrous joint-like tissue forms between the two bone ends and remains mobile for life.

CHAPTER 27

Burns

Aetiology

Burns are a common cause of injury in all countries of the world. Excessive heat is the obvious cause of burns which leads to thermal injuries. These may be caused by flames, steam, hot fluids or hot solids. Unguarded fires are a danger to children and toddlers are at particular risk from kitchen accidents. Older people may be more at risk as a consequence of impaired mobility and poor coordination. In many burn injuries alcohol intoxication is a contributory factor. The severity of a burn depends on the degree of heat and the time a tissue is exposed to the heat source. For example, a temperature of 70°C or more will cause necrosis of the full depth of the epidermis in just a few seconds.

Radiation is another possible cause, for example ultraviolet radiation may cause sunburn. Chemical burns may be caused by direct contact with a number of agents. Strong acids such as sulphuric acid from car batteries or alkalis such as cement are frequent causes. Other chemicals such as mustard gas, phosphorus or phenols will also lead to burning. If an electrical current passes through a tissue it will encounter resistance which will lead to heating and development of an electrical burn. If a current passes through the body, deep structures such as bones and muscles may be seriously injured, sometimes despite apparently minor superficial burning.

Pathophysiology

Burns often affect the skin and body surfaces but any tissue may be potentially involved. The direct effect of heat will lead to the death of cells and therefore an area of necrosis. In addition heating proteins causes them to lose their complex structure and denature. This will result in protein coagulation with consequent necrosis. (You may have noticed protein denaturation and coagulation as the clear part of an egg becomes white during cooking.) Around the coagulated burnt necrotic tissue there will be an area of constricted blood vessels with platelet coagulation known as the zone of stasis, this area may also necrose due to reduced perfusion. Around this zone there is an area of inflammation. In addition to these local effects there are several potential systemic complications of burns which are discussed below.

Superficial burns

Burns are classified by the depth of skin affected by the injury. Superficial (1st degree) burns only affect the epidermis without dermal involvement. Sunburn is a common cause of such superficial epidermal burns. Despite being superficial these burns can be extremely painful and tender if touched. The burned area is red but will blanch readily with light pressure. Blanching means the area becomes white as the pressure compresses blood vessels in the dermis. This confirms the small dermal blood vessels are intact. Vesicles (small blisters) or bullae (large blisters) do not usually develop. These burns heal rapidly as the injured epidermal cells are replaced by young cells from the germinative layer below.

Partial thickness burns

Partial thickness (2nd degree) burns injure part of the dermis and may be described as superficial or deep.

Superficial partial-thickness burns

Superficial partial-thickness burns involve the epidermis and superficial dermis. Loss of epidermis and upper dermis will expose dermal nociceptors generating a lot of pain and tenderness. Burned areas will still blanch with pressure and blisters filled with inflammatory fluid develop within 24 hours. A blister is a collection of fluid just above the germinative layer of the epidermis and they suggest partial thickness injury. Fluid loss and swelling due to local oedema may be extensive.

Healing will occur as fibroblasts and other cellular components of the dermis undergo mitosis and secrete structural components such as collagen, elastic fibres and ground substance (the tissue matrix). In addition deep epidermal cells (keratinocytes) lining sweat glands and hair follicles will divide and migrate across the surface of the burn to regenerate the epidermis. These burns will typically heal in two weeks. Epidermal regeneration will give a perfect cosmetic result providing they heal without complications such as infection. Antimicrobial creams and occlusive dressings are often used as epithelialisation progresses faster in a moist environment.

Deep partial-thickness burns

Deep partial-thickness (also referred to as deep dermal) burns extend down to involve the lower half of the dermis. These burns have a variable appearance, they may be red or white, some have mottled red and white areas. These deeper burns do not blanch as many of the dermal capillaries have been lost. Inflammatory swelling and fluid loss are again significant. As many of the nociceptors in the upper layers of the dermis are burnt away these deeper injuries are typically less painful than superficial partial thickness burns. Due to loss of upper dermal peripheral sensory receptors a pin prick may be experienced as pressure. This is because pressure receptors are located in the deep dermis and so may be preserved.

Deep partial-thickness burns take more than 3 weeks to heal as more dermis must be regenerated and the epidermal type keratinocytes are only present lining hair follicles at the deeper levels of the dermis. These deep preserved areas of epithelial cells may migrate to provide some epidermal regeneration but healing is often accompanied by hypertrophic scar formation. Infection is a common complication which further delays healing. Because of these difficulties in healing many units will surgically excise necrotic superficial tissues and then use skin grafting to close the wounds.

Full thickness burns

Full thickness (3rd degree) burns extend through the whole thickness of the dermis into the underlying subcutaneous layers. All of the epidermal and dermal elements are destroyed. The burnt skin tissues undergo coagulative necrosis and form a layer of dead tissue called an eschar. This is often surgically removed as it is an infection risk but if not the dead tissue will separate after 2-3 weeks. Full thickness injuries may appear white, black and charred or brown and leathery. They do not blanch with pressure.

Full thickness burns are less painful than partial thickness as all of the dermal sensory receptors have been necrosed. Areas of full thickness injury may be insensitive to touch as well as pain. Patients may still experience significant pain from peripheral areas of superficial or partial thickness burns. As all of the epidermis and dermis is lost in these burns, all of the potentially regenerative elements are also lost. This means full thickness burns can only regenerate from the intact skin around the periphery of the burn. As a result these burns will regenerate very slowly from the outside inwards. In practise full thickness burns will only heal by using skin grafting, unless they are very small. Without grafting healing will occur by granulation and fibrosis leaving ugly areas of contracted scars.

Body surface area involvement

Assessing the percentage of body surface area (BSA) affected by partial or full thickness burning has important consequences for fluid replacement therapy. In adults the rule of nine may be employed to approximate the percentage of skin surface involved. Another guiding principle is that the area of the patients palm and fingers is about 0.8% of BSA. The rule of nine does not apply to children who have relatively large heads and small limbs. In children charts (such as the Lund-Browder) are used. When assessing burns it is also important to check for other injuries which may be associated with the burn such as those from a fall or road traffic accident.

Principles of first aid

As always the first priorities are ABC (airway, breathing, circulation). To reduce the likelihood of inhalation injury the patient should be moved to a smoke free atmosphere as soon as possible. Inhalation of smoke and fumes may lead to respiratory arrest in which case mouth to mouth ventilation will be life saving.

Any burning should be extinguished, usually by smothering the fire. Clothes may remain hot for many seconds after a fire has been extinguished. This continued exposure to heat will continue to burn the tissues. If scalding water is spilt onto clothes this will continue to burn the skin for several minutes unless it is removed. These principles explain why clothing should be rapidly removed or doused with cold water.

Diagram 27.1
This diagram is a cross section through the skin and illustrates the epidermis, dermis and subcutaneous tissues. The arrows on the left point out the depth to which skin destruction occurs in the different classifications of burns. The presence of nociceptors in the dermis explains why injuries at this level can be so painful. Epithelial epidermal cells line the sweat gland ducts and hair follicles. This means that if the epidermis and part of the dermis are lost, the epidermis is able to regenerate from these deep preserved epithelial cells. Epidermal regeneration means the burn may heal without scar tissue formation. (It is indeed fortunate that the skin is arranged in this way, with deep reserves of epidermal cells. If this were not the case even relatively superficial injuries and burns would not be able to heal by regeneration. As a result superficial wounds would have to heal by granulation and fibrosis. This would delay the process of wound healing and make infection much more likely. Also most people would be covered in scars as a result of previous superficial injuries. Scar tissue is of course associated with poor functional and cosmetic results.)

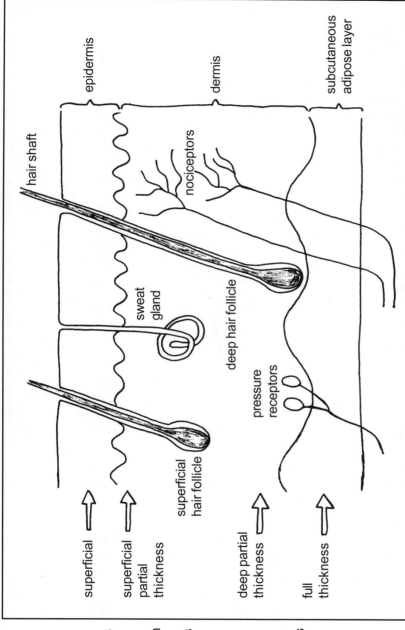

- epidermis
- dermis
- subcutaneous adipose layer
- hair shaft
- nociceptors
- sweat gland
- deep hair follicle
- superficial hair follicle
- pressure receptors
- superficial
- superficial partial thickness
- deep partial thickness
- full thickness

Diagram 27.2
The rule of nine. In adults the surface area of the body can be divided into areas of 9%. The head and neck represent 9% of BSA. Anterior and posterior aspects of the trunk represent 18% each, e.g. half of the front of the trunk is 9% of BSA. Each arm is 9% and the legs are 18% each. This means that if the front of one arm was burnt 4.5% of BSA would be involved. The front of one leg would be 9%. Genitalia and perineum compose the final 1%.

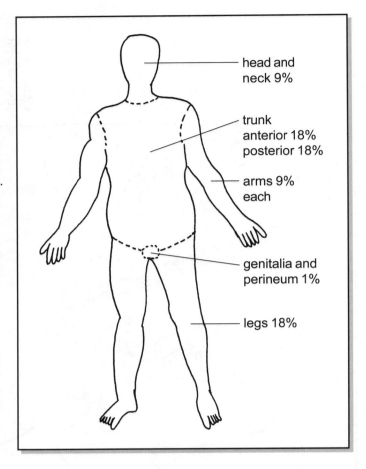

head and neck 9%

trunk
anterior 18%
posterior 18%

arms 9%
each

genitalia and perineum 1%

legs 18%

Thermal burns should be immediately immersed in cool water, probably for about 20 minutes. This provides a lot of pain relief and will conduct away the excess heat which will still be present in the tissues. Ice water should be avoided as it will cause profound vasoconstriction which will reduce the volumes of blood flowing through the injured tissues, this will mean the blood is no longer able to carry away excess heat which will allow the burning process to continue. Cool water will conduct excess heat out of the hot tissue and so will prevent ongoing tissue damage. Wet towels may be applied to the area for transfer to hospital if this is indicated. The only risk in using cool water is that it may contribute to the development of hypothermia.

Many injuries in the home are caused by people pouring water onto chip or frying pan fires. This causes the fat to explode out of the pan and may lead to severe burns as the burning fat is very hot. People should be advised to turn off the heat source and then smother the fire with a damp towel.

As infection is such a common complication in burns it is important to avoid wound contamination in the first aid situation. When a burn is removed from cool water it should be covered with a clean moist sheet. Kitchen cling-film is also an effective temporary measure to prevent wound contamination. Cling-film should be laid on a wound rather than be used to wrap around a wound. This is especially important on limbs as later swelling may lead to constriction of the blood supply.

In cases of chemical burns any powders should be brushed off the skin before wetting. The skin should then be rinsed with water. Washing with large volumes of water is better than trying to neutralize substances chemically. With acids, alkalis or burning organic chemicals the body surface should be flushed with plenty of water for 20 minutes after all of the chemicals appear to have been removed. If the eyes are exposed to burning chemicals prompt irrigation, which may need to be carried on for many minutes, can save the eyesight.

With electrical burns it is vital to make sure the current is switched off or disconnected before touching the patient, this will prevent the rescuer from also being electrocuted. It is possible for cardiac arrest to complicate electrocution.

Complications and management principles of burns

The risk of systemic complications increase with the percentage of body surface area involved. If the body surface area (BSA) involvement is over 40% the risk of severe systemic complications and death are significantly increased. Other major injuries or smoke inhalation or concurrent injuries also increase mortality. People over 60 or below 2 years of age are also at greater risk.

Hypovolaemia

Normally the epidermis forms a waterproof covering over the body. Epidermal damage can therefore allow more water to be lost to the environment. Inflamed skin surfaces 'weep' plasma onto the wound leading to loss of plasma from the blood. Intravascular volume can be further depleted after burns as extensive areas of oedema may develop. Clearly the greater the area of skin disruption the more fluids will be lost from the circulatory volume of blood. Fluid loss will lead to systemic dehydration, thirst, hypovolaemia and potentially shock. Hypovolaemia is a risk factor for the development of acute renal failure. Low circulating blood volumes will also lead to reactionary peripheral vasoconstriction reducing perfusion and therefore healing of the burn. From these potential complications it can be seen why fluid replacement therapy is so vital after significant burn injuries.

If the patient is shocked or has more than 15% BSA burns they will require intravenous fluid resuscitation. Children will require intravenous fluids if more than 10% of BSA is involved. Often a physiological crystalloid fluid, such as Ringer's or Hartmann's solutions, are given for the first 24 hours with colloids possibly being used on the second day. Fluid replacement therapy is continued depending on individual patient assessment. Urine output should be monitored and should be at least 0.5ml per Kg of body weight per hour in adults and 1 ml per Kg per hour in children. Electrolyte balance should also be monitored until the patient is fully stabilised.

After extensive burns the patient will usually be very thirsty. However, paralytic ileus may complicate large burns for the first 2 days preventing oral fluids being absorbed. Most patients are able to tolerate oral fluids after 2 days and should be encouraged to drink large volumes of fluids.

Electrolyte disturbance

Extensive tissue damage means that many individual cells will be damaged or killed. This will allow cellular contents to escape from the cytosol (the intracellular fluid in the cytoplasm) into the extracellular fluids. As intracellular fluids contain a high concentration of potassium, burn injuries may lead to hyperkalaemia. As long as renal function is good, this excess potassium can usually be excreted in the urine. However, if acute renal failure complicates burns, serum potassium levels may rise significantly with the consequent risk to cardiac physiology. These complications demonstrate how important it is to always consider electrolyte balance as well as fluid replacement.

Protein loss

As plasma exudes into the burnt area plasma proteins are lost from the circulation. This can lead to a reduction in the total amount of albumin in the plasma, a condition termed hypoalbuminaemia. Fluid replacement therapy may also dilute the albumin which is still present in the plasma. This may lead to a reduced osmolarity of the blood and contribute to oedema. Dilution of the plasma, secondary to fluid replacement therapy, may also dilute other vital electrolytes in the blood.

Pain

Burns are very painful, frightening and distressing injuries. Partial thickness burns can cause excruciating pain. Intravenous paracetamol or opioids should be given. Pain can also be reduced in the early stages of management by keeping the wound cool. Later, good wound management techniques can also be soothing. Distressed patients should be reassured with the full powers of your empathetic and interpersonal skills.

Acute oedema

In the hours and days after an acute burn injury there will be an inflammatory reaction leading to localised oedema. The oedema generated may be extensive. Oedema around the face and upper airway can lead to airway compromise. Injured arms or legs should be kept elevated until the swelling subsides.

Fluid accumulation beneath the constricted eschar of a deep burn will increase the hydrostatic pressure in the tissue fluids to the extent of closing the blood vessels. This may cut off the blood circulation to an area of tissue, fingers or a limb. Compression by oedema may also constrict the chest and abdomen leading to ventilatory compromise and even respiratory arrest. These potentially serious complications may need to be treated by escharotomy. In this procedure long incisions are made through the rigid eschar to relieve the compression beneath. As these incisions are made into necrosed skin they should not be painful. Also as only dead skin is incised they should cause no additional scaring.

Smoke inhalation

Smoke inhalation injuries and skin burns often present in the same patient. Clinically, we must maintain a high index of suspicion for this form of injury in any patient removed from a smoky or hot environment. Soot or singed hair in the nostrils indicate the patient has inhaled very hot gases or air. Inhalation of very hot gases in a fire typically leads to thermal injuries and inflammation of the upper airway. Inflammation causes oedema of the upper airway (especially the epiglottis) with consequent stridor and possible obstruction. Other indicators of upper airway involvement include difficulty swallowing and drooling of saliva. Airway oedema may require steroids to reduce the inflammatory swelling. Tracheostomy may be indicated to maintain the airway.

Toxic substances generated by combustion usually result in injuries to the lower airways. Lower airway injury may cause coughing, chest pain, wheezing and shortness of breath. Inhalation of toxic fumes from burning furniture foam or plastics in house fires may be fatal. Cyanide may be produced by some fires and will inhibit the ability of the mitochondria to produce energy. Smoke inhalation injuries will usually be supported with high concentrations of humidified oxygen.

Inhalation of hot and toxic gases which injure the lower airways also predispose to the development of pneumonia. This is a recognised complication and should be observed for carefully. Early treatment with antibiotics will reduce the likelihood of the pneumonia becoming more severe.

Carbon monoxide poisoning is another complication that may be caused by inhaling this gas in a fire. This will result in an acute reduction in the oxygen carrying capacity of the blood as a result of the formation of carboxyhaemoglobin. It is important to remember oxygen saturations may appear normal in cases of carbon monoxide poisoning as oximetry probes can not differentiate between carboxyhaemoglobin and oxyhaemoglobin. Some patients with severe carbon monoxide poisoning may require treatment in a hyperbaric oxygen chamber.

Renal involvement

If burn injuries lead to hypovolaemia this will cause reduced renal perfusion. This is a cause of acute renal failure. In significant burns a urinary catheter will usually be passed to monitor hourly volumes of urine. In addition to the risk posed to renal function by hypovolaemia there is a second potential problem.

Injuries which involve muscle tissue, such as deep or electrical burns, can cause the death of muscle cells with consequent release of myoglobin into the body fluids. This can lead to rhabdomyolysis with consequent myoglobinaemia. (Rhabdo means rod shaped or striped, like skeletal muscle fibres, myo relates to muscle and lysis means the break up of cells. Rhabdomyolysis can also develop after muscle crush injuries.). Burns may also damage red blood cells leading to the release of haemoglobin into the plasma, i.e. myoglobinaemia. Myoglobin and haemoglobin are filtered from the blood into the nephrons. Some will pass through the nephrons and enter the urine where it can be recognised in dark coloured urine which may even be treacly black. If there is too much myoglobin or haemoglobin in the glomerular filtrate these large protein based molecules will clog up the renal tubules causing acute tubular necrosis with consequent acute renal failure

Stress ulcers

Curling's ulcers are acute duodenal ulcers which may develop after significant burns. Multiple gastric erosions are another possible complication. It seems likely that these ulcers are caused by reductions in gastrointestinal mucosal blood flow caused by the sympathetic stress reaction to the injury. If patients can start eating at an early stage, or are given enteral feeding, these are less likely to develop. It is also common to give ranitidine prophylactically.

Increased nutritional requirements

After a burn injury the metabolic rate of the body increases significantly. This is partly the result of a stress induced hormonal response and partly because the body must reconstruct a lot of damaged tissue and regenerate tissue lost to necrosis. These healing processes require extensive anabolic (building up) processes. Tissue growth and regeneration require an increased intake of protein to provide the raw materials for tissue reconstruction. If burns patients are not given sufficient protein they will suffer from wasting of respiratory muscles and immune compromise, both of which contribute to pneumonia. Calorific requirements will also be significantly increased as a result of additional energy use in the wound healing process. Another factor which increases energy demand is the loss of heat from wound surfaces as a result of evaporation. As soon as the patient can eat and drink they should be given plenty of proteins and carbohydrates. If there is any delay in the patient being able to eat, enteral feeding should start at an early stage. After significant burn injury patients probably require twice as much protein and carbohydrate as normal. Energy expenditure can be reduced by keeping the patient in a warm atmosphere, ideally 30-32°C. Additional vitamins will be needed to facilitate effective wound healing and iron will help to prevent anaemia.

Hypothermia

Another physiological function of the skin which may be impaired is thermoregulation. Vasodilation can lead to excessive heat loss made worse by evaporative loss. This occurs because water evaporating from the wound surface extracts the latent heat of vaporization from the tissues and so cools the body in the same way as sweating. Keeping wet soaks or ice packs on patients for prolonged periods of time is also a risk factor for hypothermia. Cold weather is an additional obvious risk. Children are at increased risk of developing hypothermia due to their large surface area to volume ratio. Patients should be kept warm to avoid hypothermia

Wound infection

Disruption of the skin removes the normal protective covering of the body. This allows infection into the burnt area. Burns are very prone to infection and even small burns can lead to significant local infection with the risk of life threatening sepsis.

Wounds should be cleaned with soap and water at an early stage to remove any debris or superficial foreign bodies. Any devitalised tissue which can be readily removed, including larger blisters, will usually be debrided. (Small blisters should probably be left intact.) There is no consensus regarding the best dressing for burn wounds. Most experts agree that using a simple non-adherent dressing, such as paraffin gauze, plus an absorbent layer is suitable for a minor burn. All dressings must be applied using strict aseptic technique. Ongoing daily, or even twice daily, dressing changes will usually be required. During dressing changes wounds should be cleaned, debrided and fresh non adhesive dressings applied. Prophylactic antibiotics are not normally indicated as these may give rise to superinfection with resistant organisms. Antibiotics will become indicated if clinical signs of infection develop.

The presence of necrotic tissue significantly increases infection risk. This is because bacteria are able to rapidly divide in the dead tissues which supplies them with a ready made food supply. The body's immune mechanisms, such as macrophages, are not able to operate in necrosed areas. Once established, infection will rapidly migrate from necrotic to living tissues leading to a bacterial invasion which can overwhelm local defenses. This form of invasive infection leads to a condition termed burn wound sepsis with the result that the patient's life is in danger. Most infections are caused by staphylococci but streptococcus and pseudomonas may also cause problems.

Deeply burned skin forms eschars which pose a great infection liability to the patient. Most burn centres now use surgery to remove these sheets of dead tissue. If not removed these represent a significant infection risk. Surgical debridement of the dead tissue can then be followed by skin grafting. Autografting uses thin layers of the patient's own skin which avoids any rejection problems. If burns occur over joints, active or passive exercises should be performed to minimise scarring and contractures. Tetanus toxoid booster immunization should be given if required.

Infection risk explains why patients should be closely observed for clinical features such as increased pain or heat, redness or secondary swelling, increased or altered wound exudates and impaired wound healing. Systemic features of infection include pyrexia, increased malaise and leucocytosis.

Scarring and joint contractures

Deep burns cannot heal by regeneration of skin tissue. This means that without skin grafting they can only heal by granulation with subsequent fibrosis. This will lead to extensive formation of scar tissue. Once formed scar tissue starts to contract due to the action of fibroblasts and myofibroblasts. This will result in the formation of very tight contracted scars. Burn scar contractures can immobilize hands and feet and produce serious disfigurement. Such contractures will also seriously limit the mobility of joints. Contractures around the thorax can inhibit ventilation and those around limbs can compress blood vessels leading to congestion and ischaemia. Therapies aimed at prevention of scar contractures are most effective if started early in the healing process when scar tissue is still pliable, before it contracts and hardens. Scar tissue can remain inflamed and continues to remodel for up to a year after the initial injury.

CHAPTER 28

Pain

The nature of pain

Pain has been described as 'a subjective reaction to an objective stimulus'. Another way of defining pain has been 'a sensory experience evoked by tissue damage'. However, pain is more complex than a simple cause and effect system, because it involves feelings and emotions as well as sensations. The subjective nature of pain has been well summed up in the now famous McCaffery quote, 'pain is whatever the experiencing person says it is, existing whenever he or she says it does'. Algesia is another term which means pain. As usual the prefix 'an' means without, so analgesia literally means without pain. Treatments which remove or reduce pain are therefore analgesic.

The value of pain

It seems pain is generated as soon as a stimulus becomes severe enough to generate tissue damage. For example, most people report pain when the skin is heated to 45°C. This is the temperature above which tissue damage will occur if the heat is applied for a period of time. Intensity of pain is also correlated with the rate at which tissue damage occurs. From these facts it would seem reasonable to infer that pain is designed to inform us that tissue damage is occurring. So despite being an unpleasant experience, pain is essential for the maintenance of health. If we start to sustain an injury, pain will cause us to behave in such a way as to avoid further tissue damage. Once we learn what causes pain, we take measures to prevent exposure to the stimulus.

If an injury does occur, pain informs us that there is a problem. One effect of pain is to promote immobilisation, which in turn promotes healing. If a damaged tissue is mobilised as normal, it will rub against other injured areas leading to further damage and reduced healing. For example, if we did not feel pain from a broken bone, the fractured ends could grate against each other, making the damage much worse.

From a health care perspective, about 50% of patients who seek advice do so because they experience pain. This is often a good thing, as it means appropriate remedies may be prescribed. People naturally relate pain with disorder. We feel something must be wrong if we feel a pain. Conversely, some potentially serious disorders, such as most early cancers, do not generate pain. We must therefore educate people to realise that disorder may occur without pain. Pain is also useful in health care as an aid to diagnosis of an underlying pathology or injury. Many disorders generate characteristic patterns of pain which we can learn to recognise.

Inability to feel pain

Perhaps the best illustration of the usefulness of pain is seen in individuals who cannot feel pain. Very occasionally people are born who are congenitally unable to feel pain. More commonly the sensation of pain from part of the body is lost. This occurs in sensory neuropathy in diabetes mellitus, disorders causing neurological deficit, and as a result of Hanson's disease (leprosy). These patients can experience injury and not feel pain. This may result in injury and infection which may spread into the bones causing osteomyelitis.

During natural sleep, we turn frequently throughout the night if we become even mildly uncomfortable. After heroin overdose a person may lie in the same position for many hours as a result of the analgesic and hypnotic effect of the drug. This may result in deep pressure sores and rhabdomyolysis in patients who collapse on hard surfaces.

If a patient cannot feel pain in a clinical situation we need to account for this in care planning. For example, an unconscious patient will not experience pressure discomfort when lying on one side for too long. If we do not turn the patient regularly this will lead to pressure sore formation. If we have given lignocaine eye drops we should take measures to protect the eye until the sensation of pain returns. If the eye is anaesthetised, the person may get some grit between the eyelid and conjunctiva which may scratch the cornea, but not cause pain. Another interesting example is after heart transplantation. If a donated heart suffers an infarct the recipient does not feel any pain.

Components of pain

Pain is a complex phenomenon. It is sometimes useful to think of it consisting of four basic components; sensory, affective, autonomic and motor. These various components of pain may occur in varying proportions or in isolation.

Sensory component

This is the feeling of pain the individual sufferer experiences. Different terms are often used to describe pains such as sharp, achy, dull, crushing, burning, stabbing, gnawing, sickening or grating. The level of pain suffered can vary from a slight irritation to being overwhelming and intolerable.

Affective component

Affect means to do with mood or emotion. This is the way pain makes the person feel in emotional terms. Pain is upsetting, may cause anxiety and it is unpleasant and disturbing. This emotional component is sometimes described as 'hurting'.

Autonomic component

Pain has an involuntary effect on the autonomic nervous system. Initially pain leads to sympathetic stimulation, which will increase heart rate, blood pressure and breathing and it often causes sweating. Clinicians should recognise that these changes in a patient who is unable to communicate normally may well indicate the presence of pain.

Motor component

The most obvious motor effect is to withdraw the part of the body exposed to a pain. Withdrawal is a reflex and is often accompanied by a shout, scream or expletive. The reason people feel a need to vocalise when in pain may be to warn others in a group of the presence of danger. People in pain usually have a strong desire to let others know they are suffering. Some patients however, do 'suffer in silence', which is why we should always assess pain on an individual patient basis.

Descriptions of pain

Acute and chronic pain

An acute pain typically has a fairly sudden onset and the pain subsides once the cause of the pain is removed or resolves. From this it could be claimed that acute pain has a function in preventing further damage and aiding recovery by promoting rest and immobilisation.

In contrast chronic pain is persistent, even after healing is apparently complete. Onset of the problem may be acute or insidious. Unlike acute pain, chronic pain serves no function. It has been suggested that a pain becomes chronic if it persists for more that 3 months. This form of long-term pain has a destructive effect on the individual. The source of chronic pain may often be unknown, or if it is known cannot be treated or eliminated. Chronic pain may also occur in people who do not have access to health care. Over time the pain sensation often becomes more diffuse. Persistent pain may or may not increase in frequency and severity. In some cases the patient's entire world centres around modification of the pain experience.

Superficial or deep pain

Pain which arises from the skin or near the body surface is superficial. Deep pain may originate in joints, bones or body organs.

Pain threshold

This is when a stimulus first starts to generate pain. This does not vary much between individuals or over time. Apparent differences in pain perception between racial groups probably occur as a result of culturally learned attitudes to pain and its expression. Biologically, all races of people are essentially identical.

Pain tolerance

This concept is used in experiments on pain; it is the level of pain intensity which forces the individual to withdraw or ask for the stimulus to be stopped. Of course in some clinical situations, pain tolerance will be exceeded and an individual will be forced to suffer intolerable pain until we are able to intervene.

Pain perception at the peripheral level

Pain perception at this level describes the structure and function of pain sensitive neurones from their origin until they enter the central nervous system.

Nociceptors

Pain originates in specialised peripheral sensory receptors called nociceptors. These are receptors which detect noxious stimuli. All nociceptors are free nerve endings. Once a new pain impulse is generated, it travels towards the central nervous system along the dendrite of a pain specific neurone. Like other sensory neurones, the fibre which carries an impulse towards the neuronal cell body is called the dendrite. Sensory neurone cell bodies are grouped together near the spinal cord, in an area called the dorsal root ganglion. From the cell body, a short axon carries the pain impulse into the spinal cord.

Tissues which are sensitive to pain have large numbers of nociceptors; tissues which do not feel pain have no nociceptors. For example, there are numerous nociceptors in the dermis of the skin, periosteum, arterial walls, joint surfaces and in the parietal pleural and parietal peritoneal membranes. Conversely, a biopsy may be taken from the lining of the stomach which causes no pain at all. This can be explained by the absence of nociceptors in the gut lining.

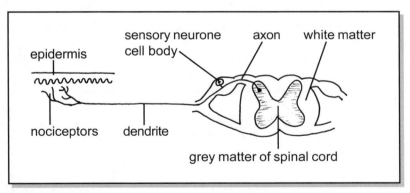

Diagram 28.1
Peripheral pathway from a dermal nociceptor into the spinal cord.

Nociception

There are basically three types of stimuli which stimulate nociceptors and may therefore give rise to pain. Thermal nociception may be initiated by things which are very hot or very cold. Secondly, strong mechanical stimuli or pressure is another group of causes; nociceptors respond vigorously if torn or cut. Thirdly, chemicals may stimulate nociceptor activity; these include acids and chemicals often associated with inflammation such as histamine and bradykinin. Chemical stimulation also explains why insect stings can be so painful.

Nociceptors only generate a nervous impulse when they are strongly stimulated. For example, it takes quite a lot of pressure to cause pain. In physiological terms this is explained by a relatively high setting of the depolarisation threshold in nociceptors. This threshold describes the level of sensation that is required to initiate depolarisation, and therefore a new nerve impulse. This high threshold prevents us feeling pain in response to the wear and tear, rough and tumble of everyday life.

A severe pain does not cause a greater degree of depolarisation than a lesser pain. The voltage level of nociceptor depolarisation, like that of all neurones, is 'all or nothing'. If pain is intense, this is communicated into the central nervous system by more impulses being generated in a particular period of time; this is referred to as frequency coding.

Local anaesthetics

These are cocaine-based preparations such as lignocaine which work on nociceptor nerve endings and dendrites. When injected onto a nerve they work by blocking the sodium ion (Na^+) channels in the axonal membranes. This blockage prevents sodium ions flowing into and out of the fibres, which in turn inhibits the ability of the affected length of fibre to polarise and depolarise. This means a nerve impulse is unable to pass along the affected length of fibre. Mixing lignocaine with a low dose of adrenaline may extend the anaesthetic effect as it reduces local blood flow by initiating vasoconstriction. As blood flow is reduced by vasoconstriction, the lignocaine is not washed away and so remains at higher local concentrations for longer.

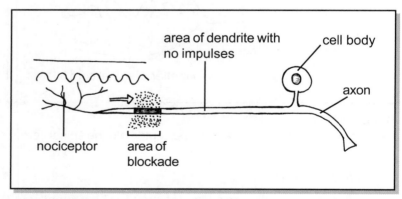

Diagram 28.2
Action of lignocaine to produce local anaesthesia as a peripheral nerve block. In this case the nociceptors generate an impulse as normal, which travels towards the spinal cord along the first part of the dendrite. However when the nerve impulse arrives at the anaesthetized section, further progression is blocked so the pain stimulus does not reach the CNS.

Aspirin

Aspirin has an analgesic effect by working at the peripheral level. Aspirin and the other non-steroidal anti-inflammatory drugs (NSAIDs) inhibit the synthesis of prostaglandins in the tissues. This reduces pain as prostaglandins work by sensitising nociceptors as part of the inflammatory response.

Basic care

Pain generated by peripheral nociceptors can be reduced by basic nursing interventions. For example, many wounds are less painful if kept moist (as opposed to dry or soggy), which is why pain can sometimes be significantly reduced by a simple change of wound dressing. Other basic interventions such as pressure relief or position change may also significantly reduce pain.

Sharp and dull pain

If we sit on a pin, or cut ourselves, the pain we feel is 'sharp' or 'pricking' in nature. We feel the pain very quickly after tissue damage is sustained, and are aware which part of the body it came from. In other words, sharp pain is well localised. Sharp pain tends to be fairly short in duration. Shortly after we have felt a sharp pain, we usually become aware of a more dull achy pain. As well as being delayed, this second form of pain is more difficult to attribute to a precise part of the body. Often we will describe an ache as coming from an area, rather than an actual location.

Fast and slow pain neurones

The theory behind sharp and dull pain is that two different forms of pain transmitting sensory neurones transmit them. Myelinated fibres called type A-delta transmit sharp pain. Myelination of these fibres allows for rapid saltatory transmission of the pain stimulus at transmission speeds of 6 to 30 metres per second. Thicker, but unmyelinated C-fibres transmit dull, achy, hurting type pains. The lack of myelin sheath results in much slower rates of neuronal transmission than would be the case in myelinated fibres. Transmission rates in C-fibres vary between 0.5 to 2 metres per second. It is for these reasons that sharp pain is also referred to as fast and dull pain as slow.

Sharp/fast pain allows for rapid reflex actions to protect the body against further injury. For example, if we touch something very hot, there will be a reflex withdrawal of the limb very quickly to prevent further tissue damage. Reflex withdrawal can only work quickly because nerve impulses are transmitted quickly, via myelinated A-delta fibres to the spinal cord. The impulse is then relayed across the spinal cord to a myelinated motor neurone which carries an impulse out from the spinal cord to an appropriate effector muscle. The combination of the sensory, relay and motor neurones forms a reflex arc. An ascending neurone also carries the pain impulse up to the brain so we become aware of it.

Pain transmission into and up the spinal cord

All information about the external world and our bodies enters the brain via sensory neurones. These are found in cranial and spinal nerves. There are 12 pairs of cranial nerves which communicate directly with the brain; these do not travel via the spinal cord. Communications from most of the body enter the spinal cord via 31 pairs of spinal nerves.

Nociceptor neurones enter the spinal cord via the dorsal nerve root, into the dorsal horn, (dorsal means posterior). All sensory neurones enter the spinal cord via the dorsal root and all motor fibres leave via the anterior root, remember 'in the back and out the front'.

Both A and C fibres enter the dorsal horn and here synapse with a short relay neurone called an interneurone. This carries the nerve impulse through part of the dorsal horn until it synapses with a third neurone which then travels diagonally across the spinal cord. This same neurone then turns upwards and joins other ascending pain neurones in a nerve bundle called the spinothalamic tract. This arrangement of neurones allows an impulse to enter the cord, cross over to the opposite side, and then be transmitted up towards the brain.

The chemical transmitter substance secreted by the fast A-delta neurones in the spinal cord is called glutamate (or glutamic acid). This is a common excitatory transmitter in the CNS with a short duration of action. However the slow C pathways use a transmitter called substance P. This was so called because it is a peptide which is a sequence of amino acids. It is believed that substance P is released more slowly than glutamate and has a longer duration of action. Like all other chemical transmitters, these are used to allow a nervous impulse to be transmitted across a synaptic gap between two neurones.

Spinothalamic tract

These nerve tracts are located in the white matter of the spinal cord and carry ascending pain transmitting neurones up to the thalamus. The spinothalamic tracts therefore connect the spinal cord with the thalamus where the sensation of pain is generated.

Pain processing in the brain stem, thalamus and sensory cortex

It is the right cerebral hemisphere of the brain which provides sensation for the left side of the body and vice versa. Unlike other sensory neurones, ascending pain fibres do not cross over at the level of the medulla and pons of the brain stem. They do not need to, as most of them have already crossed over at the level of the spinal cord. The result is that pain generated on the left side of the body is felt by the right side of the brain and vice versa.

It seems to be the thalamus, together with parts of the brain stem, which generates the sensation of pain. It seems strange to think of part of the brain

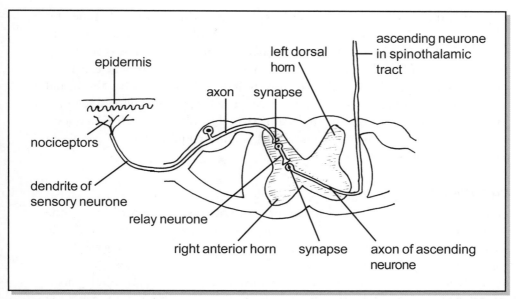

Diagram 28.3
Transmission of a pain stimulus, into, across and up the spinal cord.

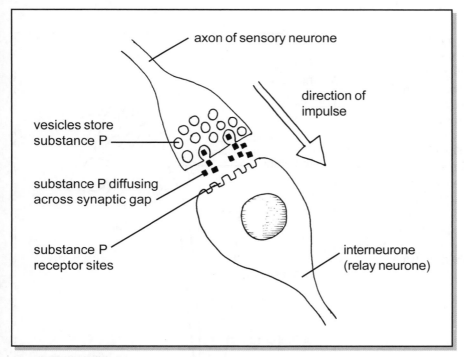

Diagram 28.4
Transmission of a pain stimulus from the axon of a C type sensory neurone
to an interneurone in the dorsal horn of the spinal cord.

generating the sensation of pain, but it is the brain which ultimately generates all experiences. Sight is generated by the occipital lobe, smell in the olfactory areas of the brain and pleasure in limbic areas. Even consciousness is generated by various parts of the brain working together. Although pain may be explained in these physiological terms this in no way reduces, what can be, the brutal reality of pain. Some areas of the brain stem and thalamus, which generate pain, also stimulate arousal in the brain. It is this arousal which generates a state of wakefulness. This explains why it is almost impossible for people in pain to get off to sleep.

Fast pain fibres

From the thalamus the sharp/fast pain neurones synapse with a further neurone communicating directly with the sensory cortex. Communication with the sensory areas of the brain is necessary if pain is to be localised to a particular part of the body. This explains why we are able to identify the precise part of the body which has been cut or stabbed with a needle. Localisation of pain is important so we can take specific, precise and localised action to avoid the cause of the pain. People who have suffered damage to the sensory cortex are still able to experience pain generated by the thalamus, but are unable to accurately localise the source.

Diagram 28.5
Fast pain fibres pass through the brain stem to the thalamus where they synapse with another fibre which communicates with the sensory cortex. The combination of the thalamus generating, and the sensory cortex localising, explains why we feel a pain in a particular part of the body. (In this case the pain is felt in the right thumb.)

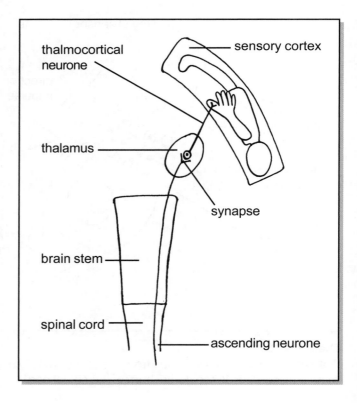

Slow pain fibres

Most of the slow C-fibres terminate at the level of the brain stem. Here they generate aching and suffering types of pain. This is important to realise when caring for patients who have sustained cerebral damage (for example after a stroke), they are still able to feel pain at the level of the brain stem. A minority of C-fibres do carry on up to the thalamus, and there is some ongoing communication with the sensory cortex. However, C-fibres which enter the thalamus do not communicate as precisely with the sensory cortex as the fast A type fibres do. This explains why aches have a more vague, or diffuse distribution in comparison to sharp pains. C-fibres also communicate with the limbic system. Limbic areas of the brain generate emotions, explaining why pain is an emotional experience; it is upsetting and causes anxiety.

Common causes of acute pain

Inflammation

Damaged tissue has been shown to contain a range of free chemicals not found in healthy tissue; these act as inflammatory mediators and derive from mast cells and the damaged tissue itself. Chemicals found in inflamed tissue include histamine, substance P, bradykinin, serotonin, prostaglandins and potassium and hydrogen ions. (It is interesting that substance P should turn up in the tissues as well as acting as a neurotransmitter.) Several inflammatory mediators act on local nociceptors to decrease their depolarisation threshold. You may remember that a nerve impulse is a wave of depolarisation moving along a nerve fibre. So a reduced depolarisation threshold means a nociceptic nerve impulse can be generated much more readily than in non-inflamed tissue. This means a stimulus such as a relatively light touch which would not normally cause pain will in an inflamed tissue. Even the pulse of arterial blood passing through an inflamed area can cause throbbing. In summary it can be said that inflammation causes hyperalgesia. Numerous inflammatory conditions will lead to pain; common examples include appendicitis, peritonitis, otitis media, cholecystitis, cystitis, pleurisy and wound infection.

Hypoxia and ischaemia

If an area is ischaemic, blood and therefore oxygen supply to the tissues will be reduced. Once oxygen supply drops below the metabolic demand of a tissue the metabolism will change from aerobic to anaerobic. Normally tissues use oxygen to generate energy, which is called aerobic metabolism (or aerobic respiration). However, if the metabolic demand of a tissue exceeds the oxygen supply then metabolism will continue without oxygen. This is termed anaerobic metabolism.

Anaerobic metabolism produces lactic acid as a waste product. As is the case with inflammatory mediators, hydrogen ions and other acids, the presence of lactic acid in the tissues will also stimulate nociceptors causing pain. Pain as a result of anaerobic respiration is seen in several disorders such as peripheral vascular disease, angina and mesenteric ischaemia. This also explains why ischaemic wounds are often more painful than non-ischaemic ones. For example, arterial leg ulcers are typically more painful than venous.

Spasm

Spasm in a hollow structure causes the pain we refer to as colic. Colicky pains are some of the worst known to pathophysiology and derive from smooth muscle. For example calculi in a ureter may cause ureteric colic and in the bile ducts biliary colic. Period and labour pains are also partly caused by colic of the uterus. You may have experienced the crampy colic originating from the colon during a bout of diarrhoea. Spasm in an organ is caused by intense muscular contraction. As a result of the increased workload of smooth muscle, anaerobic metabolism and lactic acid accumulation may occur. This localised hypoxia can be exacerbated by the muscle spasm, squeezing on local blood vessels, further reducing blood supply and drainage. Reduced rates of blood circulation will in turn reduce oxygen delivery and waste removal even more. A similar situation may occur in skeletal muscles; spasm will increase metabolic demand and compress blood vessels leading to ischaemia, hypoxia and anaerobic metabolism. This is the pain we call cramp; the remedy is to move the muscle a few times to restore normal blood circulation.

Irritation of internal membranes

Pain may originate from various internal membranes such as those which form capsules around internal organs e.g. the kidneys, liver and spleen. Pain may arise from these structures as a result of inflammation, stretching or mechanical insults.

The parietal peritoneal membrane is very sensitive and causes pain when we are hit in the stomach or stabbed. Inflammation of the parietal peritoneal membrane is also very painful. Peritonitis typically causes the patient to lie still and the overlying muscles to tighten to guard the area. Rebound or 'release pain' is typical of peritoneal irritation. Pleural pain may be severe and originates from the parietal pleura. This can cause the severe pain associated with respiratory movements seen in pleurisy. As the parietal pleura is very pain sensitive, we should always ensure that a patient receives sufficient local anaesthetic before insertion of a chest drain. When these internal membranes are inflamed the pain is made worse by movement or stretching. This is seen in meningitis where stretching of inflamed meninges causes severe pain, explaining the neck stiffness and pain seen in this disorder.

Pain from the skin

The outer layer of the skin is the epidermis. As this contains no nociceptors it is not sensitive to pain. However the underlying dermis is richly supplied with nociceptors causing it to be pain sensitive. This explains why partial thickness injuries, which remove the epidermis and part of the dermis, are so painful. Sensitive dermal nociceptors are exposed, leading to pain. This may arise as a result of a graze or burn. Subcutaneous tissues are not well supplied with nociceptors, which explains why full thickness burns are less painful than partial thickness. In a full thickness injury the dermal nociceptors are destroyed with the rest of the dermis, exposing the less sensitive underlying tissue.

Neuropathic pain

Neuropathy is a general term which relates to any disease of peripheral nerves. For example diabetic neuropathy is disease of the peripheral NS occurring as a complication of diabetes mellitus. Pain occurring as a result of neuropathy is often referred to as neurogenic. Neurogenic pain has its origin in nervous tissue. Neuralgia describes a severe pain occurring along the course of one or more nerves. This form of pain, which is usually sharp or spasm like, follows a pattern which can be explained in terms of a nerve's anatomical distribution. Neuralgic pain is often described as being 'stabbing' and can be specifically described as lancinating. For example, trigeminal neuralgia may affect nerves in the face and sciatica the sciatic nerve. Shingles is another form of neuralgic pain. Pain from toothache is caused by exposure of nerves from dental pulp which is very hot and cold sensitive. This is a sharp persistent pain. If left untreated the pain should resolve when the pulp nerves decay, but this might take months.

Common causes of chronic pain

Untreated pathology

If people have limited access to clinical attention they may suffer from ongoing pain caused by such conditions as peptic ulceration, tropical ulcers, toothache or inflammatory bowel disorders.

Untreatable pathologies

Some disorders are untreatable in particular individuals; others are very difficult to treat. For example arterial ulcers may not heal as a consequence of chronic ischaemia. Venous leg ulcers may also be painful and difficult to heal due to the presence of chronic venous hypertension. Peripheral neuropathy, phantom limb pain and mesenteric ischaemia are other examples of painful conditions which may be very difficult to treat.

Musculoskeletal

Virtually any ongoing abnormality of the musculoskeletal system can lead to chronic pain. Lower back pain is perhaps the most common. Degenerative disorders of the spinal column can lead to chronic pressure on spinal nerves. Osteoarthritis involves loss of articular cartilage and can cause very severe pain over many years. Rheumatoid arthritis may cause severe inflammation of several joints and also causes severe pain.

Cancer pain

Cancer can cause pain through a variety of mechanisms. For example progressive bone destruction can cause severe pain. This affects the periosteum and endosteum which are highly pain sensitive (as you will know if you have ever knocked your shin or broken a bone). Obstruction of the lumen of the gut or blood vessels may be caused by internal neoplasm or external pressure from a tumour and may also lead to pain. Pressure from growing tumours may cause ischaemia or venous obstruction. A tumour causing pressure on a peripheral nerve can be very painful; this may affect spinal nerves as they communicate with the spinal cord. Malignancy may also lead to inflammation, necrosis and areas of infection.

Stages of cancer pain

Early stage pain is often caused by investigations or treatments; it is short term and resolves after a few days. Intermediate stage pain may be caused by post operative contractures, nerve entrapment, cancer recurrence or metastasis. Late stage pain occurs in terminal cancer when therapy no longer controls the disease. Pain is chronic and slowly increases in intensity and without appropriate treatment the pain may become intractable. Severe chronic pain occurs in about 25% of patients who die from cancer, which is why good pain management strategies are so important during palliative care. Even without treatment, pain is not inevitable in all forms of cancer; many terminal patients have mild or no pain.

Other presentations of pain

Referred

Referred pain is when a pain originating from one part of the body is experienced in another area. Pain originating from an organ or other internal structure is often felt on the surface of the body. This phenomena can be partly explained by convergence of two sensory fibres onto one relay neurone in the dorsal horn of the spinal cord. The picture of referred pain is complicated as pain is referred more according to where structures were in the early embryo, when the nerve tracts were forming, than where a structure is now. Knowledge of typical patterns of referred pain is vital to the diagnosis of several common disorders, pain from

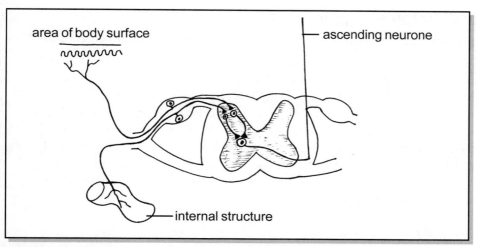

area of body surface

ascending neurone

internal structure

Diagram 28.6
A mechanism of referred pain. In this case two sensory neurones enter the dorsal horn, communicate with two relay neurones which both synapse with a single ascending neurone. When an impulse from the internal structure arrives in the thalamus the origin of the pain may be attributed to an area of body surface.

the myocardium and gall bladder being classical examples. The converse of referred pain is pain which is well localised. This form of pain is usually felt in the area of the body where it is generated. For example, pain from the urinary tract is usually well localised.

Phantom pain

A phantom pain is felt in part of the body which is no longer present. For example, a patient who has had a foot amputated may feel pain in toes which are no longer there. Phantoms occur because all of the body is mapped onto an area of the brain called the sensory cortex located in the post central gyrus of the parietal lobe. When part of the body is lost the area of the sensory cortex, which represents the missing part, seems to be unaware of the change and continues to provide the person with sensory information.

About a third of phantom limbs feel to be fixed in an uncomfortable awkward position that the patient is unable to alter. This can sometimes be 'liberated' by the patient performing movements in the mirror with the opposite side of the body. The brain may then be 'educated' into realising that the phantom is not paralysed and the symptom of the so-called cramped phantom may be relieved. This form of cerebral re-education may also reduce pain and can even cause the phantom sensations to stop completely. It may be that giving good analgesia before amputation takes place can prevent or reduce phantom pain. This claim is still controversial, but if true would indicate that phantom pain is a memory that is perpetuated in the sensory cortex.

Clinical features of pain

Acute pain

Acute pain causes stimulation of the sympathetic autonomic nervous system. It therefore causes an increase in heart rate and blood pressure. Sympathetic stimulation also leads to an increased respiratory rate, sweating and dilation of the pupils. Pain usually produces characteristic facial expressions, with a generalised agitation. However, if movement makes a pain worse, the patient will lie still or immobilise the painful part of the body. If possible a person will attempt to withdraw from a painful stimulus. Most people who are able to do so will complain if they are in pain, but we should always ask if a patient has any pain as some stoical people suffer in silence.

Chronic pain

In this situation the features of acute pain such as increased heart and respiratory rate are not present due to physiological readjustments over time. If pain persists, the body seems to be able to return the activity of the sympathetic nervous system to normal. However, people suffering chronic pain may show numerous features which could be described as psychosocial; these may include irritability, insomnia, social isolation with gross disruption of interactions with other people, feelings of helplessness and hopelessness, loss of libido (desire for sex) and depression.

Assessment of pain

Ultimately pain is a personal experience which means the only person able to state pain levels is the person suffering. Patients are the only reliable judges of their own pain. This is why a pain assessment scale should be used. We ask the patient to assess their own level of pain on a scale, usually 0 to 10, where 10 represents the worst pain imaginable and 0 represents no pain at all. This approach is particularly useful for monitoring the effectiveness of analgesics. If reported pain was 5 before giving analgesia and 1 after 30 minutes, the treatment has been reasonably effective. Pain scales also allow us to plot changes in patient's pain over time.

Longer term, persistent or intermittent pains may be assessed using the PQRST of pain. This is done by asking questions based on the following thinking:

P Provoking factors; what makes it worse or relieves.
Q Quality of the pain; e.g. deep, superficial, crushing, sharp, dull, gnawing, burning.
R Region and radiation; where is the pain and where does it go.
S Severity and intensity; on a pain rating scale.
T Times; related to onset, duration, frequency.

Age and pain

Traditionally it had been assumed that fetal and neonatal pain does not exist. These assumptions had profound clinical application. For example, in the past neonates were not given anaesthetic agents, but only muscle relaxants, during invasive procedures including surgery. Later this position changed and the reality of child and neonatal pain became well accepted. We now know what is obvious; children and newborn babies feel pain, just as adults do. It seems reasonable to assume that health care professionals have inflicted outrageous levels of pain on children in the past.

It is now known that the human fetus possesses an active central nervous system from at least the eighth week of development. This means that unborn children may well feel pain from this time in the first trimester. Further evidence for this comes from studies of stress hormones in fetal blood and the obvious withdrawal movements a fetus makes in the uterus, away from a painful stimulus. Many infants scream lustily immediately after delivery by caesarean section under maternal general anaesthesia. This means babies are not anaesthetized when the mother is, so could therefore feel pain.

Scientifically then the evidence for fetal pain is clear. However, it is not generally admitted to exist and is not usually accounted for. The situation is analogous to the one suffered by neonates in the past, a situation where pain is assumed not to exist because the individual can not sit up and report it to us in clear English. If fetal pain were to be accounted for this would mean anaesthetising a fetus before termination of pregnancy was to be carried out. However, if such anaesthetics were given this would admit the humanity of the fetus which would be inconvenient.

Other groups of people may also be incapable of communicating their pain; this may occur in patients with dementia or psychiatric illness. The only way to be safe is to assume that all people feel pain just as we do. This would mean we should provide an equivalent level of anaesthesia or analgesia to a person who cannot communicate with us, as we would give to a patient who can.

Pain inhibition physiology

The process of physiologically modifying the amount of pain felt is referred to as modulation. Modulation of pain impulses and experience takes place in the spinal cord and brain.

Central descending inhibition of pain

Activity in two specific parts of the hypothalamus is able to stimulate activity in an area of the midbrain and upper pons called the periaqueductal grey matter. (This long name just means the nerve cell bodies around the aqueduct for cerebrospinal fluid that runs through the midbrain.) From this area of the upper brain stem, neurones communicate down to an area in the lower pons and upper medulla called the raphe nucleus. From the raphe nucleus, neurones travel down specialised tracts in the spinal cord called the dorsolateral columns. Neurones from these columns communicate with specific interneurones in the dorsal horn of the spinal cord, which in turn communicate with afferent pain transmitting neurones which are carrying pain impulses into the dorsal horns of the spinal cord. (Afferent refers to pathways which carry impulses through the CNS from the periphery.)

The reason this complex sounding anatomy is important is that the structures discussed above form the bodies own inbuilt analgesic system. Activation of these structures seems to be initiated by the mind, when it realises that it would be inappropriate to feel pain in a particular situation.

Once in the dorsal horn these neurones, which carry descending impulses, inhibit the transmission of pain impulses across the spinal cord. Transmission in both A and C type fibres is inhibited. In other words the central nervous system has a built in pain suppression system, which can prevent the initial entry of pain into the spinal cord. This dedicated pain suppression arrangement is called the analgesia system.

Diagram 28.7
Components of the analgesic system. Initial activation of the hypothalamus by higher brain stimulation activates neurones which carry impulses from the hypothalamus to the periaqueductal grey matter. From here a further neurone carries the impulses down to the raphe nucleus. From the raphe nucleus, neurones descend in the dorsolateral columns into the anterior horn of the spinal cord.

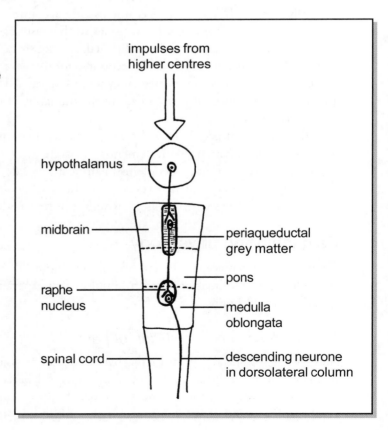

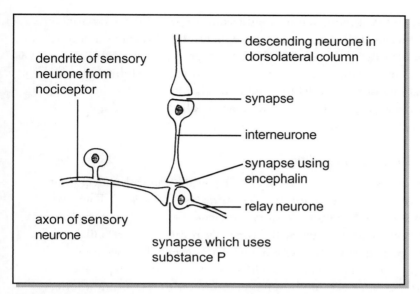

Diagram 28.8
A nerve fibre from the descending dorsolateral tract communicates with an interneurone which, in turn, inhibits the transmission of pain across the spinal cord. In this case, release of encephalin from the interneurone inhibits the release of substance P from a C fibre and so inhibits ascending pain transmission. (As well as inhibiting pain transmitting neurotransmitters, encephalin also has some post synaptic inhibition effect.) In the absence of encephalin afferent pain impulses may pass readily from the periphery to the spinothalamic tracts.

The transmitter substance involved in inhibition of a pain impulse across the spinal cord is encephalin, one of the endorphins. This transmitter binds to specialised encephalin receptors. In addition to being present in the dorsal horn, encephalin receptors are found in the other areas of the analgesic system discussed above. Encephalin stimulates the activity of the analgesic system.

It is the presence of these encephalin receptors in the bodies own analgesic system which allows us to benefit from opioid analgesics (such as codeine, morphine and diamorphine). Opium molecules have the same molecular shape as endorphin molecules. This means that when we give opiate drugs they are able to bind with the endogenous encephalin receptors and stimulate them. This increases the amount of post synaptic activity in the analgesic system, which will decrease the degree of afferent pain transmission, so reducing pain. So, opioid drugs artificially stimulate the bodies inbuilt analgesic system by binding into encephalin receptor sites.

In experimental studies, electrical stimulation of the upper areas of the analgesic system renders conscious animals insensitive to pain. What this indicates is that the bodies analgesic system is capable of 'switching off' pain. Given that pain is designed to protect the body this may seem a strange system to have, as it will tolerate further tissue damage. However, it seems that this whole analgesic system is designed to promote survival. In a fight or flight situation, tissue damage is likely to be sustained. If pain from such an injury inhibits affective action, the probability of survival will be reduced. For example if pain from a twisted ankle means we cannot run away, we may be killed by a wild animal or enemy.

Observations about descending inhibition

In stressful situations there seems to be something in the mind that decides it is inappropriate to feel pain when affective action needs to be taken. There are numerous examples of this from combat situations, where soldiers have sustained severe injuries but not felt any pain at the time. Even during sport, an injury may not produce pain during the excitement of the event, but become very painful afterward. This is also seen in accident and emergency departments. People who know they must get into hospital may travel with significant injuries giving rise to little pain. Once they are in hospital however, and the mind knows they no longer need to take affective action the pain starts to return.

Dr. David Livingstone, an early African explorer was once attacked by a lion and severely bitten. Fortunately he survived the attack and reported that at the time he did not feel pain. He concluded that God had given a great gift to animals, that they could not feel much pain when lions were killing them. This level of analgesia presumably came about as the mind of Livingstone realised that he was in a life or death survival situation and that to feel pain at the time would only reduce the chances of his survival.

Clinical applications of descending inhibition

It may well be that patients who have more control over what is happening to them enjoy more descending inhibition. This is consistent with descending inhibition operating when the individual needs to take appropriate action. Conversely, stress and anxiety make pain worse, and these emotions are partly caused by feelings of a lack of control. People who feel in control, even in a nasty situation, have less stress and anxiety than those who feel helpless and unable to act. It is for these reasons we should try and give patients as much control over their situation and treatments as possible. We need to be prepared to give up control and pass it to our patients.

One obvious application of this principle is patient controlled analgesia (PCA); because the patient has control, they often require lower doses of analgesia than if we are in control of giving pain relief. We also need to try and give patients more control during clinical procedures and investigations. For example, we need to make it clear that we will stop or suspend a procedure (if it is at all possible) if they request us to do so.

Ascending inhibition of pain (gate theory)

In the dorsal horn of the spinal cord, nerve fibres carrying information about touch inhibit the activity of interneurones which carry pain impulses. This means that if part of the body hurts, we can reduce the transmission of pain across the cord by rubbing the painful area. The correct name for this aspect of physiology is the gate theory of afferent inhibition. Afferent refers to impulses entering the central nervous system, in this case the touch and rubbing impulses. Gate implies that entry into the CNS is limited; impulses must enter through a 'gate'. If rubbing impulses block the entrance to the 'gate', pain cannot get through at the same time. In the same way, if a room only has one door and several people are leaving, we cannot leave at the same time, because the doorway is temporarily blocked.

Clinical applications of ascending inhibition

Rubbing around a painful area immediately after an injury can help considerably in pain reduction. In other situations, massage is a way of generating peripheral touch stimuli which may also reduce the transmission of pain through the dorsal horn. Massage can also promote relaxation and so help to lower levels of anxiety, which in turn may reduce pain. Traditional treatments for pain such as hot and cold compresses probably also work in the same way, this time the blocking impulses are temperature based as opposed to mechanical.

Another treatment based on ascending competitive inhibition is transcutaneous electrical nerve stimulation (TENS). This involves taping electrode pads to the surface of the patient's skin and then allowing them to control the strength of electrical stimulation of the area. The patient can then turn the intensity up or down, according to analgesic effect and comfort. In this case the blocking impulses at the gate would be generated by the electrical current. It is possible that acupuncture, at least in a few anatomical positions, may have a gating effect.

Placebo effect

A placebo is an effect that occurs because the patient believes it will happen. Placebo effects can be positive or negative. For example if we give a treatment that the patient believes will be beneficial, this belief has a helpful effect which is independent of any direct physiological action. If we give an analgesic, and the patient believes the treatment will work, there will be beneficial effects which are independent of the actual pharmacological action of the treatment.

So when we give an injection of morphine, perhaps 70% of the beneficial effect is attributable to the pharmacology of the drug and 30% to a positive placebo effect. If we tell the patient that a drug we are giving is useless, this will rob them of the positive placebo effect. In order to take full advantage of the placebo effect we have to tell the patient that a treatment is effective. If they believe us, and believe in us, they will enjoy a positive placebo effect. As well as this, if our patients have confidence in us, this will reduce their levels of anxiety, which will in turn reduce the amount of pain they feel. Having said this, we never lie to or seek to mislead patients in any way, but we probably could be more positive than we are more of the time.

Treat or remove the cause of pain whenever possible

Pain should be treated as far as possible by removing the cause. For example, a patient in bed may be in pain because they are lying in a position which is uncomfortable for their back. It would make more sense to change the patient's position than to give them intravenous morphine. Also if someone has a painful splinter, it would be better to pull it out rather than give nerve block analgesia. Immobilisation of fractures significantly reduces pain as it prevents broken edges of bone grating against each other and protruding into other tissues. Traction also has a similar beneficial effect. Pain from a dislocated finger or shoulder is best treated by restoring the joint. Pain caused by myocardial ischaemia can be temporarily relieved by rest, stopping smoking and taking nitrate based vasodilators. In the longer term myocardial ischaemic pain can be reduced by surgical interventions to improve myocardial perfusion. Most ischaemic pains can be reduced by not smoking. Pain caused by wound infection can be reduced by removing necrotic material from wounds and using good local wound management strategies. Antibiotics will also reduce the level of infection and so reduce the pain. Muscle cramps and spasms can be extremely painful and are normally treated by stretching and then relaxing the muscle involved. Pain from dental caries is best treated by filling or removing the offending tooth. Pain from appendicitis can be cured by removing the inflamed appendix.

Final Thoughts

If you have managed to work through this book you have my congratulations. Like me, I expect you found some of the material fascinating, how the body functions, how things can go wrong and how there can be physiological compensation. If this book has in any way improved your understanding and therefore the care you are able to give to one person, I would count that success.

Ultimately of course, despite being interesting, pathology is the enemy as it represents human suffering and death. We must never lose sight of the individual person in our care. Each person is unique and must be respected as an individual with holistic needs. Our science is only a part of the care he or she needs. The caring concern of another human being can be just as therapeutic as our more technical and pharmacological interventions.

In the first century Jesus of Nazareth told a story about a man on a journey. While on his personal journey he found another man who had been severely attacked and left with serious injuries. The traveller saw the injured man and had compassion for him, while exposing himself to personal risk he bandaged his wounds, pouring on oil and wine. At further inconvenience and expense to himself he conveyed the man to a safe place and facilitated his recovery. This story, which is one of many, gives us an example which we may choose to follow as we journey through life.

Index